Probabilistic Models of the Brain

Neural Information Processing Series

Michael I. Jordan and Sara A. Solla, editors

Probabilistic Models of the Brain: Perception and Neural Function

Edited by
Rajesh P. N. Rao
Bruno A. Olshausen
Michael S. Lewicki

A Bradford Book
The MIT Press
Cambridge, Massachusetts
London, England

The MIT Press is pleased to keep this title available in print by manufacturing single copies, on demand, via digital printing technology.

Library of Congress Cataloging-in-Publication Data

Probabilistic models of the brain: perception and neural function / edited by Rajesh P. N. Rao, Bruno A. Olshausen, Michael S. Lewicki
      p. cm. (Neural information processing series)
    "A Bradford book."
    Includes bibliographical references and index.
    ISBN 978-0-262-18224-9 (hc. : alk. paper)—978-0-262-52627-2 (pb.)
    1. Brain–Mathematical models. 2. Neurology–Statistical Methods. I. Rao, Rajesh P. N. II. Olshausen, Bruno A. III. Lewicki, Michael S. IV. Series.
    [DNLM: 1.Brain Mapping–methods. 2. Models, Neurological. 3. Models, Statistical. 4. Neurons–physiology. 5. Visual Perception–physiology. WL 335 P9615 2002]
    QP376.P677 2002
    612.8'2'011–dc21   2001042806

Contents

Series Foreword

The yearly Neural Information Processing Systems (NIPS) workshops bring together scientists with broadly varying backgrounds in statistics, mathematics, computer science, physics, electrical engineering, neuroscience and cognitive science, unified by a common desire to develop novel computational and statistical strategies for information processing, and to understand the mechanisms for information processing in the brain. As opposed to conferences, these workshops maintain a flexible format that both allows and encourages the presentation and discussion of work in progress, and thus serve as an incubator for the development of important new ideas in this rapidly evolving field.

The Series Editors, in consultation with workshop organizers and members of the NIPS Foundation Board, select specific workshop topics on the basis of scientific excellence, intellectual breadth, and technical impact. Collections of papers chosen and edited by the organizers of specific workshops are built around pedagogical introductory chapters, while research monographs provide comprehensive descriptions of workshop-related topics, to create a series of books that provides a timely, authorative account of the latest developments in the exciting field of neural computation.

Michael I. Jordan, Sara A. Solla

Preface

A considerable amount of data has been collected over the past several decades on the cellular, physiological, and anatomical properties of the brain. However, with the exception of a few notable early efforts, it is only in recent years that concerted attempts have been made to link the distinctive properties of the brain to concrete computational principles. In our view, an especially promising computational approach has been the use of probabilistic principles such as maximum likelihood and Bayesian inference to derive efficient algorithms for learning and perception. Our enthusiasm for this approach is based in part on some of its recent demonstrated successes, for example:

- The application of efficient coding algorithms to natural signals has been shown to generate receptive field properties similar to those observed in the nervous system.

- The instantiation of these algorithms in the form of "analysis-synthesis" loops has suggested functional models for the reciprocal feedforward-feedback connections between cortical areas.

- The theory of Bayesian belief propagation in probabilistic networks has yielded robust models for perceptual inference and allowed for a functional interpretation of several intriguing visual illusions and perceptual phenomena.

This book presents a representative sampling of some of the current probabilistic approaches to understanding perception and brain function. The book originated from a workshop on *Statistical Theories of Cortical Function* held in Breckenridge, Colorado, as part of the Neural Information Processing Systems (NIPS) conference in December, 1998. The goal of the workshop was to bring together researchers interested in exploring the use of well-defined statistical principles in understanding cortical structure and function. This book contains chapters written by many of the speakers from the NIPS workshop, as well as invited contributions from other leading researchers in the field. The topics include probabilistic and information theoretic models of perception, theories of neural coding and spike timing, computational models of lateral and cortico-cortical feedback connections, and the development of receptive field properties from natural signals.

While books with the words "brain" and "model" (or any of its cognates) in their title abound, one of the attributes that we feel sets the present book apart from many of its predecessors is its emphasis on the use of well-established probabilistic principles in interpreting data and constructing models. A second unique attribute is the attempt to present within a single volume both top-down computational models and bottom-up neurally-motivated models of brain function. This allows the similarities between these two types of approaches to be appreciated. To facilitate these connections, chapters containing related topics have been cross-referenced by the authors as much as possible. The introductory chapter provides an overview of the field and summarizes the contents of each chapter. A list of open problems and contentious issues is included at the end of this chapter to encourage new researchers to join in the effort and help infuse new ideas and techniques into the field.

We expect the book to be of interest to students and researchers in computational and cognitive neuroscience, psychology, statistics, information theory, artificial intelligence, and machine learning. Familiarity with elementary probability and statistics, together with some knowledge of basic neurobiology and vision, should prove sufficient in understanding much of the book.

We would like to thank Sara Solla, Michael Jordan, and Terry Sejnowski for their encouragement, the reviewers of our book proposal for their comments, and the NIPS workshops co-chairs for 1998, Rich Zemel and Sue Becker, for their help in organizing the workshop that was the seed for this book. We are also grateful to Michael Rutter, formerly of MIT Press, for his role in initiating the project, Bob Prior of MIT Press for seeing the project through to its completion, and Sergio Lucero for his excellent work in assembling the chapters in LaTeX.

Introduction

Each waking moment, our body's sensory receptors convey a vast amount of information about the surrounding environment to the brain. Visual information, for example, is measured by about 10 million cones and 100 million rods in each eye, while approximately 50 million receptors in the olfactory epithelium at the top of the nasal cavity signal olfactory information. How does the brain transform this raw sensory information into a form that is useful for goal-directed behavior? Neurophysiological, neuroanatomical, and brain imaging studies in the past few decades have helped to shed light on this question, revealing bits and pieces of the puzzle of how sensory information is represented and processed by neurons at various stages within the brain.

However, a fundamental question that is seldom addressed by these studies is *why* the brain chose to use the types of representations it does, and what ecological or evolutionary advantage these representations confer upon the animal. It is difficult to address such questions directly via animal experiments. A promising alternative is to investigate computational models based on efficient coding principles. Such models take into account the statistical properties of environmental signals, and attempt to explain the types of representations found in the brain in terms of a *probabilistic model* of these signals. Recently, these models have been shown to be capable of accounting for the response properties of neurons at early stages of the visual and auditory pathway, providing for the first time a unifying view of sensory coding across different modalities. There is now growing optimism that probabilistic models can also be applied successfully to account for the sensory coding strategies employed in yet other modalities, and eventually to planning and executing goal-directed actions.

This book surveys some of the current themes, ideas, and techniques dominating the probabilistic approach to modeling and understanding brain function. The sixteen chapters that comprise the book demonstrate how ideas from probability and statistics can be used to interpret a variety of phenomena, ranging from psychophysics to neurophysiology. While most of the examples presented in the chapters focus on vision, this is not meant to imply that these models are applicable only to this modality. Many of the models and techniques presented in these chapters are quite general, and therefore are applicable to other modalities as well.

The probabilistic approach

The probabilistic approach to perception and brain function has its roots in the advent of information theory, which inspired many psychologists during the 1950's to attempt to quantify human perceptual and cognitive abilities using statistical techniques. One of these was Attneave, who attempted to point out the link between the redundancy inherent in images and certain aspects of visual perception [2]. Barlow then took this notion a step further, by proposing a self-organizing strategy for sensory nervous systems based on the principle of *redundancy reduction* [3, 4]—i.e., the idea that neurons should encode information in such a way as to minimize statistical dependencies. The alluring aspect of this approach is that it does not require that one pre-suppose a specific goal for sensory processing, such as "edge-detection" or "contour extraction." Rather, the emphasis is on formulating a *general* goal for sensory processing from which specific coding strategies such as edge detection or contour integration could be derived.

Despite the elegance of Attneave's and Barlow's proposals, their ideas would not be put seriously to work until much later. [1] Most modeling work in sensory physiology and psychophysics over the past 40 years has instead been dominated by the practice of attributing *specific* coding strategies to certain neurons in the brain. This approach is probably best exemplified by Marr and Hildreth's classic theory of edge-detection [11], or the plethora of Gabor-filter based models of visual cortical neurons that followed [10, 6, 8]. It is also prevalent in the realms of intermediate and high level vision, for example in schemes such as codons [14], geons [5], and the medial axis transform [13] for representing object shape. In contrast to the probabilistic approach, the goal from the outset in such models is to formulate a specific computational strategy for extracting a set of desired properties from images. Nowhere is there any form of learning or adaptation to the properties of images. Instead, these models draw upon informal observations of image structure and they rely heavily upon mathematical elegance and sophistication to achieve their goal.

Interest in the probabilistic approach was revived in the 1980s, when Simon Laughlin and M.V. Srinivasan began measuring the forms of redundancy present in the natural visual environment and used this knowledge to make quantitative predictions about the response properties of neurons in early stages of the visual system [9, 15]. This was followed several years later by the work of Field [7], showing that natural images exhibit a characteristic $1/f^2$ power spectrum, and that cortical neurons are well-adapted for representing natural images in terms of a *sparse code* (where a small number of neurons out of the population are active at any given time). Then drawing upon information theory, as well as considerations of noise and the $1/f^2$ power spectrum, Atick [1] and van Hateren [16] formulated efficient coding theories for the retina in terms of whitening of the power spectrum (hence removing correla-

---

1. There were some early attempts at implementing these principles in self-organizing networks (e.g. [12]), but these fell short of being serious neurobiological models.

tions from signals sent down the optic nerve) in space and time. This body of work, accumulated throughout the 1980's and early 1990's, began to build a convincing case that probabilistic models could contribute to our understanding of sensory coding strategies. Part II of this book contains eight recent contributions to this area of inquiry.

The probabilistic approach has also been applied beyond the realm of sensory coding, to problems of perception. In fact, the idea that perception is fundamentally a problem of inference goes back at least to Hermann von Helmholtz in the nineteenth century. The main problem of perception is to deduce from the patterns of sensory stimuli the properties of the external environment. What makes this problem especially difficult is that there is ambiguity at every stage, resulting from lack of information, inherent noise, and the multitude of perceptual interpretations that are consistent with the available sensory data. Even something as simple as the interpretation of an edge can be complicated: Is it due to a reflectance change on the object? Is it a shadow that arises from the object's 3-dimensional structure? Or does it represent an object boundary? Determining which interpretation is most likely depends on integrating information from the surrounding context and from higher level knowledge about typical scene structure.

The process of inference is perhaps most compellingly demonstrated by the famous Dalmatian dog scene (reproduced in Figure 7.1), in which the luminance edges provide little or no explicit information about the object boundaries. Like a perceptual puzzle, each part of the image provides clues to the best interpretation of the whole. The question is how to combine these different sources of information in the face of a considerable degree of uncertainty. One framework for addressing these problems in the context of perceptual processing is that of Bayesian Inference (Szeliski, 1989; Knill and Richards, 1996).

What makes Bayesian inference attractive for modeling perception is that it provides a general framework for quantifying uncertainty and precisely relating what one set of information tells us about another. In Bayesian probability theory, uncertainty is represented by probability distribution functions, and Bayes' rule specifies the relation between the distributions (and therefore the uncertainties) and the observed data. A discrete distribution might represent uncertainty among a set of distinct possible interpretations, such as the probability of a word given a sound. A continuous distribution represents uncertainty of an analog quantity, such as the direction of motion given a time-varying image. By quantitatively characterizing these distributions for a given perceptual task, it is then possible to make testable predictions about human behavior. As we shall see in the chapters of Part I of this book, there is now substantial evidence showing that humans are good Bayesian observers.

Contributions of this book

The chapters in this book fall naturally into two categories, based on the type of approach taken to understand brain function. The first approach is to formulate probabilistic theories with a predominantly *top-down* point of view—i.e., with an emphasis on computational algorithms rather than the details of the underlying neural machinery. The goal here is to explain certain perceptual phenomena or analyze computational tractability or performance. This has been the predominant approach in the psychology, cognitive science, and artificial intelligence communities. Part I of the book, entitled *Perception*, comprises eight chapters that embody the top-down approach to constructing probabilistic theories of the brain.

The second approach is the formulate theories of brain function that are motivated by understanding neural substrates and mechanisms. The goal of such theories is twofold: (a) to show how the distinctive properties of neurons and their specific anatomical connections can implement concrete statistical principles such as Bayesian inference, and (b) to show how such models can solve interesting problems such as feature and motion detection. Part II of this book, entitled *Neural Function*, presents eight such models.

The first three chapters of Part I present an introduction to modeling visual perception using the Bayesian framework. Chapter 1 by Mamassian, Landy, and Maloney serves as an excellent tutorial on Bayesian inference. They review the three basic components of any Bayesian model: the likelihood function, the prior, and the gain function. Likelihood functions are used to model how visual sensors encode sensory information, while priors provide a principled way of formulating constraints on possible scenes to allow unambiguous visual perception. Gain functions are used to account for task-dependent performance. Mamassian, Landy, and Maloney illustrate how Bayesian models can be investigated experimentally, drawing upon a psychophysical task in which the observer is asked to judge 3D surface structure. They show how the assumptions and biases used by the observer in inferring 3D structure from images may be modeled in terms of priors. More importantly, their work provides a compelling demonstration of the utility of the Bayesian approach in designing and interpreting the results of psychophysical experiments.

This approach is carried further in Chapter 2 by Schrater and Kersten, who explore the Bayesian approach as a framework within which to develop and test predictive quantitative theories of human visual behavior. Within this framework, they distinguish between mechanistic and functional levels in the modeling of human vision. At the mechanistic level, traditional signal detection theory provides a tool for inferring the properties of neural mechanisms from psychophysical data. At the functional level, signal detection theory is essentially extended to pattern inference theory, where the emphasis is on natural tasks and generative models for images and scene structure. Drawing upon examples in the domain of motion processing and color constancy, Schrater and Kersten show how ideal observers can be used to test theories at both mechanistic and functional levels.

Jacobs then uses the Bayesian approach in Chapter 3 to explore the question of how observers integrate various visual cues for depth perception. Again, the emphasis is on evaluating whether or not observers' cue integration strategies can be characterized as "optimal" in terms of Bayesian inference, in this case by using an *ideal observer* as the standard of comparison. Jacobs shows that subjects integrate the depth information provided by texture and motion cues in line with those of the ideal observer, which utilizes the cues in a statistically optimal manner. He also shows that these cue integration strategies for visual depth are adaptable in an experience-dependent manner. Namely, subjects adapt their weightings of depth-from-texture and depth-from-motion information as a function of the reliability of these cues during training.

The next two chapters of Part I focus on the computation of motion within a probabilistic framework. Chapter 4, by Weiss and Fleet, describes a Bayesian approach to estimating 2D image motion. The goal is to compute the posterior probability distribution of velocity, which is proportional to the product of a likelihood function and a prior. Weiss and Fleet point out that there has been substantial confusion in the literature regarding the proper form of the likelihood function, and they show how this may be resolved by properly deriving a likelihood function starting from a generative model. The generative model assumes that the scene translates, conserving image brightness, while the image is equal to the projected scene plus noise. They then show that the likelihood function can be calculated by a population of units whose response properties are similar to the "motion energy" units typically used as models of cortical neurons. This suggests that a population of velocity tuned cells in visual cortex may act to represent the likelihood of a velocity for a local image sequence.

Chapter 5 by Freeman, Haddon, and Pasztor describes a learning-based algorithm for finding the scene interpretation that best explains a given set of image data. To illustrate their approach, they focus on the optical flow problem, where the goal is to infer the projected velocities (scene) which best explain two consecutive image frames (image). Freeman, Haddon, and Pasztor use synthetic scenes to generate examples of pairs of images, together with their correct scene interpretation. From these data, candidate scene explanations are learned for local image regions and a compatibility function is derived between neighboring scene regions. Given new image data, probabilities are propagated in a Markov network to infer the underlying optical flow in an efficient manner. They first present the results of this method for a toy world of irregularly shaped blobs, and then extend the technique to the case of more realistic images.

The final three chapters of Part I address questions at the level of computational theory. In Chapter 6, Nadal reviews recent results on neural coding and parameter estimation based on information theoretic criteria, exploring their connection to the Bayesian framework. He analyzes the amount of information conveyed by a network as a function of the number of coding units, and shows that the mutual information between input stimuli and network output grows at best linearly for a small number of units, whereas for a large number of units the growth is typically logarithmic. He also proposes some future directions to extend information theoretic approaches (in particular, the *infomax* approach) to the analysis of efficient sensory-motor coding.

In Chapter 7, Yuille and Coughlan examine the fundamental limits of vision from an information theoretic point of view. Their goal is to clarify when high-level knowledge is required to perform visual tasks such as object detection, and to suggest trade-offs between bottom-up and top-down theories of vision. This is especially helpful in clarifying the need for cortical feedback loops in perception. As a specific application of their theory, Yuille and Coughlan analyze the problem of target detection in a cluttered background and identify regimes where an accurate high-level model of the target is required to detect it.

Chapter 8 by Papageorgiou, Girosi, and Poggio presents a new paradigm for signal analysis that is based on selecting a small set of bases from a large dictionary of class-specific basis functions. The basis functions are the correlation functions of the class of signals being analyzed. To choose the appropriate features from this large dictionary, Papageorgiou, Girosi, and Poggio use Support Vector Machine (SVM) regression and compare this to traditional Principal Component Analysis (PCA) for the tasks of signal reconstruction, superresolution, and compression on a set of test images. They also show how multiscale basis functions and basis pursuit de-noising can be used to obtain a sparse, multiscale approximation of a signal. Interestingly, one of their results shows that the L_ϵ norm, which measures the absolute value of error past a certain threshold, may be a more appropriate error metric for image reconstruction and compression than the L_2 norm in terms of matching humans' psychophysical error function.

Part II of the book makes the transition from top-down to bottom-up probabilistic approaches, with an emphasis on neural modeling. The first three chapters of Part II discuss models of orientation selectivity. Chapter 9, by Piepenbrock, presents a model that explains the development of cortical simple cell receptive fields and orientation maps based on Hebbian learning. What makes this model stand apart from most models of orientation maps is that the learning is driven by the viewing of natural scenes. The underlying assumption is that visual experience and the statistical properties of natural images are essential for the formation of correct cortical feature detectors. In the model, interactions between cortical simple cells lead to divisive inhibition—a nonlinear network effect that may be interpreted as a cortical competition for input stimuli. The degree of competition is controlled by a model parameter that critically influences the development outcome. Very weak competition leads to large global receptive fields, whereas only strong competition yields localized orientation selective receptive fields that respond to the edges present in the natural images. The model implies that the early visual pathways serve to recode visual stimuli step by step in more efficient and less redundant ways by learning which features typically occur in natural scenes.

In Chapter 10, Wainwright, Schwartz, and Simoncelli present a statistical model to account for the nonlinear and adaptive responses of visual cortical neurons based on the idea of divisive normalization. The basic idea behind divisive normalization is that the linear response of a filter, characterizing the localized receptive field of a neuron, is rectified (and typically squared) and then divided by a weighted sum of the rectified responses of neighboring neurons. Wainwright, Schwartz, and Simoncelli show that natural image statistics, in conjunction with Barlow's redundancy reduction hypothesis, lead to divisive normalization as the appropriate nonlinearity for removing statistical dependencies between the responses of visual cortical neurons to natural images. The model can also account for responses to non-optimal stimuli, and in addition, adjusting model parameters according to the statistics of recent visual stimuli is shown to account for physiologically observed adaptation effects.

In Chapter 11, Zemel and Pillow build upon previous work showing how neural tuning curves (such as those of orientation selective neurons) may be interpreted in a probabilistic framework. The main idea of this approach is to interpret the population response as representing the probability distribution over some underlying stimulus dimension, such as orientation. Here, they show how the population response can be generated using a combination of feedforward and feedback connections. In addition, they include the preservation of information explicitly in the objective function for learning the synaptic weights in the model. Zemel and Pillow show that their model can support a variety of cortical response profiles, encode multiple stimulus values (unlike some previous models), and replicate cross-orientation effects seen in visual cortical neurons in response to stimuli containing multiple orientations. They also describe several testable predictions of their model involving the effect of noise on stimuli and the presence of multiple orientations.

The next four chapters of Part II focus on how probabilistic network models can also incorporate the actual spiking properties of cortical neurons. Chapter 12 by Lewicki shows how a spike-like population code may be used for representing time-varying signals. The model is derived from two desiderata: 1) coding efficiency and 2) a representation that does not depend on phase shifts. The second goal is important, because it avoids the traditional approach of blocking the data which often produces inefficient descriptions. Encoding is accomplished by maximizing the likelihood of the time-varying signals over a distributed population of relative event times. The resulting representation resembles coding in the cochlear nerve and can be implemented using biologically plausible mechanisms. The model is also shown to be equivalent to a very sparse and highly overcomplete basis. Under this model, the mapping from the data to the representation is nonlinear but can be computed efficiently. This form also allows the use of existing methods for adapting the kernel functions.

Chapter 13 by Olshausen focuses on the relation between sparse coding and neural spike trains. He proposes that neurons in V1 are attempting to model time-varying natural images as a superposition of sparse, independent events in both space and time. The events are characterized using an overcomplete set of spatiotemporal basis functions which are assumed to be translation-invariant in the time domain (as in Lewicki's model). When adapted to natural movies, the basis functions of the model converge to a set of spatially localized, oriented, bandpass functions that translate over time, similar to the space-time receptive fields of V1 neurons. The outputs of the model are computed by sparsifying activity across both space and time, producing a non-linear code having a spike-like character—i.e.,, continuous, time-varying images are represented as a series of sharp, punctate events in time, similar to neural spike trains. Olshausen suggests that both the receptive field structure and the spiking nature of V1 neurons may be accounted for in terms of a single principle of efficient coding, and he discusses a number of possibilities for testing this hypothesis.

In Chapter 14, Ballard, Zhang, and Rao present a model for spike-based communication between neurons based on the idea of synchronized spike volleys. In this model, neurons are used in a "time-sharing" model, each conveying large numbers of spikes that are part of different volleys. The phase between a neuron's successive spikes is unimportant but groups of neurons convey information in terms of precisely-timed volleys of spikes. Ballard, Zhang, and Rao show how such a model of spike-based neural communication can be used for predictive coding in the cortico-thalamic feedback loop between primary visual cortex and the lateral geniculate nucleus (LGN).

Chapter 15 by Hinton and Brown explores the hypothesis that an active spiking neuron represents a probability distribution over possible events in the world. In this approach, when several neurons are active simultaneously, the distributions they individually represent are combined by multiplying together the individual distributions. They also describe a learning algorithm that is a natural consequence of using a product semantics for population codes. Hinton and Brown illustrate their approach using a simulation in which a non-linear network with one layer of spiking hidden neurons learns to model an image sequence by fitting a dynamic generative model.

The final chapter (16), by Rao and Sejnowski, deals with the issues of cortical feedback and predictive coding. They review models which postulate that (a) feedback connections between cortical areas instantiate statistical generative models of cortical inputs, and (b) recurrent feedback connections within a cortical area encode the temporal dynamics associated with the generative model. The resulting network allows predicting coding of spatiotemporal inputs and suggests functional interpretations of nonclassical surround effects in the visual cortex on the basis of natural image statistics. Rao and Sejnowski show that recent results on spike timing dependent plasticity in recurrent cortical synapses are consistent with such a model of cortical feedback and present comparisons of data from model simulations to electrophysiological data from awake monkey visual cortex.

Open questions

The enterprise of developing probabilistic models to explain behavioral and neural response properties exhibited by the brain is still very much in its infancy. Research in the last five years, of which this book represents only a part, has so far provided just a glimpse of the potential of the probabilistic approach in understanding brain function. The strength of the probabilistic approach lies in its generality—for example, it is rich enough to provide a general global framework for vision, from low-level feature-detection and sensory coding (Part II of the book) to higher-level object recognition, object detection, and decision making (Part I of the book).

We leave the reader with a list of important questions and issues that motivated some of the early research in the field and that continue to provide the impetus for much of the recent research, including the research described in this book:

- How does the brain represent probabilities? How does it combine these probabilities to perform inference?

- How broadly can the principle of statistically efficient coding of natural signals be applied before some other principle, such as task-related adaptation, becomes more important?

- How good is the characterization of perception as Bayesian inference? What are the alternatives?

- What role do feedback pathways play in inference?

- Should neurons be modeled as deterministic or stochastic elements? Are mean-field models or stochastic sampling models more appropriate?

- How does the brain deal with "noise?" How many bits of precision can a spike encode? More generally, what exactly does a spike mean?

- Are neurons integrators or coincidence detectors? How important is input synchrony? What role do cortical oscillations have in probabilistic theories of the brain?

- What do probabilistic theories predict about the function of lateral inhibitory connections, recurrent excitatory connections, cortico-cortical feedback connections, and subcortical connections in the brain?

These are, no doubt, daunting questions. However, as probabilistic methods for inference and learning become more sophisticated and powerful, and as discoveries in neuroscience and psychology begin to paint an increasingly detailed picture of the mechanisms of perception, action, and learning, we believe it will become possible to obtain answers to these intriguing questions.

Rajesh P. N. Rao
University of Washington, Seattle

Bruno A. Olshausen
University of California, Davis

Michael S. Lewicki
Carnegie Mellon University, Pittsburgh

References

[1] Atick, J. J. Could information theory provide an ecological theory of sensory processing. *Network*, 3:213–251, 1992.

[2] Attneave, F. Some informational aspects of visual perception. *Psychological Review*, 61(3):183–193, 1954.

[3] Barlow, H. B. Possible principles underlying the transformation of sensory messages. In W. A. Rosenblith, editor, *Sensory Communication*, pages 217–234. Cambridge, MA: MIT Press, 1961.

[4] Barlow, H. B. Unsupervised learning. *Neural Computation*, 1:295–311, 1989.

[5] Biederman, I. Recognition by components: A theory of human image understanding. *Psychological Review*, 94:115–145, 1987.

[6] Daugman, J. G. Two-dimensional spectral analysis of cortical receptive field profiles. *Vision Research*, 20:847–856, 1980.

[7] Field, D. J. Relations between the statistics of natural images and the response properties of cortical cells. *J. Opt. Soc. Am. A*, 4:2379–2394, 1987.

[8] Heeger, D. Optic flow using spatiotemporal filters. *International Journal of Computer Vision*, 1(4):279–302, 1987.

[9] Laughlin, S. A simple coding procedure enhances a neuron's information capacity. *Z. Naturforsch.*, 36:910–912, 1981.

[10] Marcelja, S. Mathematical description of the responses of simple cortical cells. *Journal of the Optical Society of America*, 70:1297–1300, 1980.

[11] Marr, D., Hildreth, E. Theory of edge detection. *Proceedings of the Royal Society of London, Series B*, 207:187–217, 1980.

[12] Goodall, M. C. Performance of a stochastic net. *Nature*, 185:557–558, 1960.

[13] Pizer, S. M., Burbeck, C. A., Coggins, J. M., Fritsch, D. S., Morse, B. S. Object shape before boundary shape: scale-space medial axes. *Journal of Mathematical Imaging and Vision*, 4:303–313, 1994.

[14] Richards, W., Hoffman, D. D. Codon constraints on closed 2D shapes. *Computer Vision, Graphics, and Image Processing*, 31:265–281, 1995.

[15] Srinivasan, M. V., Laughlin, S. B., Dubs, A. Predictive coding: A fresh view of inhibition in the retina. *Proc. R. Soc. Lond. B*, 216:427–459, 1982.

[16] van Hateren, J. H. Spatiotemporal contrast sensitivity of early vision. *Vision Research*, 33:257–267, 1993.

Part I: Perception

1 Bayesian Modelling of Visual Perception

Pascal Mamassian, Michael Landy, and Laurence T. Maloney

Introduction

Motivation

Through perception, an organism arrives at decisions about the external world, decisions based on both current sensory information and prior knowledge concerning the environment. Unfortunately, the study of perceptual decision-making is distributed across sub-disciplines within psychology and neuroscience. Perceptual psychologists and neuroscientists focus on the information available in stimuli, developmental researchers focus on how knowledge about the environment is acquired, researchers interested in memory study how this knowledge is encoded, and other cognitive psychologists might be primarily interested in the decision mechanisms themselves. Any perceptual task evidently involves all of these components and, at first glance, it would seem that any theory of perceptual decision making must draw on heterogeneous models and results from all of these areas of psychology.

Many researchers have recently proposed an alternative (see chapters in [8]). They suggested that Bayesian Decision Theory (BDT) is a convenient and natural framework that allows researchers to study all aspects of a perceptual decision in a unified manner. This framework involves three basic components: the task of the organism, prior knowledge about the environment, and knowledge of the way the environment is sensed by the organism [6]. In this chapter, we summarize the key points that make the Bayesian framework attractive as a framework for the study of perception and we illustrate how to develop models of visual function based on BDT.

We emphasize the role played by prior knowledge about the environment in the interpretation of images, and describe how this prior knowledge is represented as prior distributions in BDT. For the sake of terminological variety, we will occasionally refer to prior knowledge as "prior beliefs" or "prior constraints", but it is important to note that this prior knowledge is not something the observer need be aware of. Yet,

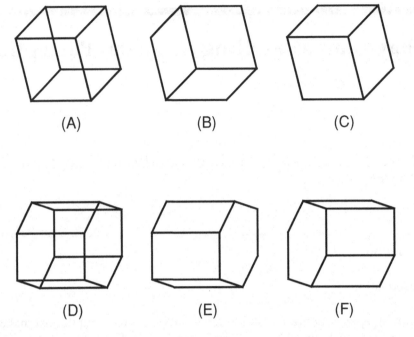

Figure 1.1: Multistable figures. Figures A and D typically engender one of two interpretations (B or C for A, and E or F for D). When viewed long enough, the interpretation will alternate between B and C and between E and F. The interpretation might vary when the figure is repeatedly presented or when the observer blinks or changes fixation.

as we shall see, these implicit assumptions can be revealed through psychophysical experimentation.

To introduce the Bayesian approach, we illustrate how to model a simplified problem of three-dimensional perception. The problem is not realistic but our intent in presenting it is to introduce the terminology, concepts, and methods of Bayesian modelling. Following the example, we illustrate how the framework can be used to model slightly more realistic problems concerning the perception of shape from shading and from contours. We conclude with a general discussion of the main issues of the Bayesian approach. Other tutorials on Bayesian modelling of visual perception with more technical details include Knill, Kersten & Yuille [7], Yuille & Bülthoff [18], and Maloney [9].

Before introducing Bayesian modelling, we first remind the reader what makes three-dimensional perception difficult.

Visual perception as an ill-posed problem

Consider the line drawing in Fig. 1.1A. Even though this line drawing is consistent with an infinite number of polyhedra, human observers usually report only two distinct interpretations, illustrated in Figs. 1.1B and C. Similarly, Fig. 1.1D is usually interpreted as shown in Figs. 1.1E or F. If Fig. 1.1A is viewed long enough, the observer will usually experience alternation between the interpretations suggested in Figs. 1.1B and C, but only one interpretation is seen at any point in time.

Two questions arise: (1) Why are only two of an infinite number of possible interpretations seen? (2) And why do we see only one interpretation at a time rather than, say, a superposition of all of the possible interpretations?

A proper answer to the first question requires that we explain why the visual system favors certain interpretations over others *a priori*. Within the Bayesian framework, this mechanism will prove to be the prior distribution. An answer to the second question will lead us to consider how perceptual decisions are made within the Bayesian framework.

Because space perception is ill-posed with many possible scenes consistent with the available sensory information, Bayesian modelling will prove to be particularly appropriate (for a recent review of visual space perception, see [5]).

A Simple Example: 3D Angle Perception

In this section, we introduce the key concepts of Bayesian modelling by means of a simple example. We will not attempt here to model the interpretation of the line drawings in Fig. 1.1. That would require too much investment in mathematical notation (to represent figures made out of lines in space) and would serve to obscure rather than display the elements of Bayesian modelling. Instead, we consider a perceptual task that is extremely simple, rather unrealistic, but plausibly related to perceptual interpretation of the drawings in Fig. 1.1: estimation of the angle formed by two intersecting lines in space given only the projection of the lines onto a single retina.

Task

The problem is illustrated in Fig. 1.2: Given two intersecting lines in an image forming angle φ, what is the angle θ between the two lines in three-dimensional space? Just as for Fig. 1.1, the observer looks at a two-dimensional image and has to make an inference about some three-dimensional property of the scene.

At the outset, our problem appears impossible. We do not even know whether the two lines intersect in space! Even if we somehow knew that they did, we still don't know how to go from the proximal angle φ to the distal angle θ. Clearly there can be no deterministic rule that takes us from proximal to distal angles, for there are many values of distal angle θ that all lead to the same value of the proximal angle φ. But perhaps we can, given the proximal angle φ, rank the possible values of the distal angle θ as candidates by some measure of plausibility.

To do so, we need to understand how the scene was generated. Let's imagine that

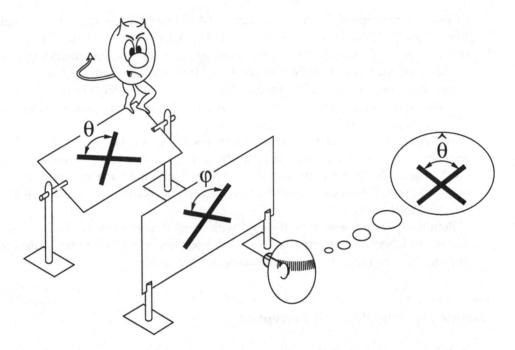

Figure 1.2: Perception of 3D angles. The angle θ between two line segments in 3D space projects as an angle φ in the image. A demon spins the physical stimulus about a horizontal axis, resulting in a random value of slant. The task of the observer is to infer θ given φ.

the scene is completely under the control of a "Demon" who first draws the angle on a transparent sheet of acrylic (Fig. 1.2), perpendicular to the line of sight of the observer, and then gleefully spins the sheet of acrylic about a horizontal axis. The spin is so forceful that we can assume that the acrylic sheet ends up at any slant angle σ as likely as any other. While the angle is drawn and the sheet spun, the observer waits patiently with eyes closed. The angle that the Demon drew is symmetric around the vertical axis before and after the spin as illustrated in Fig. 1.2. At the Demon's command, the observer opens his or her eyes and, challenged by the Demon, must specify the true angle θ given that only the projection φ is seen.

   Given this generating model, we can say quite a lot about the relation between φ and the possible θs that might have given rise to it. As the acrylic sheet gets more slanted relative to the line-of-sight, the projected angle φ in Fig. 1.2 increases to 180 degrees (when the sheet is horizontal) and then decreases back to the true value, when the acrylic sheet is upside down. The projected angle φ is always greater than or equal to the true angle θ. We can say more than this, though. Given the known value of φ and what we know about the generating model, we can compute the probability that any particular value of the unknown θ was the angle that the Demon drew. This probability distribution is the first element of Bayesian modelling that we introduce and it is the *likelihood function*.

Likelihood function

Let us assume that the angle φ between the two lines in the image is measured to be 135 degrees. What is the likelihood that any given world angle θ, say, 95 degrees, was the angle that the Demon chose to draw? To answer this question, we can imagine the following simulation. We take our own acrylic sheet with two lines painted on it separated by 95 degrees and we then spin it ourselves, repeatedly, simulating what the Demon did, over and over. Following each simulation of the Demon's spin, we measure the resulting angle φ. If the projected angle is approximately[1] the angle φ that we measured (say, 135 degrees plus or minus 5 degrees), we decide that the simulation is a "hit", otherwise it is a "miss". Repeating this procedure 1000 times, we end up with 5 hits and 995 misses. We conclude that the probability of obtaining an image angle of approximately 135 degrees given a world angle of 95 degrees is about 0.005.

If we repeat our simulation experiment for all possible values of the world angle, we obtain a histogram estimation of the *likelihood function* (Fig. 1.3). The likelihood is a function of both the known image angle φ and the unknown world angle θ.

Note that θ is a random variable whereas φ is considered as a fixed parameter (cf. [1]). For this reason, we prefer to think of the likelihood function as a function of the distal angle θ indexed by the proximal angle φ. It is important to understand that the likelihood function is not a probability distribution function since the integral over all values of the distal angle θ need not be 1; it is the integral over all values of the proximal angle φ that must equal 1. We introduce the following notation for the likelihood function:

$$\text{likelihood}_\varphi(\theta) = p(\varphi \mid \theta) \tag{1.1}$$

The Demon is still waiting for a response. Given the likelihood function in Fig. 1.3, it would be foolish to guess that the Demon drew an angle as small as, say, 10 degrees. The likelihood that a world angle of 10 degrees would lead to the observed value of φ (135 degrees) is very small relative to larger angles. The likelihood increases for world angles up to 135 degrees at which point the likelihood drops to zero. (Recall that the reason for the zero values above 135 degrees is that the projected angle is always larger than the world angle so it is impossible for a world angle larger than 135 degrees to produce an image angle of 135 degrees. The largest likelihood is therefore reached for a world angle equal to 135 degrees.) The world angle that is most likely to have given rise to the observed φ is 135 degrees.

If we choose this angle as our estimate of the response variable, we follow the strat-

---

1. Note that angle is a continuous variable, so we are dealing with a continuous distribution. The probability of any particular value (e.g. an image angle of precisely 135 degrees) is zero. Such distribution functions are not easily estimated using Monte Carlo simulations without approximating them as discrete distributions (e.g. binning the angles into bins of width 10 degrees).

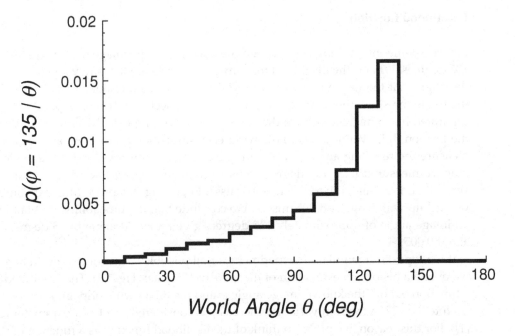

Figure 1.3: The likelihood function (when the image angle is 135 degrees). The likelihood characterizes the chances that a particular world angle projects as a given image angle.

egy called Maximum Likelihood Estimation (MLE) [17]. We choose, as our response, the world angle that had the highest probability of generating the observed sensory information. This decision rule is close in spirit to the Likelihood Principle proposed by Helmholtz [4].

The likelihood function captures all of the sensory information we have. What happens if we have extra knowledge or beliefs beyond the simple geometrical knowledge included in the likelihood function? Suppose that we know that our Demon has a marked bias toward world angles near 90 degrees and an aversion toward smaller or larger angles.

Prior distributions

We represent our knowledge about the Demon's preference for some world angles over others as a *prior distribution*, a probability distribution function on the response variable:

$$\text{prior}(\theta) = p(\theta) \tag{1.2}$$

Figure 1.4 shows one such prior distribution chosen to be a Gaussian distribution with a mean of 90 degrees and a standard deviation of 30 degrees. The value of the standard deviation in effect represents how strong the Demon's preference for 90 is.

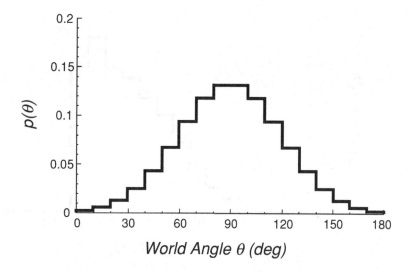

Figure 1.4: Prior distribution (discretized Normal distribution with a mean of 90 deg and a standard deviation of 30 deg). The prior distribution represents the prior belief of the observer as the frequency of occurrence of various world angles.

When the standard deviation is very small, the resulting Gaussian will be almost a spike at 90. If this distribution accurately captured the Demon's behavior, then we would know the Demon almost always picked an angle of 90 degrees or very close to it. Even without sensory information, we would expect to be able to make a very good estimate of the world angle. If, on the other hand, the standard deviation is very large, the resulting Gaussian tends to a uniform distribution. This case represents a very slight preference of the Demon for 90 degrees such that knowledge of the prior is not helping us much in our estimation task. We shall assume for now that the Demon's preference is well captured by a Gaussian with standard deviation of 30 degrees as shown in Fig. 1.4: the bias toward 90 is strong but not so strong as to tempt us to ignore the sensory information embodied in the likelihood function.

So far, we have encountered two elements found in any Bayesian model: the likelihood function and the prior. The former represents everything we know about the process that turns the state of the world into sensory information. The latter describes what we know about the relative plausibility of different states of the world. Both represent knowledge in probabilistic terms, permitting us to combine sensory information and prior knowledge about the world using probability calculus.

Bayes' theorem and the posterior distribution

The Demon is still waiting for an answer. We next need to combine likelihood and prior to compute a posterior distribution, our estimate of the probability of different

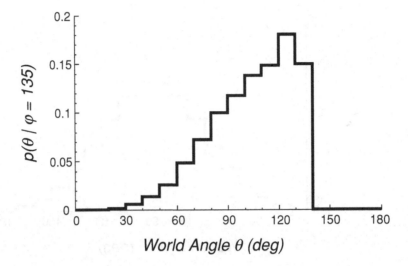

Figure 1.5: Posterior distribution (given that the image angle was 135 degrees). The posterior distribution represents the likelihood of occurrence of the response variable weighted by prior beliefs.

states of the world (here, θ) given everything we know. The following formula describes how to compute the posterior distribution:

$$\text{posterior}_\varphi(\theta) = C \times \text{likelihood}_\varphi(\theta) \times \text{prior}(\theta) \tag{1.3}$$

where C is a constant chosen so that the posterior is indeed a probability distribution function (i.e., the integral over all possible values of θ is one). Intuitively, the posterior of one world angle θ is simply the likelihood weighted by the prior probability of occurrence of θ. The formula is derived from Bayes' Theorem, a simple mathematical result concerning computations with conditional probabilities:

$$p(\theta \mid \varphi) = p(\varphi \mid \theta) \times p(\theta)/p(\varphi) \tag{1.4}$$

The left-hand side is the posterior, $p(\varphi \mid \theta)$ is the likelihood, and $p(\theta)$ is the prior.

Comparing the last two equations, we note that C equals the inverse of $p(\varphi)$, but it is easy to avoid computing it (or even thinking about it) since (1) it is the constant needed to make the posterior distribution a distribution, and (2) given the uses to which the posterior is put, it often turns out that the normalization by C is not necessary.

The posterior distribution is our estimate of the probability distribution of the unknown angle θ after both the sensory data and the prior distribution are taken into account. Fig. 1.5 shows the posterior distribution when the likelihood function was computed as in Fig. 1.3 and the prior probability was chosen as in Fig. 1.4 . Note that the peak of the posterior distribution is located between the peaks of the likelihood function (Fig. 1.3) and the prior distribution (Fig. 1.4).

In effect, the two sources of information we have are being pooled. The likelihood function would lead us to pick values of θ near 135 degrees as our maximum likelihood guess, the prior would lead us to favor a guess nearer 90 degrees, reflecting knowledge of the Demon's preference. The two pieces of information average out to a posterior whose peak falls around 125 degrees, about 22% of the way from the likelihood peak to the prior peak.

We could imagine redoing this example with different values of the standard deviation of the prior. When the standard deviation is smaller, the peak of the posterior moves toward the peak of the prior (i.e., 90 degrees), when it is larger, the peak of the posterior moves toward the peak of the likelihood function (i.e., 135 degrees). The standard deviation of the prior is effectively controlling the relative importance of prior and sensory information. When the Demon's preference toward 90 is known to be very strong, we should favor our prior knowledge and downweight conflicting sensory data. Alternatively, we should favor the sensory data when the prior is weak.

Intelligent selection of the distributional form for the prior is an important part of modelling. Within the Bayesian framework, the prior encodes all we know about the state of the world independently of the current sensory input.

Still, the Demon is becoming impatient. The posterior distribution is what we have, but what we need is an estimate of θ, a "best guess". That's what the Demon wants from us.

Gain, loss, and the decision rule

The decision rule links the posterior distribution with the action taken by the observer. The action can be an explicit motor act, such as orienting the hand appropriately to grasp an object, or an estimate of some aspect of the world such as the angle θ. One possible criterion for choosing an action is to pick the mode of the posterior distribution, the most probable value of θ according to the posterior distribution. If we used such a *Maximum a Posteriori (MAP) Rule*, our response to the Demon's challenge would be "125 degrees". This rule is widely used in the Bayesian literature and it is a plausible choice of decision rule.

Within the framework of Bayesian Decision Theory the choice of decision rule is remarkably simple and principled. It begins by assuming that, for every action we might take, there are consequences that depend upon the true state of the World: a numerical gain or loss, where a loss is merely a negative gain. In the example we have been pursuing, we have neglected to describe the consequences of our actions. Let us remedy this deficiency now.

Suppose that, if we guess the Demon's angle θ to within, say, 5 degrees, he goes away (+100, a gain). If we miss by more than 5 degrees, he draws a new angle, spins the acrylic sheet anew, and continues to torment us (−50, a loss). We shall call such a specification of gain and loss a *gain function*. We can then choose the action that maximizes our expected gain (cf. also chapter 6 by Nadal). The *Bayes decision rule* is precisely the choice of action α that, given the posterior, maximizes expected gain:

$$\text{expected\_gain}_\varphi(\alpha) = \int_\theta \text{posterior}_\varphi(\theta) \times \text{gain}(\alpha, \theta) d\theta \tag{1.5}$$

The particular gain function we chose in this example is an example of a *discrete Dirac* or *Delta* gain function which takes on two values only. The larger gain is obtained when the angle estimate (the action) is within a small interval surrounding the correct angle, otherwise the lesser gain is obtained. If the small interval is infinitesimally small, then, it turns out that the Bayes decision rule corresponding to the Delta gain function is precisely the MAP rule. When the interval is small but finite, as in our example, the Bayes decision rule is approximately the MAP rule. Thus, if we wish to be rid of the Demon as quickly as possible, we should pick the most probable value of θ according to the posterior distribution. Any other choice prolongs, on average, our encounter with the Demon.

But suppose that the gains and losses are different from those just specified. What if the Demon appears with his acrylic sheet and announces that, today, he will force the observer to pay him, in dollars, the square of the difference in degrees between his estimate and the true value of θ. A five degree error costs $25, a 10 degree error, $100. This gain/loss function is the *least-square loss function*, a very commonly used loss criterion in statistical estimation. The Observer's immediate question is likely to be "Is the MAP still the best rule to use?" The answer turns out to be no. The rule which minimizes his expected loss now is to pick the *mean* of the posterior distribution, not the mode. The Bayes rule associated with the least-square loss function is the mean. The mean of the posterior distribution in Fig. 1.5 is 105 degrees, significantly less than the MAP estimate, which was 125.

We have already noted that the prior distribution is responsible for the shift of the peak of the posterior probability away from the peak of the likelihood function. If the prior distribution is uniform (i.e. there is no evidence for any bias for the Demon's behavior), the maximum of the posterior equals the maximum of the likelihood. In this limit case, the maximum a posteriori (MAP) rule is identical to the maximum likelihood estimate (MLE) rule.

While the Delta gain function and the associated MAP rule are appealing for their simplicity, this decision rule is sometimes prone to favor unstable interpretations such as scenes viewed from accidental viewpoints [3, 18]. One possible cure to this problem is to choose a loss function that gracefully increases when the estimate of the world angle α deviates from the real world angle θ. The least-square loss function described above is one such function.

It is important to emphasize that there is not one computation applied to the posterior distribution that defines uniquely the Bayes rule. Rather, the rule varies as the gains and losses vary. The Bayes rule is always: *do whatever you must to maximize expected gain*.

The Bayesian framework allows us to model the consequences of gains and losses on behavior and to represent performance in different tasks in a common framework so long as the effect of a change of task can be modeled as a change in possible gains and losses. See Berger [1] or Maloney [9] for a more detailed discussion.

One important property of the decision rules we have discussed so far is that the same action will be chosen whenever the same stimulus φ is seen. This must be contrasted with the variable behavior of any biological organism. There are at least two approaches to modelling this variability. The first approach is to recognize that we have neglected to model photon noise and sources of noise in the visual system. Introduction of these as contributors to the likelihood component of a Bayesian model would introduce variability into human responses to identical stimuli. The second approach is to abandon the Bayes rule as a realistic decision rule. For instance, Mamassian & Landy [11] have modeled human response variability with what they termed a "non-committing" rule. According to this non-deterministic rule, an action is chosen with a probability that matches its posterior probability. Actions with high posterior probabilities are selected more often than those with low posterior probabilities, but any action may potentially be chosen. This decision is also known as *probability matching* [13] and is often observed in human and animal choice behavior when the gain function is the Delta gain function described above. It is important to note that this rule is not optimal (the MAP rule always leads to higher gain). Even though the MAP Rule is optimal in this case, humans and other animals persist in probability matching to a remarkable degree. In fact, it might be a better strategy for an animal since it allows exploration of the state space for learning (for an introduction to learning by exploration, see [16]).

Discussion

In this section, we have defined the three fundamental steps in Bayesian modelling of visual perception (Fig. 1.6). The first step is to define the prior distributions to represent what we know about the probability of encountering different states of the world. The second step is to compute the likelihood function by determining all the ways the stimuli could have been generated and their frequency of occurrence. Using Bayes' theorem, likelihood and priors can be combined to produce a posterior distribution, i.e., the best estimate of the probability of each possible state of the world given the sensory data and the prior distribution. The third and last step is to settle on a decision rule that transforms the posterior distribution into an action. In a full Bayesian model, this decision rule is computed from Bayes' rule and is fully described by the gain function.

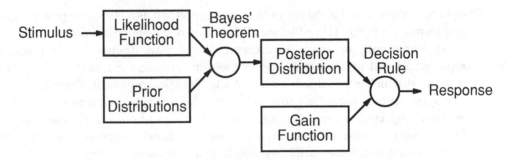

Figure 1.6: Flowchart of the steps involved in Bayesian modelling.

The Study of Human Priors: Perception of Embossed Surfaces

Issues

In the previous part of the chapter, we have provided a model of perceptual decision making based on sensory information, *a priori* knowledge, and the choice of a decision rule. The critical question is, of course, "Are Bayesian models appropriate for human vision?" While it is too early to answer this question conclusively, a first test of the model is to analyze the compatibility of the model with human data. At this point, it is important to keep in mind that even if visual processing could be perfectly represented as a Bayesian model, the modeler's choice of distribution, likelihood, gain function, or decision rule may be different from what is actually embodied in visual processing. Our first endeavor should therefore be to learn more about the form of the prior distributions, gain functions, and decision rules that accurately model human vision.

Assuming for now that we know how to compute the likelihood function and the decision rule, we shall use Bayesian models to investigate how prior knowledge is encoded in the visual system. As a first guess, it is convenient to model prior knowledge as a Gaussian distribution (or von Mises distribution for periodic variables such as angles; cf. [12]). The advantage of the Gaussian distribution is that it is fully parameterized by only two parameters, namely its *mean* and *variance*. This prior encodes a preference in favor of the mean value and values near it. The variance of the Gaussian is inversely related to the strength of the evidence in favor of the prior mean. As the variance increases, the prior distribution converges to the uniform distribution. It is important to note that while the Gaussian distribution is everywhere non-zero, other non-Gaussian priors can be zero across an interval; in this case, no amount of sensory data can beat the prior.

In this section, we consider simple visual tasks that are sufficiently ambiguous that we can hope to observe the influence of prior distributions in visual performance.

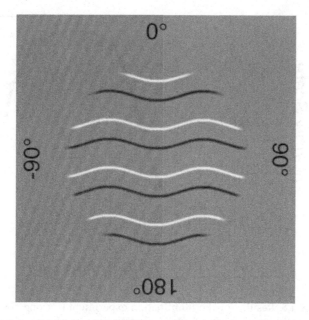

Figure 1.7: Stimulus used in the illumination experiment. This figure was presented at different orientations in the image plane. Observers indicated whether they perceived the wide or narrow strips bulging in relief.

We summarize here our work on the perception of shaded embossed surfaces with parallel contours [10, 11, 12].

Assumption of illumination from above-left

Light sources are usually located above our head. It is commonly believed that this regularity of the illumination position is at the origin of the change in perceived relief of figures that are turned upside-down [2, 14]. We have been interested in quantifying this prior assumption used by the visual system [10]. We report the results of this experiment with reference to the Bayesian framework developed in the previous part of this chapter.

Stimuli were shaded embossed surfaces as shown in Fig. 1.7. These stimuli can be interpreted as planar frontal surfaces with either narrow or wide strips bulging towards the observer. When the figure is rotated in the image plane, the perception alternates between these two interpretations. The fact that the very same figure can be interpreted in two different ways with a mere rotation indicates that the visual system is using additional knowledge beyond the stimulus information. We presented the figure at different orientations to human adult observers and asked them whether they perceived the bulging strips as being narrow or wide. Each orientation was presented multiple times to estimate the variability of responses for each orientation.

Results for one observer are shown in Fig. 1.8. Let us call *narrow score* the proportion of times the stimulus was interpreted as formed by narrow strips bulging. The

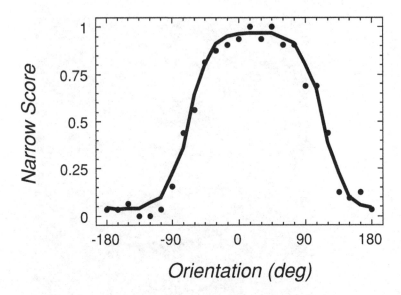

Figure 1.8: Results for the illumination experiment (for one observer). The dots indicate the proportion of times an observer perceived the narrow strips in relief, and the solid line shows the performance of the model.

plot shows the narrow score as a function of the orientation of the figure in the image plane. It is clear from the plot that responses depended strongly on the orientation of the stimulus. When the bright contours of the figure are interpreted as edges facing the light source and dark contours in shadow, the peak narrow score should occur when the stimulus orientation is zero. Remarkably, the center of the peak of the narrow score is shifted to the right of zero, corresponding to a stimulus most consistent with light coming from above and slightly to the left of the observer (for a similar demonstration of an above-left illumination bias, see [15]).

The smooth curve in Fig. 1.8 shows the best fit of the Bayesian model to the human data. The model has knowledge about the shape of the object, the illumination and viewing conditions. The object is modeled as a flat surface with strips in relief. The narrow strips are either raised or lowered relative to the background flat surface and the orientation of the edge between the strip and the background defines the *bevel angle* (positive values correspond to the narrow strips being in relief). The illumination conditions are modeled with an ambient and a point light source of different intensities. In addition, the illumination model includes commonly used shading assumptions (uniform Lambertian reflectance). Finally, the viewpoint is modeled as the orientation of the viewing direction relative to the surface, thereby disregarding the distance between viewer and object.

The object, illumination, and viewing models have degrees of freedom that can be described as free parameters. Each parameter has its own prior distribution. For most parameters, we have no *a priori* knowledge and hence assume uniform prior distributions for these parameters. To model the prior assumptions that we anticipated to exist, we gave the corresponding parameter a non-uniform distribution, generally a Gaussian distribution specified by a mean (the value toward which observers were biased) and a variance (inversely related to the effectiveness). In this way, we allowed for biases on the thickness of the strips in relief (i.e., bevel angle), the light source tilt (i.e., light direction from approximately above) and the surface tilt (i.e., view-from-above, discussed in the next section).

The model calculates the posterior probability $p(narrow \mid stimulus)$ by first calculating that probability for each possible combination of illumination and viewpoint parameters, and then summing them:

$$\int p(narrow, illumination, viewpoint \mid stimulus) \, d(illumination) d(viewpoint) \qquad (1.6)$$

The integrand is expanded using Bayes' theorem into a likelihood and a prior term. The prior probability term, $p(narrow, illumination, viewpoint)$, is further expanded by assuming that illumination and viewpoint parameters are independent. Finally, the output of the model is obtained after application of the non-committing decision rule. That is, the proportion of times observers respond "narrow" is the same as the calculated posterior probability that the stimulus arose from an object with bulging narrow strips.

Each parameter can now be estimated from the best fit of the model to the human data. The advantage of the model is that each parameter has a straightforward meaning. The best-fitted parameter for the light source direction indicates a bias of approximately 25 degrees to the left of the vertical. The effectiveness of this bias on the light source position and the bias for the viewpoint can be estimated by looking at the variance of the corresponding prior distributions. In addition, there was a very slight bias to prefer narrow rather than wide strips in relief.

Assumption of viewpoint from above

Using the line drawing shown in Fig. 1.9, we showed that observers have a bias to interpret contour drawings as if they were viewing the object from above [11]. In this experiment, observers reported whether the line drawing appeared to be the projection of a surface patch which was egg-shaped or saddle-shaped. Again, these images were shown at various orientations in the image plane, and observers indicated whether they initially perceived the object as egg- or saddle-shaped. We rely on the initial interpretation, averaged across multiple presentations of the same stimulus, to determine the observer's propensity to perceive the stimulus in one way or the other.

The data in Fig. 1.10 clearly showed that responses again depended strongly on the stimulus orientation. The preference for a viewpoint located above the scene can be modeled as a preference for the normal to the surface to point upwards [11]. This preference can therefore be modeled as a bias on the tilt of the surface normal, with the preferred tilt equal to 90 degrees. The bias on the surface normal results in a bias

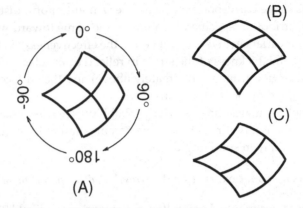

Figure 1.9: Stimuli used in the viewpoint experiment. The line drawing shown in A can be interpreted as an egg-shaped patch or saddle-shaped patch depending on its orientation in the frontal plane. Figure B tends to be seen as egg-shaped more often, whereas C is more often seen as saddle-shaped. Each stimulus was presented at different orientations in the image plane. Observers indicated whether they perceived an egg-shaped or saddle-shaped patch.

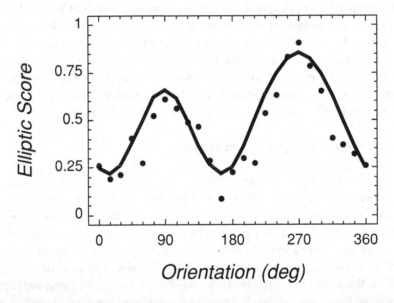

Figure 1.10: Results for the viewpoint experiment (averaged over 7 observers). The elliptic score (i.e. the proportion of times observers indicated Fig. 1.9A was egg-shaped) is shown as a function of the orientation in the image plane. The best fit of the Bayesian model is shown as a solid line.

to interpret contours that are convex-upward in the image as being convex toward the observer.

We again fit a Bayesian model using exactly the same strategy as in the illumination case above. Here, the scene description included parameters related to the surface shape (same-sign principal curvatures correspond to egg-shaped surfaces), the viewpoint (i.e. the surface orientation as defined by its slant, tilt and roll), and the way surface contours were painted on the surface patch (defined by their orientation relative to the principal lines of curvature). Most parameters were given uniform prior distributions except for the surface tilt (corresponding to our suspected bias for a viewpoint above the object), the surface curvature (for a good fit we required a bias for perceiving 3D contours as convex) and the surface contour orientations (which were biased to be closely aligned with the principal lines of curvature). Again, the non-committing rule was used. From the best fit of a Bayesian model that included these prior constraints, we estimated the standard deviation of the prior distribution on surface tilt orientation to be approximately 30 degrees.

The prior assumption on the surface tilt probably plays a role in the interpretation of the Necker cube shown in Fig. 1.1A. We have already noted that only two interpretations out of an infinite number are preferred by human observers (Figs. 1.1B and 1.1C). With prolonged viewing, observers alternate between these two interpretations with a frequency that can be well-modeled by a Gamma distribution. The mean time spent in each interpretation, however, is different. One direct prediction from the results of this section is that the preferred cube interpretation will be the one for which most of the normals to its faces point upwards.

Interaction of prior assumptions

In the last two sections, we have seen that the interpretation of ambiguous figures is guided by two assumptions: a preference for the illumination to be located above (and to the left) of the observer and a similar preference to have the viewpoint located above the scene. In this section, we look at stimuli for which both of these assumptions can be used to disambiguate the figure. For some orientations of each stimulus the two prior constraints were in agreement as to the preferred interpretation of the stimulus, and in others they were in conflict. An example stimulus is shown in Fig. 1.11 [12].

These stimuli can again be perceived as embossed surfaces with either narrow or wide strips in relief. The data show that the observer's interpretation changed as the figure was rotated in the frontal plane (Fig. 1.12).

The human performance was well modeled by a Bayesian model that included both the illumination and the viewpoint priors described in the previous sections. The model was of exactly the same form as the previous two, including parameters for the surface shape (i.e. the bevel angle), the illumination and viewpoint. Again, the non-committing rule was used and the parameters of the prior distributions were varied to best fit the data. The best fit of the model allowed us to extract the parameters of the prior distributions. The light direction bias was 10 degrees to the left of the vertical (the viewpoint bias was set to 90 degrees for the surface tilt). The standard deviation of the illumination prior was about 40 degrees, whereas the

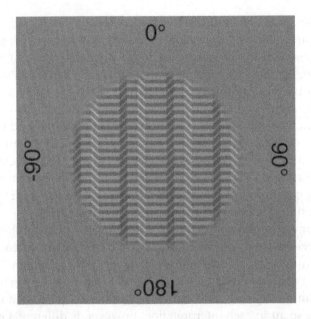

Figure 1.11: Stimuli used for the interaction of priors experiment. Depending on its orientation in the frontal plane, this figure can be interpreted as an embossed surface with narrow or wide strips in relief. Both shading and contour cues to shape are present in the stimulus.

standard deviation of the viewpoint prior was about 80 degrees. In addition, there was a very slight bias to prefer narrow over wide strips in relief.

In the first part of this chapter, we argued that the standard deviation of a prior distribution is inversely related to the effectiveness of this prior. We tested whether this effectiveness could be affected by changing properties of the stimulus. We repeated the prior interaction experiment for stimuli for which the stimulus contrasts of the shading and surface contours were independently varied. We fit each contrast condition separately. We found that increasing the shading contrast decreased the standard deviation of the illumination prior, and similarly, increasing the contour contrast decreased the standard deviation of the viewpoint prior. These results are consistent with the notion that the effectiveness of a prior distribution reflects the reliability of the particular cue with which it is associated (see chapter 3 by Jacobs for a related finding). It is important to realize that we have treated these prior distributions as variable things, dependent on aspects of the stimulus itself. The apparent cue reliability that drives this change can be estimated from ancillary measures extracted from the stimulus (e.g., the contrast of the shading or contour edges in our example).

Discussion

In this part of the chapter, we have summarized three studies that looked at the 3D perception of ambiguous images. We used the Bayesian framework developed

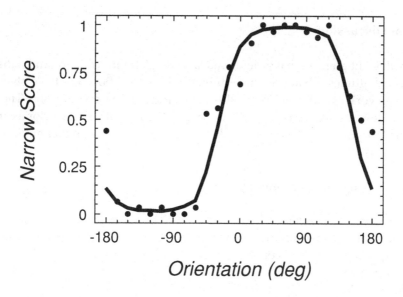

Figure 1.12: Results for the interaction of priors experiment (averaged over 8 observers). The figure gives the proportion of trials observers indicated that the narrow strips were seen bulging as a function of the image plane orientation of the stimulus. The solid line shows the best fit of the Bayesian model.

in the first section of this chapter to focus on the prior assumptions used by the visual system. We found a preference for the illumination to come from above-left and for the viewpoint to be located above the scene. The Bayesian models allowed us to explain human performance quantitatively.

We also looked at a situation in which the consequences of two prior assumptions must be combined. We found that our framework was still applicable in predicting human performance, but only if we allowed the standard deviation of the prior distributions to be affected by the stimulus properties. In this experiment, different parts of the stimuli changed contrast but the task of the observer was kept constant. Therefore, we did not change the gain function or the decision rule to try to explain the shifts of human criteria with stimulus contrast. In addition, while the likelihood changed with the stimulus contrast, this change was not large enough to explain the criteria shifts. Only a change in the prior distribution could reasonably explain the changes in human performance. More specifically, we found that the prior confidence value as measured by the variance of the prior distribution was inversely related to the contrast of the stimulus attributes relevant for this prior. This finding is important because it forces us to reconsider a basic tenet of Bayesian modelling that prior constraints are pieces of knowledge that are independent of the stimuli and of the task with which observers are confronted. This issue is further discussed in the next section.

General Discussion

In this chapter, we have described a general framework to study the resolution of ambiguities arising in three-dimensional perception. We have shown how the framework can be implemented by describing a few applications. The framework is Bayesian in the sense that it emphasizes the role played by prior assumptions. In this last part of the chapter, we discuss some of the issues that are inherent in this framework.

Is this really Bayesian modelling?

The models we discussed in the previous section were cited as examples of Bayesian modelling of depth disambiguation. In fact, they stray fairly far from a strict Bayesian interpretation of a decision making problem. We now describe the Bayesian and non-Bayesian components of our models, and discuss our motivation for departing from the strict Bayesian approach.

Our models begin in the Bayesian spirit by defining prior distributions on various parameters that give rise to the stimulus situation. These parameters describe the objects of the physical environment, the illumination conditions and the viewing geometry. More specifically in our examples, objects are parameterized by the bevel angle, reflectances of the various surfaces, principal surface curvatures, orientation of the surface contours relative to those surface curvatures, and surface shape. The illuminant is simply characterized by the position of the light sources and their intensities. Finally, the viewing geometry is parameterized as the orientation of the observed object relative to the viewer (the viewing distance should also be included in perspective projection). When we have no reason to expect observers to have a particular bias, we give the corresponding parameter a uniform prior distribution. In contrast, where biases are expected, the prior is modeled as a non-uniform distribution where the modes of the distribution match the biases. Typically, we anticipate a single bias along each dimension, so that the prior distribution is unimodal (e.g. Gaussian). For instance, among all possible light source directions in the frontal plane, only one direction is preferred. Moreover, we showed how these biases can be estimated experimentally [11, 12]. So far, this is pretty much the Bayesian methodology.

However, we depart from a strict Bayesian methodology in a number of ways. Let us first consider the likelihood function. The likelihood characterizes the mapping from world to retinal image. When the stimulus has very low contrast, photon statistics will affect the image registered on the retina. Moreover, internal noise will also affect the way stimuli are represented at successive stages in the visual system (see chapters 2 by Schrater & Kersten and 4 by Weiss & Fleet). These external and internal sources of noise will cause the proximal stimulus to be stochastic and as a result, the computed likelihood will vary from trial to trial, and the observer's decision will vary when the same distal stimulus is repeatedly presented. In contrast, our likelihood function is deterministic. Either this set of object, illumination and viewing parameters gives rise to this image or it does not. We argued that with our high-contrast stimuli, external noise is negligible and internal noise alone can not reasonably explain the large variations in subjects' responses.

Our second departure from a strict Bayesian approach is the way we treat the decision rule. In a sense, this follows directly from our choice of a deterministic likelihood function. If the decision rule is a Bayes rule, it is also deterministic. Examples of Bayes rules include the maximum likelihood and the MAP rules. When the likelihood and decision rules are both deterministic, the observer will give the same response to trials that use the same stimuli. This prediction was clearly violated in our psychophysical experiments. Therefore, instead of following a Bayes rule, we chose a stochastic rule that we termed a "non-committing decision rule". According to this rule, the observer first computes the posterior probability of each possible scene given the image and then chooses each response with probability equal to its estimated posterior probability. If, for instance, there are only two possible scenes whose posterior probabilities are 0.7 and 0.3 respectively, then the observer will choose the first scene with a probability equal to 0.7. This rule is suboptimal (unless the gains are such that incorrect answers are not penalized) and hence is not a Bayes rule. However, it is a behavior that is commonly found in humans and animals, and is referred to as *probability matching* [13].

Finally, we depart from a Bayesian approach by the way we treat prior constraints. We looked at the effect of context on prior constraints by varying the stimulus contrast along different parts of an image. We found that the effect of the prior associated with the shading cue to depth increased with shading contrast (and similarly for the contour cue to depth). We fit the model to the data separately for each contrast condition, allowing the parameters for the priors (light-from-above and viewpoint-from-above) to vary between fits. That is, we allowed the prior distributions to depend on the stimulus. This is distinctly *not* a Bayesian operation. If the priors depend on the stimulus, then they are not "prior"! Nevertheless, the results of this exercise were quite interesting. The variance of the prior distributions, as we have discussed, is inversely related to their effectiveness in biasing the overall estimate. We found that this effectiveness was a monotonic function of contrast. This makes sense, even though it is entirely contrary to the notion that these were parameters of prior distributions.

In summary, we depart from the traditional Bayesian approach by the way we treat the three basic components of any Bayesian model. We believe that the reasons for these departures were well-motivated for the experiments presented in this chapter. Future research will tell us whether our choices are valuable in other contexts.

Future directions

The Bayesian-inspired models of visual perception described in this chapter provide an explicit account of the interaction between sensory information and prior assumptions, as well as the decision rule used by the observer in a given task. Each component of the models is justifiable and experimentally testable. Therefore, Bayesian models appear psychologically more relevant than previous models that relied on *ad-hoc* components such as the "smoothness constraint" (in fact, other frameworks such as regularization are just special cases of the Bayesian framework; [18]). In spite of its great appeal, Bayesian modelling is still in its infancy. We now discuss some future directions of research.

The first issue deals with the interaction between the likelihood function and the prior distributions. In this chapter, we have chosen a likelihood function that faithfully takes all the information in the image and that is not affected by noise. This choice implies a highly peaked likelihood function and a moderate influence of the prior distributions on the posterior distribution. Alternatively, the same posterior distribution could have been obtained by a more shallow likelihood function and a greater influence of the prior distributions (cf. the influence of external noise on the likelihood function in [7]). More work is needed to understand better how different contextual situations (such as different amounts of external noise) affect the likelihood function and the prior distributions (cf. chapter 7 by Yuille & Coughlan).

Another issue deals with the origin and stability of prior constraints. Do prior constraints directly reflect the statistical regularities of the environment? If so, we can foresee that priors will be conditional on context (e.g. a forest prior vs. a city prior). When more than one prior can be applied in a certain context, then these priors will have to compete (for an example on shape from shading, cf. [18]). Another related question is whether priors can be updated when the environmental conditions change. Updating a prior constraint means that the visual system has the ability to sample and memorize an extremely large number of scenes (cf. [19]). This strategy is impractical unless some sort of approximation is used to build the new priors. Finding biologically plausible implementations of Bayesian models and their approximations is an area of active research (see the chapters in the second part of this book).

One final important issue deals with the importance of the task with which the visual system is faced. It is obvious that different tasks correspond to different decision rules. Some motor tasks might put the organism more at risk than purely visual exploration tasks, thereby affecting the cost of making the wrong decision. However, it is perhaps less obvious that the task could also affect the prior constraints used. Different tasks might indeed direct the attention of the visual system to different components of the stimulus and their associated priors. Future research should look at the level(s) within the visual system at which the choice of task has influence.

To conclude, we have reviewed the main principles underlying Bayesian modelling of three-dimensional perception. The framework entails the derivation of the likelihood function, the description of prior assumptions and the choice of a decision rule. We believe that this framework provides a powerful tool to study the mechanisms involved in human visual perception and that it can have important generalizations in others areas of cognitive neuroscience.

Acknowledgments

Funding was partially provided by the Human Frontier Science Program grant RG0109/1999-B, AFOSR grant 93NL366 and NIH grant EY08266.

References

[1] Berger, J. O. (1985). *Statistical Decision Theory and Bayesian Analysis* (Second Ed.). New York, NY: Springer-Verlag.

[2] Brewster, D. (1826). On the optical illusion of the conversion of cameos into intaglios and of intaglios into cameos, with an account of other analogous phenomena. *Edinburgh Journal of Science, 4*, 99–108.

[3] Freeman, W. T. (1996). The generic viewpoint assumption in a Bayesian framework. In D. C. Knill & W. Richards (Eds.), *Perception as Bayesian Inference* (pp. 365–389). Cambridge, UK: Cambridge University Press.

[4] von Helmholtz, H. (1865–67). *Handbuch der physiologischen Optic*. Hamburg, Germany: L. Voss.

[5] Hershenson, M. (1999). *Visual Space Perception: A Primer*. Cambridge, MA: MIT Press.

[6] Kersten, D. (1999). High-level vision as statistical inference. In M. S. Gazzaniga (Ed.), *The New Cognitive Neurosciences*. Cambridge, MA: MIT Press.

[7] Knill, D. C., Kersten, D. & Yuille, A. L. (1996). Introduction: A Bayesian formulation of visual perception. In D. C. Knill & W. Richards (Eds.), *Perception as Bayesian Inference* (pp. 1–21). Cambridge, UK: Cambridge University Press.

[8] Knill, D. C. & Richards, W. (1996). *Perception as Bayesian Inference*. Cambridge, UK: Cambridge University Press.

[9] Maloney, L. T. (2001). Statistical decision theory and biological vision. In D. Heyer & R. Mausfeld (Eds.), *Perception and the Physical World*. Chichester, UK: Wiley.

[10] Mamassian, P. & Goutcher, R. (2001). Prior knowledge on the illumination position. *Cognition, 81*, B1-B9.

[11] Mamassian, P. & Landy, M. S. (1998). Observer biases in the 3D interpretation of line drawings. *Vision Research, 38*, 2817–2832.

[12] Mamassian, P. & Landy, M. S. (in press). Interaction of visual prior constraints. *Vision Research*.

[13] Myers, J. L. (1976). Probability learning and sequence learning. In W. K. Estes (Ed.), *Handbook of Learning and Cognitive Processes: Approaches to Human Learning and Motivation*, Volume 3 (pp. 171–205). Hillsdale, NJ: Erlbaum.

[14] Rittenhouse, D. (1786). Explanation of an optical deception. *Transactions of the American Philosophical Society, 2*, 37–42.

[15] Sun, J. & Perona, P. (1998). Where is the sun? *Nature Neuroscience, 1*, 183–184.

[16] Sutton, R. S. & Barto, A. G. (1998). *Reinforcement Learning: An Introduction.* Cambridge, MA: MIT Press.

[17] Szeliski, R. (1989). *Bayesian Modeling of Uncertainty in Low-Level Vision.* Boston, MA: Kluwer.

[18] Yuille, A. & Bülthoff, H. H. (1996). Bayesian decision theory and psychophysics. In D. C. Knill & W. Richards (Eds.), *Perception as Bayesian Inference* (pp. 123–161). Cambridge, UK: Cambridge University Press.

[19] Zhu, S. C. & Mumford, D. (1997). Prior learning and Gibbs reaction-diffusion. *IEEE Transactions on Pattern Analysis and Machine Intelligence, 19*, 1236–1250.

2 Vision, Psychophysics and Bayes

Paul Schrater and Daniel Kersten

Introduction

Neural information processing research has progressed in two often divergent directions. On the one hand, computational neuroscience has advanced our understanding of the detailed computations of synapses, single neurons, and small networks (cf. [27]). Theories of this sort have benefited from the scientific interplay between testable predictions and experimental results from real neural systems. As such, this direction is aimed most directly at the mechanisms implementing visual function.

On the other hand, theoretical neural networks have been subsumed as special cases of statistical inference (cf. [34, 3, 26]). This direction is well-suited to large scale systems modeling appropriate to the behavioral functions of perceptual and cognitive systems. We've seen considerable progress in the solution of complex problems of perception and cognition–solutions obtained without specific reference to neural or biological mechanisms. However, in contrast to small-scale neuron-directed modeling, behavioral theories face a different experimental challenge–namely, how can quantitative models be refined by experiment? The neural implementation of a model of statistical pattern recognition typically has too many independent variables to test neurophysiologically, and behavioral tests are unsatisfying because most of the parameters are unmeasureable.

The purpose of this chapter is to suggest that the development of neural information processing theories based on statistical inference is actually a good thing for psychology, and in particular for visual psychophysics. The proper level of abstraction avoids the premature introduction of unmeasureable neural parameters that are too numerous or difficult to test behaviorally. Yet, as is the case for thermodynamics and models of molecular motion, the bridge between statistical pattern theories and neural networks can be made when required.

The principle concern of psychologists is behavior. In vision, we use the term behavior broadly to include perceptual psychophysics, experimental studies of visual cognition, and visual motor control . One can also distinguish two often divergent directions in the study of visual behavior in questions that address: 1) neural mechanism and 2) functional tasks. These questions can often be rephrased in the form of questions that address what the visual system can do when pushed to extremes, in contrast to what it does do in natural circumstances.

What people can do. There is a long tradition of relating the phenomena of visual perception and psychophysical performance to underlying neural mechanisms. Probably the most famous and successful example is color trichromacy which was deduced from psychophysical experiments of Helmholtz, Maxwell and others in the 19th century. The neurophysiological basis in terms of discrete retinal receptor types wasn't firmly established until the middle of the 20th century. Another example is the intriguing correspondence between the wavelet-like patterns that humans detect best and the receptive field profiles of simple cells in V1 [7, 43, 20]. For tests of mechanism, the behavioral tasks can be rather unnatural and the stimuli often bear little resemblance to the kinds of images we typically see. Signal detection theory has played an important role in relating behavior to mechanism [15]. It provides a bridge between theory and experiment as applied to neural mechanisms. In this first case, statistical or signal detection theories provide the means to account for the information available in the task itself–a step often neglected in drawing conclusions about mechanism from psychophysical measurements.

What people do do. There is also an ecological tradition in which we seek to understand how visual function is adapted to the world in which we live. Answering the question "How well do we see the shapes, colors, locations, and identities of objects?" is an important component in providing answers to the more general question "How does vision work?". The challenge we address below is arriving at a quantitative model to answer the "How well do we see ..." question for natural visual tasks. Statistical inference theory, and in particular the specific form we describe below as pattern inference theory, plays a role in the analysis of both kinds of perceptual behavior–but is particularly relevant for developing quantitative predictive models of visual function.

In this chapter, we describe a framework within which to develop and test predictive quantitative theories of human visual behavior as pertains to both mechanism and function. What are we asking for in a quantitative theory? A complete quantitative account of a human visual task should include models both of function, and of the mechanisms to realize those functions.

Problems of vision: ambiguity and complexity

At the functional level, one would like a model whose input is a natural image or sequence and whose output, shows the same performance as the human along some dimension. Further, the model should also predict the pattern of errors with respect to ground truth. Below we will describe a recent study which compared the perceived surface colors under quasi-natural lighting conditions with those of a Bayesian estimator.

Any such modeling effort immediately runs into two well-known *theoretical problems* of computer vision: ambiguity and complexity. How can a vision system draw reliable conclusions about the world from numerous locally ambiguous image measurements? The ambiguity arises because any image patch can be produced from many different combinations of scene variables (e.g. object and illumination properties). In addition, *all* of the scene variables, both relevant and irrelevant for the observer's task, contribute to natural image measurements. In general, image measurement space is high-dimensional, and building models that can deal with these problems leads to complex models that are difficult to analyze and for which it is difficult to determine what are the essential features. One possible solution is the historical one–take an empirical approach to human vision, and develop models to summarize the data from the ground up.

However, the complex high-dimensional nature of the relevant scene parameters leads to an *empirical problem* as well: psychophysical testing of models of human perception under natural conditions could rapidly become hopelessly complex. For example, with over a dozen cues to depth, a purely empirical approach to the problem of cue integration is combinatorially prohibitive. Thus, we are faced with two formidable problems in vision research. First, how do we develop relevant and analyzable models for vision, and second, how do we test these models experimentally?

Developing theories

For the modeling problem, we will argue that it is crucial to specify the correct level of analysis, and we distinguish modeling at the functional level from modeling at the level of mechanisms. The functional level constitutes a description of the *information* required to perform for particular task without worrying about the specific details of the computations. It addresses issues of the observer's prior knowledge and assumptions about scene structure, image formation, and the costs associated with normal task demands. On the other hand, the mechanistic level is concerned with the specific details of neural computations.

Functional level modeling

At the functional level, we wish to model a natural visual task, like apple counting. Given the natural task, the solution we propose is to let the ideal (Bayesian) observer for the task serve as a default model. The modeling strategy is to hypothesize that human vision uses all the information optimally. Of course, human vision is not optimal, but starting from the optimal observer yields a coherent research strategy in which models can be modified to discard the same kinds and amount of information as the human visual system. This approach departs from the historical bottom-up approach to modeling, but we suggest that it may be ultimately simpler than trying to determine how to "smarten up" a suboptimal model based on experiment. Here the main focus is how often the human is ideal or "ideal-like". By ideal-like we mean that peformance parallels ideal in all but a small number of dimensions (e.g. additive internal noise). Below we discuss an approach to information modeling we call "pattern inference theory", that is an elaboration of signal detection theory that provides the generative and decision theoretic tools to model the informational limits to natural tasks [22, 21, 25].

Two main strategies at the functional level can be distinguished: a) model the complexity of the visual inference, and compare the model with human performance, but don't try to directly model the information that is present in natural scenes [44]; b) model the physical information, and measure how well this model accounts for human performance. It is this second strategy we illustrate below with an example from color constancy [4]. Having a general purpose model for counting apples in trees may be in the distant future, but part of that model will involve understanding how surface colors for apples can be distinguished from those of leaves. Because of interreflections, any given point of the retinal image will often have wavelength contributions from direct and indirect light sources (i.e. from apples and leaves), that need to be discounted to infer the identity and properties of objects.

Mechanism level modeling

At the mechanism level we are interested in how visual stimuli are actually processed, what features in the image are measured, what kinds of representations does the visual system use. One would like an account of the neural systems, the spatial-temporal filtering, neural transformations and decision processes leading to the output. Here the modeling methods are more diffuse, encompassing optimal image encoding ideas [32, 47, 40] and more traditional analyses of the utility of image measurements for some task (e.g. the optic flow field for inferring egomotion).

In these kinds of study the model is typically not generated through an ideal observer analysis of a natural task. Nevertheless, we can profitably use the ideal observer approach to test mechanistic models. Here, deviations from ideal provide insight into biological limitations. The immediate focus of interest is how much human performance differs from ideal, because it is the differences which are diagnostic of the kinds of mechanisms used by the visual system. For example, we know that light discrimination departs from the ideal at high light levels, long durations, and large regions [2]. We also know that human pattern detection competes well with ideal observers when the patterns match the receptive field profiles of simple cells [7, 43, 20].

The way in which spatial resolution departs from ideal can be explained in large part by optical, sampling, and neural inefficiencies [14].

In addition, having an understanding of the ideal observer for the task used in the laboratory to test the mechanistic hypotheses is crucial. Psychophysically testing hypotheses of mechanism leads to a problem in addition to that of complexity: inferring mechanisms from psychophysics must take into account how performance depends on the information for the task. In particular, *opposite conclusions can be drawn from psychophysical results depending on how the information is modeled.* (cf. [10, 23, 24, 9]) As we illustrate below, ideal observer analysis, a part of a signal detection theory, provides the solution to this problem of information normalization.

As an example of the difference between functional and mechanistic levels, consider the following question. What are the crucial features of leaf texture as distinct from apples that would lead to reliable segmentation? This kind of question can be addressed at the functional level by specifying generative texture models [47] for the task and testing whether the most statistically reliable features for discrimination are used by the human observer. However, one could imagine a finer grain analysis to test whether the particular features hypothesized by the information model are indeed processed in terms of particular spatial filters. At this level, laboratory manipulations can be geared towards analysing mechanisms of visual processing. In the context of our apple counting problem, part of a complete explanation will be to understand how motion parallax can help to segment apple from leaf surfaces–but underneath this level, is the question of the kind of motion mechanism human vision might use to support such functional inferences.

Testing models using ideal observers

One of the major points of this chapter is that the modeling problem naturally breaks into two: determining how a useful signal (e.g. objects, distances, shapes, etc) gets *encoded* into intensity changes in the image, and second, determining the limits to *decoding* the image to infer the signals. The encoding problem, which involves modeling both the regularities and structure in the signal domain as well as the image formation process, has been frequently neglected in studies of human vision (but see [33]). We discuss this problem more completely in the section on Pattern Inference Theory below. On the other hand, the decoding problem involves finding decoding strategies that clearly depend on how the signals were encoded. In the study of decoding, the fundamental object is the optimal decoder, comparedto which all other decoders can be described in terms of the information about the signals they discard. Thus studying the decoding problem relies on theories of ideal observers, or more generally of optimal inference. If we describe human perception as a process of decoding images, then the ideal observer can be used to describe human performance in terms of deviations from optimality. Returning to the question of how to test our models experimentally, the preceding suggests the strategy of comparing human to ideal performance. We will discuss how this comparison can be used to test theories and give two examples of such tests below.

In the next section, we outline the elements of a Bayesian approach to vision applicable to both the analysis of mechanism and function. In the following section, we apply these elements to questions of mechanism and in particular we illustrate information normalization in the analysis of motion measurements. The last section shows how information modeling has been used to provide a quantitative account of an aspect of functional vision, color matching results for simple natural images.

Bayesian Perception and Pattern Inference Theory

Because observers use their visual systems to do things, theories of visual perception cannot be built in isolation from functional visual tasks. We see the consequences of this statement as including the following principles: 1) vision is inference; 2) vision has relevant knowledge of scene structure prior to performing a task; 3) the affordances (value of the outcomes) of a completed task determine the costs and benefits of acquiring visual knowledge. A fundamental approach that quantifies these principles is a theoretical apparatus we call *Pattern Inference Theory*, which is a conjunction of Bayesian Decision Theory with *Pattern Theory*. As an elaboration of signal detection theory, we choose the words *pattern* and *inference* to stress the importance of modeling complex natural signals, and of considering tasks in addition to detection, respectively.

We have elsewhere [22, 46] argued that Pattern Inference Theory provides the best language for a quantitative theory of visual perception at the level of the naturally behaving (human) visual system. The term, "Pattern Theory" was coined by Ulf Grenander to describe the mathematical study of complex natural patterns [16, 17, 30, 46]. In our usage, Pattern Inference Theory is a probabilistic model of the observer's world and sensory input, which has two components: the objects of the theory, and the operations of the theory. The objects of the theory are the set of possible image measurements I, the set of possible scene descriptions S, and the joint probability distribution of S and I: $p(S, I)$. The operations are given by the probability calculus, with decisions modeled as cost functionals on probabilities. The richness of the theory lies in exploiting the structure induced in $p(S, I)$ by the regularities of the world (laws of physics) and by the habits of observers. This emphasizes a central role for the modeling of representations and their transformations. Pattern Inference Theory also assumes a central role, in perception, of generative (or synthetic) models of image patterns, as well as prior probability models of scene information. Our example below compares two generative models of color, one based on direct, and a second on direct plus indirect lighting. An emphasis on generative models, we believe, is essential because of the inherent complexity of the causal structure of high-dimensional image patterns. One must model how the multitude of variables, both needed and unneeded, interact to produce image data in order to understand how to decode those patterns.

How can we describe the processes of visual inference as image decoding by means of probability computations (i.e. from the point of view of pattern inference theory)? To do so requires a probabilistic model of tasks. We consider a task as specifying four ingredients: 1) the relevant or primary set of scene variables S_{prim}, 2) the irrelevant or secondary scene variables S_{sec}, 3) the scene variables which are presumed known S_f, and 4) the type of decision to be made. Each of the four components of a task plays a role in determining the structure of the optimal inference computation[1].

Bayesian decision theory provides a precise language to model the costs of errors determined by the choice of visual task [45, 6]. The ideal observer that minimizes average error finds the $S_{prim}*$ which minimizes the following risk:

$$R(S_{prim}; I, S_f) = - \int_{S_{sec}*} P(S_{sec}, S_{prim} \mid I, S_f) \, dS_{sec} \qquad (2.1)$$

with respect to the posterior probability, $P(S_{sec}, S_{prim} \mid I)$. In practice, the posterior probability $P(S_{sec}, S_{prim} \mid I, S_f$ is factored into two terms (and a constant denominator) using Bayes theorem: the likelihood, $P(I \mid S_{sec}, S_{prim})$, which is determined by the generative model for the image measurements (see figure 2.1), and the prior probability, $P(S_{prim})$. A simple Bayesian maxim summarizes the above calculation: Condition the joint probability on what we know, and marginalize over what we don't care about[2]. As seen in the color constancy section below, we have prior knowledge of the illuminant spectrum, we measure the shape and image color, we don't care about the illumination direction, and we want to estimate the surface color properties that minimize color judgment errors.

---

1. The cost or *risk* $R(\Sigma; I)$ of guessing Σ when the image measurement is I is defined as the expected *loss*:

$$R(\Sigma; I) = \int_S L(\Sigma, S) P(S \mid I) dS$$

with respect to the posterior probability, $P(S \mid I)$. The best interpretation of the image can then be made by finding the Σ which minimizes the risk function. The loss function $L(\Sigma, S)$ specifies the cost of guessing Σ when the scene variable is S. One possible loss function is $-\delta(\Sigma - S)$. In this case the risk becomes $R(\Sigma; I) = -P(\Sigma \mid I)$, and then the best strategy is to pick the most likely interpretation. This is standard *maximum a posteriori estimation* (MAP). A second kind of loss function assumes that costs are constant over all guesses of a variable. This is equivalent to marginalization of the posterior with respect to that variable.
2. This Bayesian maxim is due to James Coughlan

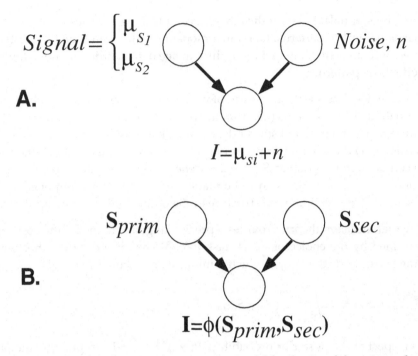

$$Signal = \begin{cases} \mu_{S_1} \\ \mu_{S_2} \end{cases} \qquad Noise,\ n$$

A.

$$I = \mu_{si} + n$$

$$\mathbf{S}_{prim} \qquad \mathbf{S}_{sec}$$

B.

$$\mathbf{I} = \phi(\mathbf{S}_{prim}, \mathbf{S}_{sec})$$

Figure 2.1: Panel A illustrates the generative model for the signal detection task. Signal detection theory provides tools particularly appropriate for the behavioral analysis of visual mechanisms. Panel B illustrates the general form of the generative model for the pattern inference theory task. Pattern inference theory is an elaboration of signal detection theory which seeks to take into account the specific generative aspects, $\phi()$ of natural image formation, and the full range of natural tasks. Pattern Inference Theory is of particular relevance for modeling natural visual function.

Pattern inference theory, ideal observers, and human vision

In order for the pattern inference theory approach to be useful, we need to be able to construct predictive theories of visual function which are amenable to experimental testing.

How do we formulate and test theories of vision at the functional level within a Bayesian pattern inference theory framework? Tests of human perception can be based on hypotheses regarding constraints contained in: the two components of the generative model, 1) the prior $p(S)$ and 2) the likelihood $p(I|S)$; 3) the image model $p(I)$; 4) the posterior $p(S|I)$; or 5) the loss function. The first four can be called information constraints, whereas the fifth can be called a decision constraint. These levels can be translated into tests of: 1) prior knowledge and assumptions of scene structure; 2) model of the observer's image formation process; 3) what image measurements and image coding does the observer do; 4) the information about a scene available to the observer given an image; 5) the decisions and strategies used by the observer.

It is at the level of the posterior that provides the most complete quantitative model of the information available to an observer to perform a task. Whether this information is used optimally or not depends on whether the observer's loss function is matched to the particular task. Thus it is important to investigate more than one task that uses the same posterior in order to attribute a loss of information to the observer's posterior rather than a loss due to an inappropriate loss function. In all cases, we want to design our experiments to focus on the constraint hypotheses. For example, if we are interested in testing hypotheses about the observer's prior distribution on light source direction, then the experimenter could focus on simple ambiguous scenes whose interpretation depends on the light source direction. In these scenes the prior is expected to dominate.

However, the fact that testing at the level of information constraints uses information common to many decisions has a practical side-effect: we can define subdomains of S and I that are more easily implemented in the laboratory, and yet use the same posterior. This allows the experimenter to focus on testing the interesting predictions of the hypotheses.

As we've noted above above, in psychophysical experiments, one can: a) test at the functional or constraint level–what information does human vision avail itself of?, or; b) test at the mechanism level–what neural subsystem can account for performance? Because of its emphasis on modeling natural pattern representations and transformations, Pattern Inference Theory is of primary relevance to hypotheses testable at the former level, (e.g. hypotheses about the representations appropriate for inference). Signal detection theory (SDT) is of primary importance for the latter as we will see in the motion example below, where SDT provides the tools for rigorous tests of neural representation. In both cases, using an ideal observer allows a simple and meaningful comparison to be made between human and ideal performance.

The primary use of an ideal observer in an experimental setting is to provide a measure of the information available to perform a task that can be used to normalize the performance of any other human or model observer. Reporting human and model performance relative to ideal performance allows a straight forward comparison of the results from completely different tasks and visual cues. In other words, it allows comparisons like "Is the visual system better at processing edges or shading information?" [42]. A standard way of performing this normalization is to compute efficiency, which is a measure of the effective number of samples used by the observers [11, 2].

This normalization function also provides a criterion by which to judge whether two models are functionally equivalent, and when a model can be firmly rejected. If two models produce the same efficiency curves for all relevant changes in task and stimuli, then the two models are equivalent. Notice, however, that two models can be equivalent by this criterion and yet could employ very different computations at the level of mechanism. This also allows us to construct models that are functionally equivalent to the human visual system. Everywhere human performance deviates from ideal, we modify the ideal observer to discard equivalent information and no more. Notice that this construction has a test of the viability of a model for human performance built into it. Anytime a human observer can out-perform a model observer on a task, that model can be eliminated as a possible model for the human visual system.

In the next section we will look at an in-depth example of an application of the ideal observer approach to the problem of the determining the mechanisms used by the visual system to detect motion.

Ideal Observer Analysis: Mechanisms of Motion Measurement

Experimental studies of human perceptual behavior are often left with a crucial, but unanswered question: To what extent is the measured performance limited by the information in the task rather than by the perceptual system itself? Answers to this question are critical for understanding the relationship between perceptual behavior and its underlying biological mechanisms. Signal detection theory provided an answer through ideal observer analysis.

To show the power and limitations of this approach consider an example of a recent application (by one of the authors) of classical signal detection theory to the problem of visual motion measurement.

A model for motion detection

When a person moves relative to the environment, the visual image projected onto the retina changes accordingly. Within small regions of the retina and for short durations this image change may be approximated as a two-dimensional translation. The set of such translations across the visual field is termed the Optic Flow field. Having described a simple approximation of the otherwise complicated time-varying retinal image, the question remains whether the human visual system uses such an approximation. A number of physiological and psychophysical experiments have established that the mammalian visual system does contain mechanisms sensitive such local image translations [31], but these studies did not specify how local image translations might be measured by the visual system. One approach, initially due to Heeger [19] and later refined [18, 41] , uses fundamental properties of translating signals to derive an estimator for the velocity of the translation. Consider an image sequence $I(x, y, t)$. If in a window of space and time $W(\vec{x}, t)$ (e.g. gaussian) the image motion can be described as a translation, then $I(x, y, t) \approx \sum_{ij} w_{ij}(\vec{x} - \vec{x}_i, t - t_j)I(\vec{x} -$

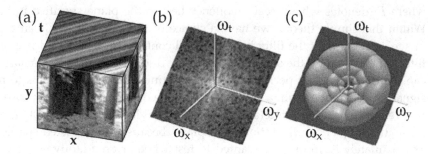

Figure 2.2: A translational motion detector. **(a)**, Space-time luminance pattern of an image translating to the right. This is a representation of the intensity information in the retinal image (the x- y plane) over time (t). The rightward motion can be inferred from the oriented pattern on the x-t face. **(b)**, The Fourier amplitude spectrum of the luminance pattern, represented by the intensity of points in a three-dimensional spatio-temporal frequency domain. Non-zero Fourier amplitudes are constrained to lie on a plane through the origin. The orientation of this plane uniquely specify the direction and speed of translation. **(c)**, Construction of a translation detector [39], illustrated in the Fourier domain. Pairs of balls symmetric about the origin indicate the Fourier amplitude spectra of band-pass filters whose peak frequencies lie in the plane. A translation detector can be constructed by summing the squared outputs of such filters.

$\vec{v}_{ij}t, t)$. It is easy to show that the spatio-temporal (3-D) Fourier transform of one windowed region is given by

$$\mathcal{F}\{w_{ij}(\vec{x} - \vec{x}_i, t - t_j)I(\vec{x} - \vec{v}_{ij}t, t)\} = S(\vec{\omega}_x, \omega_t)$$
$$= W(\vec{\omega}_x, \omega_t) \otimes (S_I(\vec{\omega}_x)\delta([\vec{\omega}_x \ \omega_t]^T[\vec{v}_{ij} \ 1])) \quad (2.2)$$

Note that the delta function term is an equation for a plane in the Fourier domain specified by $[\vec{\omega}_x \ \omega_t]^T[\vec{v}_{ij} \ 1] = 0$. Thus the equation says that local image translations in the Fourier domain are characterized by the spatial spectrum of the image projected onto a plane whose orientation is uniquely specified by the velocity of the translation, which is convolved by the Fourier transform of the windowing function. For a Gaussian windowing function, the result is easy to state: translations are specified by blurred planes (or pancakes) in the Fourier domain. Figure 2.2a and b illustrate this without the windowing function. Given this description, a simple velocity detector can be constructed by pooling the outputs of spatio-temporal filters whose peak frequencies lie on a common plane (e.g. see figure 2.2c). Because the phase spectrum is not required for the velocity estimates, a noise resistant [39] detector can be built by pooling the outputs of filters that compute the *energy* within a region of spatio-temporal frequency (e.g. like complex cells in V1). For a windowed signal S, the output R of the detector is given by

$$R = \sum_j \sum_{\vec{\omega}_x, \omega_t} a_j |F_j(\vec{\omega}_x, \omega_t)|^2 |S(\vec{\omega}_x, \omega_t)|^2 \quad (2.3)$$

where F_j denotes whose peak frequency lies on the plane specified by the signal. Within this simple theory, we have a choice of the weights a_j. Given a particular image, only some of the filter bands F_j will contain the signal, and responses from filters not containing the signal will be solely due to noise. Thus a "smart" detector can improve detection performance by adjusting its pooling weights to match the signal. On the other hand, a good non-adaptive detector can be built by optimizing the weights for the expected (average) signal. This leads to a detector that pools over all spatial frequency orientations in a plane, because the expected spatial signal is approximately isotropic. We wanted to test whether an adaptive or fixed pooling power detector is a good model of human motion detection.

Notice the putative motion detection mechanisms have not been motivated from within signal detection theory. Rather they were motivated via a simple approximation and signal processing issues.

Testing the model

Finding a task for which the model is ideal

Signal detection theory can be used to assess the feasibility of such a model. To do so, we use the fact that the model we are interested in is an ideal observer for *some* task and stimuli. The idea is that if we have human observers perform the optimal task for the model, then if the model is a good description: 1) Humans should be good at the task 2) the model should predict errors on related tasks. Schrater et. al. [35] have recently shown that the putative motion detectors are ideal observers for detecting a class of novel stochastic signals added to Gaussian white noise. The stochastic signals are produced by passing Gaussian white noise through the filters used to construct the motion detector. In general, a detector which computes the Fourier energy within a filter is an ideal observer for stochastic signals generated by passing Gaussian white noise through the filter. Thus, by varying the number and placement of filters, we can produce motion stimuli that are consistent with a single translational velocity and have various spatial frequency spectra, or stimuli that are consistent with multiple velocities. Examples of some filters and stimuli are shown in figure 2.3.

So how do we go about testing our model by detecting these stochastic stimuli? The ideal observer analysis gives immediate simple testable predictions: 1) Under the adaptive model as we vary the spatial structure of the motion stimulus, human performance should be constant relative to the ideal for each stimulus. 2) Under the fixed model, we should see predictable variations in performance. 3) If the model is false, we should be terrible at the task.

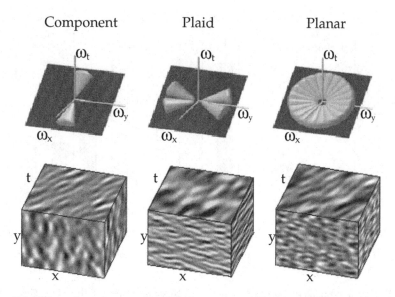

Figure 2.3: Filter sets and examples of their corresponding signals. The top row depicts level surfaces (65% of peak response) of the three different filter sets used to generate stimuli. The bottom row depicts space-time luminance patterns of signals produced by passing spatio-temporal Gaussian white noise through the corresponding filter sets. **(a)** The "component" stimulus, constructed from a spatially and temporally band-pass filter. The x-y face of the stimulus shows structures that are spatially band-pass and oriented along the x axis. The orientation of structures on the x-t face indicates rightward motion. **(b)** The "plaid" stimulus, constructed from two "component" filters lying in a common plane. The x-y face of the stimulus shows a mixture spatial of spatial structures with dominant orientations close to the y axis. **(c)** The "planar" stimulus, constructed from a set of 10 "component" filters lying in a common plane. The stimulus is spatially band-pass and isotropic (x-y face), and exhibits rightward motion (x-t face).

Testing the predictions

Translating these predictions into the detection task, the adaptive model predicts that any configuration of Fourier energy on the plane should be equally detectable. To test this prediction, we had observers vary the total energy of one of the three signals shown in figure 2.3 added to white noise until just detectable. The thresholds are plotted as signal power to noise power ratios in figure 2.4a. Note that the thresholds are lowest for detecting the "planar" signal with energy spread equally across a plane, followed by "plaid", with two bands, followed by the "component" filter, with only one band. However, unlike the non-stochastic stimuli used in previous signal detection experiments, here the signal to noise energy measure does not capture the subject's relative performance on the three stimuli. Looking at the threshold data, we might be tempted to conclude that planar stimuli are most easily detected and "component" and "plaid" stimuli are comparable in detectability. In fact, if we

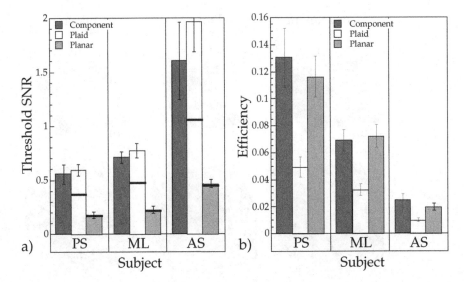

Figure 2.4: (a) Detection performance of three subjects for the three stochastic signals of Fig. 2.3. Threshold signal to noise ratio (SNR) for 81.1% detectability. SNR is calculated as the ratio of the signal power to the background noise power. Heavy black lines indicate predictions for ideal summation, derived from the component condition thresholds. **(b)** Detection efficiencies for the three stimulus types. Efficiencies are plotted in proportions, with 1.0 reflecting perfect performance; that is, performance matching that of an ideal observer tuned to the structure of the signal in the stimulus (different for each stimulus type). The differences between the efficiencies of the pattern stimuli (plaid and planar stimuli) and the component stimulus provide a quantitative measure of summation of the pattern's components.

correctly normalize the observers thresholds by the ideal observers' thresholds for each stimulus to compute an efficiency measure, then we find that the "planar" and "component" stimuli are about equally detectable, whereas the "plaid" stimulus is much less detectable. Efficiencies are plotted in figure 2.4b.

The results suggest that the human visual system has band-pass filters similar to the "component" stimulus filter (and similar to V1 complex cells), and similar to the "planar" stimulus filter, but not to partial tilings of the plane. Thus the predictions of the fixed detector model have been confirmed, while the predictions of the adaptive detector have been contradicted. Notice also that the information normalization provided by the ideal observers is not superfluous. An attempt to compare detection performance across stimuli in terms of common stimulus measures (e.g. Fourier energy or power spectral height) for detectability would lead to erroneous conclusions. In addition, note that the efficiencies on these stimuli are about 10%, which is not extremely high (e.g. > 50% has been found for some other detection tasks [7]) but do not rule out the model either. It is likely, however, that the model does not capture all the important elements of motion detectors in the visual system (e.g. opponency).

From ideal observer to human observer model

The question remains how much of human motion detection can be accounted for by the simple fixed detector that pools over an entire plane. To address this question, we can turn from looking at the ideal observer for each stimulus and instead try to predict the inefficiencies in human performance using the fixed detector model.

To do this, we compared the detectability predicted by the fixed model on a set of five stochastic stimuli, three new and the "planar" and "plaid" stimuli above. The new stimuli were created by passing spatio-temporal white noise through three configurations of filters, illustrated in Fig. 2.5. The first is a plaid signal, similar to the plaid used above. The second is a "planar triplet", created by adding a component band to the plaid, in the same plane as the plaid, and the third is a non-planar triplet, created by adding a component band out of the plane of the plaid. Detection thresholds were measured using the same method as above. The model predicts improved summation for the planar triplet, relative to the plaid, but no improved summation for the non-planar triplet. We computed predictions for the detection thresholds of each of the stimuli by implementing a specific fixed power dectector model. The detector optimally summed energy over the band of frequencies contained in the planar stimulus from experiment 1. We assumed that the output of this detector was corrupted by the internal noise levels estimated from subjects' detection thresholds for the component stimulus in experiment 1. Figure 2.5 shows observer's thresholds compared to the model predictions for the five pattern stimuli used. Given the assumptions built into the model concerning the exact spatio-temporal frequency band covered by the planar power detector, the match is surprisingly good. That is, not only do the qualitative results follow the predictions of the planar power detector model, but the quantitative results are well fit by a pre-defined instantiation of the model (without fitting the parameters of the model to the data).

Although signal detection theory worked well in the analysis of mechanisms of motion detection, we need a theoretical framework for which the signals can be any properties of the world useful for the visual behavior; for example, estimates of object shape and surface motion are crucial for actions such as recognition and navigation, but they are not simple functions of light intensity. Natural images are high-dimensional functions of useful signals, and arriving at decoding functions relating image measurements to useful signals is a major theoretical challenge. However, both of these problems are expressible in terms of Pattern theory.

So, in the next section, we focus on the first problem: How can we model the computations that have to be solved? This modeling problem can be broken down into synthesis: a) modeling the structure of pattern information in natural images; and analysis, b) modeling the task and extracting useful pattern structures.

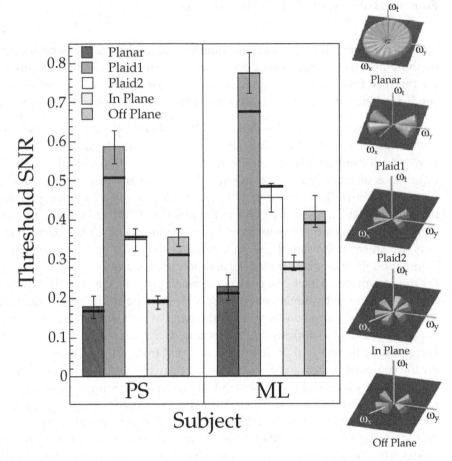

Figure 2.5: Threshold SNRs for detecting the five types of pattern stimuli replotted from experiments 1& 2, where Plaid1 in the legend denotes the plaid from the first experiment and Plaid2 from the second. Plaid1 differs from Plaid2 in that its energy is more diffusely spread over frequency. Black bands indicate the predictions of a planar filter, based on subjects' detection thresholds for the component stimulus used in experiment 1.

Bayesian Models: Color Constancy

Robust object recognition relies on the estimation of object properties that are approximately invariant with respect to secondary variables such as illumination and viewpoint. Material color is one such property, and the phenomenon of perceptual color constancy is well-established (cf. [6] for a Bayesian analysis). For practical and scientific reasons, most laboratory studies of human color constancy have been limited to simple flat surfaces, or to the lightness dimension (see [1] and [5]).

Extracting color invariants from real surfaces is a more theoretically complex task, the wavelength information received by the eye being a function of the surface shape, material properties, and the illumination. Adding to this complexity is the fact that wavelength information also depends on reflected light from nearby surfaces. Until recently, it was not at all clear whether human vision makes use of knowledge of 3D surface structure to infer surface color properties, which as we will see, involves a rather subtle computation. A recent study by Marina Bloj and colleagues has shown that human vision can indeed take into account 3D shape when inferring surface color [4]. In addition, their ideal observer analysis of the physical information available provided a quantitative account of human color matches.

Figure 2.6 illustrates the basic finding. A card consisting of a white and red half is folded such that the sides face each other. If the card's shape is seen as it truly is (a corner), the white side is seen as a white card, slightly tinted pink from the reflected light. However, if the shape of the card is made to *appear* as though the sides face away from each other (convex or "roof" condition), the white card appears magenta– i.e. more saturated towards the red[3]. Bloj et al. made quantitative measurements in which observers picked a comparison surface whose color best matched the white side of the target (see figure 2.7).

Notice that this is a simplified version of the natural task of determining the reflectance and illumination of an object in the presence of other objects. The problem is interreflections. The interreflections can be modeled pairwise. Then the color is determined by the illuminant, the reflectance functions of the surfaces, and the configuration of surfaces (geometry). Let us look at how to model the physics given a pair of surfaces.

Look at the illustration of two surfaces in figure 2.6. When two surfaces are concave with respect to a light source, the interreflections off of both surfaces provide a secondary source of illumination with different characteristics for both surfaces. As the angle between these surfaces decreases, the amount of inter-reflected light re-reflected off the other surface increases, and hence the spectrum of the reflected light off both surfaces changes. On the other hand, as we increase the inter-surface angle, the amount of inter-reflected light decreases until it reaches zero at 90 degrees. Because of the perspective ambiguity in interpreting a folded card as convex or concave, there are two interesting subcases of this continuum, one where the angle is acute and one where the angle is obtuse. These two cases are experimentally the most interesting because they yield completely different shape and reflectance attributions to the observation that one of the two surfaces was pink.

---

3. The apparent switch in shape from corner to roof can be accomplished either by using a pseudoscope, a pair of dove prisms which effectively reverse the stereo disparities, or by using a monocular cue, such as linear perspective (see http://vision.psych.umn.edu/www/kersten-lab/kersten-lab.html).

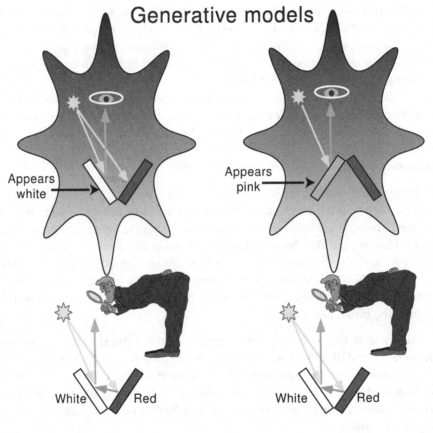

Generative models

Corner, white surface &
illumination with inter-reflection

Roof, pink surface &
illumination without inter-reflection

Figure 2.6: The white side of the folded card appears to either be pink or magenta, depending on the assumed shape of the card, i.e. whether the card is concave like a corner, or convex like a roof. The illumination model for a corner involves direct as well as inter-reflections, whereas the illumination model for the roof interpretation involves only direct lighting.

Let's see how to model the information for optimal inference. The primary variable of interest is the reflectivity ($S_{prim} = \rho$) (measured in units of chroma). The likelihood is determined by either the one-bounce (corner) or zero-bounce model (roof condition) of mutual illumination. They assume that the shape is fixed by stereoscopic measurements, i.e. condition on shape ($S_f = roof\ or\ corner$). The one-bounce model yields the intensity equation for surface 1 (the "white surface"):

$$I_1(\lambda, x, \rho, E, \alpha_1, \alpha_2) = E(\lambda)\rho_1(\lambda)[\cos \alpha_1 + f_{21}\rho_2(\lambda) \cos \alpha_2] \tag{2.4}$$

where the first term represents the direct illumination with respect to the surface and the second term represents indirect (mutual) illumination due to light reflected from the red side (surface 2) [8]. $f_{21}(x)$ is the form factor describing the extent to which surface 2 reflects light onto surface 1 at distance x from the vertex [13]. The angles α_1 and α_2 denote the angle between the surface normal and the light source direction for surfaces 1 and 2 respectively.

For the zero-bounce generative model (roof condition):

$$I_1(\lambda, x, \rho, E, \alpha) = E(\lambda)\rho_1(\lambda)\cos\alpha_1 \tag{2.5}$$

These generative models provide the likelihood function. Observers do not sense I_1, but have a measure of color called chroma, modeled by the capture of the light by the retinal cones followed by a transformation, which we will denote as a function $C(\alpha, x, \rho, E) = f(\vec{K}(\lambda) \cdot I_i(\lambda, x, \rho, E, \alpha))$, where $\vec{K}$ denotes the three cone action spectra, and $\cdot$ denotes inner product. Thus the likelihood of observation C_{obs} being due to a color patch $C^i(\alpha, x, \rho^i, E)$ in the presence of some additive measurement noise is given by:

$$p(C_{obs}|\rho^i, x, \alpha, E) = K\exp(\frac{-0.5 * (C_{obs} - f(\vec{K} \cdot I_i))^2}{\sigma^2}) \tag{2.6}$$

Now marginalize this conditional probability with respect to illumination direction and space (i.e. $S_{sec} = \{\alpha, x\}$) assuming uniform priors, and assume a priori (built-in) knowledge of the illuminant spectrum $E(\lambda)$ of daylight. Matching errors to the i_{th} patch are predicted by:

$$P(\rho_1^i|C_{obs}) \propto \sum_\alpha \sum_x \exp(-|C_{obs} - C^i(\alpha, x)|^2/2\sigma^2) \tag{2.7}$$

assuming a uniform prior on C_{obs} where σ is determined by the matching noise. (See [4] for details).

Experimental and theoretical matches are shown in figure 2.7. To a first approximation, the separation and spread of the observers' matches are predicted well by an observer which is ideal apart from an internal matching variability determined by σ. In other words, human matches are "ideal-like."

There are a number of important points to be made here. Note that the surfaces and lighting were carefully chosen to provide the bare minimal model for the natural visual task of inferring surface reflectance in the presence of interreflections. This reduction in complexity is important in that it allowed a highly controlled experimental test of the basic question. In addition, note that the one additional noise parameter that was used to model the observer's deviations from ideal is in fact not a free parameter (i.e. it was not fit to the data). Instead, the noise parameter was estimated from a separate color matching experiment.

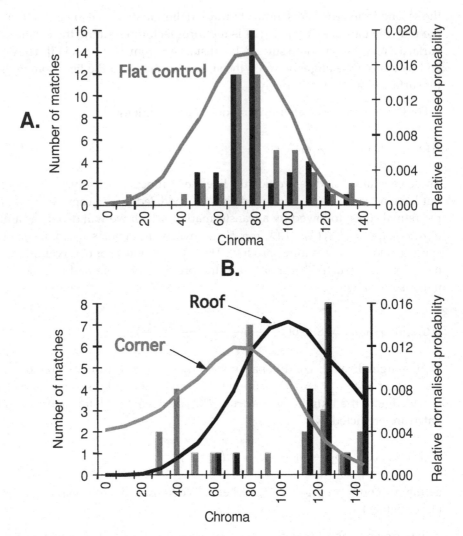

Figure 2.7: Panel A shows the distribution of human subject matches to a flat card, neither roof nor corner condition. Variability of matches is modeled as the standard deviation, σ of "matching noise." Panel B shows the distribution of matches under the two experimental conditions. Figure adapted from Bloj et al. (1999). Reprinted with permission from Nature.

Summary and Conclusions

We have discussed the problem of developing and testing quantitative models of human visual behavior. To that end we distinguished modeling function from modeling mechanism. The ideal observer plays a key role for both levels as:

- The information normalization tool for tests of visual mechanism.
- The default model for functional models of natural vision.

In testing models of vision, we emphasized the fundamental role of the ideal observer in interpreting human and model performance. The ideal observer provides a fundamental measure of the information available to perform a task, and thus serves to normalize human performance with respect to the task. Ideal observers can be used to define a task-independent measure of performance (efficiency), provide a measure of the functional equivalence of models, and serve as a default model to be modified by experiment. We described experiments of Schrater et al. supporting neural mechanisms specialized for the measurement of local image velocities, which are equivalent to specific sums of sets of complex cells in cortical area V1 [35].

By assuming that vision can be described as a process of decoding scene properties from images, we can use the approach of Pattern Inference Theory to develop ideal observers that serve as the starting point and comparator for a models of functional vision. A key point is the importance of modeling the generative or forward process of natural image pattern formation (or encoding). The results of Bloj et al. [4] showed that the visual system takes into account knowledge of inter-reflected light in determining surface color. From this perspective, theories of human visual performance can be developed iteratively from the ideal observer down (cf. [29]). This may be a more tractable strategy than to build models of system function bottom-up from mechanism components.

Acknowledgement

Supported by NSF SBR-9631682 and NIH RO1 EY11507-001.

References

[1]   Adelson, E. H. (1999). Lightness Perception and Lightness Illusions. In M. Gazzaniga, M. S. (Ed.), *The New Cognitive Neurosciences*(pp. 339-351). Cambridge, MA: MIT Press.

[2]   Barlow, H. B. A method of determining the overall quantum efficiency of visual discriminations. *J. Physiol. (Lond.).* 160, 155- 168. 1962.

[3]   Bishop, C. M. (1995). *Neural Networks for Pattern Recognition.* Oxford: Oxford Univeristy Press.

[4]   Bloj, M. G., Kersten, D., & Hurlbert, A. C. (1999). Perception of three-dimensional shape influences colour perception via mutual illumination. *Na-*

ture, **402**, 877-879.

[5] Kraft, J. M., & Brainard, D. H. (1999). Mechanisms of color constancy under nearly natural viewing. *Proceedings of the National Academy of Sciences USA*, **96**, 307-312.

[6] Brainard, D. H., & Freeman, W. T. (1997). Bayesian color constancy. *J Opt Soc Am A*, **14**, (7), 1393-411.

[7] Burgess, A. E., Wagner, R. F., Jennings, R. J., & Barlow, H. B. (1981). Efficiency of human visual signal discrimination. *Science*, **214**, 93-94.

[8] Drew, M., & Funt, B. (1990). Calculating surface reflectance using a single-bounce model of mutual reflection. *Proceedings of the 3rd International Conference on Computer Vision* Osaka: 393-399.

[9] Eagle, R. A., & Blake, A. (1995). Two-dimensional constraints on three-dimensional structure from motion tasks. *Vision Res*, **35**, (20), 2927-41.

[10] Eckstein, M. P. (1998). The lower efficiency for conjunctions is due to noise and not serial attentional processing. *Psychological Science*, **9**, 111-118.

[11] Fisher, R. A. (1925). *Statistical Methods for Research Workers*, Edinburgh: Oliver and Boyd.

[12] Freeman, W. T. (1994). The generic viewpoint assumption in a framework for visual perception. *Nature*, **368**, 542-545.

[13] Foley, J., van Dam, A., Feiner, S., & Hughes, J. (1990). *Computer Graphics Principles and Practice*, (2nd ed.). Reading, Massachusetts: Addison-Wesley Publishing Company.

[14] Geisler, W. Sequential Ideal-Observer analysis of visual discriminations. *Psychological Review*. 96,(2), 267-314. 1989.

[15] Green, D. M., & Swets, J. A. (1974). *Signal Detection Theory and Psychophysics*. Huntington, New York: Robert E. Krieger Publishing Company. 1974.

[16] Grenander, U. (1993). *General Pattern theory*, Oxford Univ Press.

[17] Grenander, U. (1996). *Elements of Pattern theory*. Baltimore: Johns Hopkins University Press.

[18] Grzywacz, N. M. & Yuille, A. L. A model for the estimate of local image velocity by cells in the visual cortex. *Proc. Royal Society of London A*, **239**, 129–161, (1990).

[19] Heeger, D. J. Model for the extraction of image flow. *J. Opt. Soc. Am. A*, **4**, 1455–1471, (1987).

[20] Kersten, D. (1984). Spatial summation in visual noise. *Vision Research*, **24**, 1977-1990.

[21] Kersten, D. (1999). High-level vision as statistical inference. In Gazzaniga, M. (Ed.), *The New Cognitive Neurosciences* Cambridge, MA: MIT Press.

[22] Kersten, D., & Schrater, P. W. (2000). Pattern Inference Theory: A Probabilistic Approach to Vision. In Mausfeld, R., & Heyer, D. (Ed.), *Perception and the*

Physical World(pp. Chichester: John Wiley & Sons, Ltd.)

[23] Knill, D. C. (1998). Discrimination of planar surface slant from texture: human and ideal observers compared. *Vision Res*, **38**, (11), 1683-711.

[24] Knill, D. C. (1998). Surface orientation from texture: ideal observers, generic observers and the information content of texture cues. *Vision Res*, **38**, (11), 1655-82.

[25] Knill, D.C., and Richards, W. (Eds). (1996). *Perception as Bayesian Inference*. Cambridge University Press. .

[26] Knill, D. C., & Kersten, D. K. (1991). Ideal Perceptual Observers for Computation, Psychophysics, and Neural Networks. In Watt, R. J. (Ed.), *Pattern Recognition by Man and Machine*(pp. 83-97). MacMillan Press.

[27] Koch, C., & Segev, I. (1998). Methods in Neuronal Modeling : From Ions to Networks. Cambridge, MA: MIT Press, 671 pages.

[28] Liu, Z., Knill, D. C., & Kersten, D. Object Classification for Human and Ideal Observers. *Vision Research*. 35,(4), 549-568. 1995.

[29] Liu, Z., & Kersten, D. (1998). 2D observers for human 3D object recognition? *Vision Res*, **38**, (15-16), 2507-19.

[30] Mumford, D. (1996). Pattern theory: A unifying perspective. In Knill, D. C., & W., R. (Ed.), *Perception as Bayesian Inference*(pp. Chapter 2). Cambridge: Cambridge University Press.

[31] Nakayama, K. Biological image motion processing: a review. *Vis. Res.*, **25**, 625–660, (1985).

[32] Olshausen, B. A., & Field, D. J. Emergence of simple-cell receptive field properties by learning a sparse code for natural images. *Nature*. 381, 607-609. 1996.

[33] Richards, W. E. (1988). *Natural Computation*. Cambridge, Massachusetts: MIT Press.

[34] B. Ripley. *Pattern Recognition and Neural Networks*. Cambridge University Press. 1996.

[35] Schrater, P. R., Knill, D. C., & Simoncelli, E. P. (2000). Mechanisms of visual motion detection. *Nature Neuroscience*, **1**, 64 - 68.

[36] Schrater, P. (1998). Local Motion Detection: Comparison of Human and Ideal Model Observers. Ph.D. thesis, Philadelphia: University of Pennsylvania.

[37] Schrater, P. R., & Kersten, D. (1999). Statistical Structure and Task Dependence in Visual Cue Integration. Workshop on Statistical and Computational Theories of Vision – Modeling, Learning, Computing, and Sampling, Fort Collins, Colorado.

[38] Simoncelli, E. P., Adelson, E. H., & Heeger, D. J. (1991). Probability Distributions of Optical Flow. Mauii, Hawaii: *IEEE Conf on Computer Vision and Pattern Recognition*.

[39] Simoncelli, E. P. (1993). Distributed Analysis and Representation of Visual Motion. Ph.D., Cambridge, MA: Massachusetts Institute of Technology, Department of Electrical Engineering and Computer Science,

[40] Simoncelli, E. P. (1997). Statistical Models for Images: Compression, Restoration and Synthesis. Pacific Grove, CA.: IEEE Signal Processing Society.

[41] Simoncelli, E. P. & Heeger, D. A model of neuronal responses in visual area MT. *Vis. Res.*, **38**, 743–761, (1998).

[42] Tjan, B., Braje, W., Legge, G. E., & Kersten, D. (1995). Human efficiency for recognizing 3-D objects in luminance noise. *Vision Research*, **35**, (21), 3053-3069.

[43] Watson, A. B., Barlow, H. B., & Robson, J. G. (1983). What does the eye see best? *Nature*, **31**,, 419-422.

[44] Weiss, Y., & Adelson, E. H. (1998). Slow and smooth: a Bayesian theory for the combination of local motion signals in human vision (A.I. Memo No. 1624). M.I.T.

[45] Yuille, A. L., & Bülthoff, H. H. (1996). Bayesian decision theory and psychophysics. In D.C., K., & W., R. (Ed.), *Perception as Bayesian Inference*(pp. Cambridge, U.K.: Cambridge University Press.

[46] Yuille, A. L., Coughlan, J. M., & Kersten, D. (1998). Computational Vision: Principles of Perceptual Inference. *http://vision.psych.umn.edu/www/kersten-lab/papers/yuicouker98.pdf*

[47] Zhu, S.C., Wu, Y., and Mumford, D. (1997). Minimax Entropy Principle and Its Application to Texture Modeling. Neural Computation. **9**(8).

3 Visual Cue Integration for Depth Perception

Robert A. Jacobs

Introduction

The human visual system obtains information about the depth of an object from a large number of distinct cues. Cues to depth result from object rotation, observer motion, binocular vision in which the two eyes receive different patterns of light, texture gradients in retinal images, and many other factors. A remarkable feature of human perception is that we are not overwhelmed by this wealth of information. Instead, we seem to effortlessly integrate information provided by each cue into a unified percept that is highly accurate. Moreover, we do this in a wide variety of visual environments. It is important to note that no single cue is necessary for depth perception or dominates our perception of depth (Cutting and Vishton, 1995). Moreover, no individual cue has been demonstrated to be individually capable of supporting depth perception with the robustness and accuracy shown by human observers. Clearly, our remarkable abilities to perceive visual depth are based on our abilities to integrate information provided by a variety of depth cues. In this chapter, we examine two important aspects of visual cue integration for depth perception. First, we address the question of whether or not observers integrate information based on multiple cues in an efficient manner. This can be evaluated by examining the degree to which their cue integration strategies can be characterized as statistically "optimal" in a Bayesian sense. Next, we look at the role that visual learning may play in cue integration. We address the question of whether or not observers' cue integration strategies for visual depth are adaptable in an experience-dependent manner.

In principle, there are many possible ways in which observers might integrate information provided by the available cues in a visual environment. Clark and Yuille (1990) proposed that cue integration strategies can be placed along a continuum that is defined by strong fusion models at one end and weak fusion models at the other end. Strong fusion models combine information from multiple cues in an unrestricted manner. In some circumstances, strong fusion models may use relatively simple mechanisms. For example, cue vetoing is a nonlinear combination rule in which depth estimates are based on one or more cues in a visual scene that are ranked highest in a hierarchical ordering (Bülthoff and Mallot, 1988). Empirical evidence consistent with a cue veto mechanism is provided by the Ames room illusion where perspective and other cues appear to veto a 'familiar size' cue (i.e. the adults in the far corners of the room are about equally tall). In other circumstances, strong fusion models may use more complicated combination strategies that allow cues to interact in highly nonlinear ways. Computationally, such models are often implemented using a coupled Markov random field approach (Marroquin, Mitter, and Poggio, 1987). Experimental evidence consistent with these models has been provided by several investigators. Rogers and Collett (1989) found that observers judged shape in accordance with disparity information when binocular disparity and motion parallax were placed in conflict, though strong interaction between motion and stereo information was implied by the percept of nonrigid motion. Nawrot and Blake (1989, 1991, 1993) found that retinal disparity can disambiguate depth relations in otherwise ambiguous kinetic depth effect displays, and that adaptation effects and perceptual priming effects can transfer between stereoscopic and kinetic depth displays.

In contrast to strong fusion models, weak fusion models compute a separate estimate of depth based on each depth cue considered in isolation; these estimates are then linearly averaged to yield a composite estimate of depth. Surprisingly, weak fusion models for depth perception have received a considerable degree of empirical support across a wide variety of experimental conditions (e.g., Bruno and Cutting, 1988; Dosher, Sperling, and Wurst, 1986; Landy, Maloney, Johnston, and Young, 1995). For instance, it has been found that increases in the number of depth cues available in a stimulus display lead to increases in the amount of depth perceived, and also to improvement in the consistency and accuracy of depth judgments (Bruno and Cutting, 1988; Bülthoff and Mallot, 1988; Dosher, Sperling, and Wurst, 1986; Landy, Maloney, and Young, 1991). Moreover, many researchers have found that linear cue combination models accurately account for observers' depth judgments. Bruno and Cutting (1988), for example, varied in a factorial design the availability of four depth cues (occlusion, relative size, height in the visual field, and motion perspective). Data from direct and indirect scaling tasks were consistent with the hypothesis that subjects used a nearly linear additive procedure analogous to a weak fusion model.

In this chapter, we examine two important aspects of visual cue integration for depth perception. First, we address the question of whether or not observers' cue integration strategies can be characterized as "optimal" where the optimality criteria are based on Bayesian statistics. This is done by comparing observers' perceptions to those of a computational model known as an *ideal observer*. The ideal observer is a statistical model that uses a Bayesian statistical procedure in order to integrate depth perceptions based on individual visual cues into a single, unified depth percept. From a Bayesian statistical viewpoint, the ideal observer achieves the best possible performance. In the experiment reported below, it was found that subjects combined the depth information provided by texture and motion cues in a statistically optimal manner. Because subjects' depth judgments closely matched those of the ideal observer, this means that their visual systems efficiently integrated the depth information available in the visual environment. A gentle introduction to Bayesian modeling of visual perception can be found in the chapter by Mamassian, Landy, and Maloney in this book. Bayesian models are also discussed in the chapters by Schrater and Kersten, Weiss and Fleet, and Freeman, Haddon, and Pasztor.

A second issue addressed in this chapter is the role of visual learning in cue integration. We study the question of whether or not observers' cue integration strategies for visual depth are adaptable in an experience-dependent manner. Previous studies have shown that observers' visual cue combination strategies are flexible in that these strategies adapt so as to make greater or lesser use of different cues in different visual environments (Backus and Banks, 1999; Jacobs and Fine, 1999; Young, Landy, and Maloney, 1993). For example, people rely on depth-from-stereo information more than depth-from-motion information when viewing nearby objects but not when viewing distant objects (Johnston, Cumming, and Landy, 1994; Cutting and Vishton, 1995). Maloney and Landy (1989) argued that the weight assigned to a depth judgment based on a particular cue should reflect the estimated reliability of that cue in the current scene under the current viewing conditions. If so, and if observers' cue integration strategies are adaptable, then it ought to be the case that changes in the reliability of a visual cue should result in changes in observers' cue integration strategies. In the experiment reported below, it was found that subjects adapted their weightings of depth-from-texture and depth-from-motion information as a function of training experience. Subjects adjusted their cue combination rules to use a cue more heavily after training in which that cue was reliable versus after training in which the cue was unreliable.

Optimal Visual Cue Integration

In this section, we compare the depth judgments of human observers to those of an ideal observer by analyzing the results of a depth-matching experiment. We were interested in knowing whether or not human observers use the depth information available in a visual environment efficiently for the purpose of cue integration.

Previous researchers have speculated that the weight assigned to a visual cue should be proportional to the reliability of that cue (Maloney and Landy, 1989). Unfortunately, there is relatively little available empirical data that directly evaluates this hypothesis in a quantitative manner (see Knill, 1998, for a notable exception). Previous studies have tended to be qualitative in nature. For example, Young, Landy,

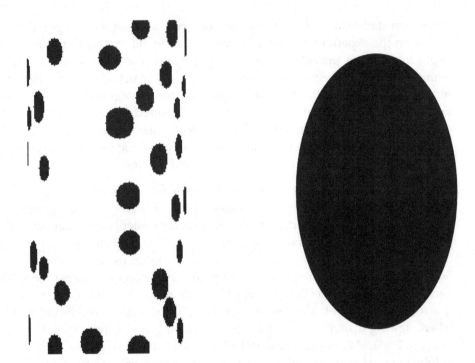

Figure 3.1: On the left is an instance of a texture-informative stimulus depicting a simulated elliptical cylinder. The height of the ellipse on the right is equal to the depth of the depicted cylinder.

and Maloney (1993) used a perturbation technique in order to analyze observers' depth perceptions based on texture and motion cues. They found that when either cue was corrupted by added noise, subjects tended to rely more heavily on the uncontaminated cue. While this result suggests that observers' combination rules are sensible, the experiment does not provide sufficient detail in order to assess whether or not these rules are statistically optimal. Our goal was to conduct an experiment that would permit us to quantitatively compare human observers' depth perceptions with those of an ideal observer. From a methodological viewpoint, an important feature of the experiment was the use of a subset of trials in which the visual stimulus contained only one of the visual cues of interest, as well as a subset of trials in which the stimulus contained all of the cues of interest. The ideal observer was provided with a subject's data from the single-cue trials, and was required to predict his or her data on the multiple-cue trials.

In each trial of the depth-matching experiment a display of a simulated elliptical cylinder (i.e. the horizontal cross-section of the cylinder was an ellipse) appeared on the left side of a video screen, and an ellipse appeared in the center of the screen (see Figure 3.1). The width of the ellipse was constant, and was equal to the width of the cylinder. However, subjects could increase or decrease the height of the ellipse by pressing keys on the keyboard. Subjects were instructed to adjust the height of the ellipse so that it matched the depth of the depicted cylinder. On training trials, subjects then received feedback; immediately after making a response the "target" ellipse was shown on the right side of the screen. The height of the target ellipse was equal to the depth of the depicted cylinder (meaning that the shape of the target ellipse was equal to the shape of the horizontal cross-section of the depicted cylinder). On test trials, subjects were not shown the target ellipse.

Twenty cylinders were used in the experiment. The shapes of these cylinders were identical in height (320 pixels) and width (160 pixels), though they differed in depth (from 80 to 270 pixels). On one-third of the trials the shape of the cylinder was primarily given by visual texture information (texture-informative stimuli), on one-third of the trials it was given by motion information (motion-informative stimuli), and on the remaining trials it was given by both sources of information (texture-and-motion informative stimuli). In texture-informative visual stimuli, a texture cue to the shape of a cylinder was created by mapping a homogeneous and isotropic texture consisting of circular spots to the cylinder's surface using a texture mapping algorithm (Hearn and Baker, 1997). The left side of Figure 3.1 shows an instance of a texture-informative stimulus. In motion-informative stimuli, a motion cue to the shape of a cylinder was created by moving small points of light horizontally along the cylinder's surface in either a clockwise or anticlockwise direction. Note that the cylinder did not rotate; rather the points moved along the simulated surface of static cylinders. Thus, the stimuli were different from kinetic depth effect stimuli. The motion cue in the stimuli used here is an instance of a constant flow field (Perotti, Todd, Lappin, and Phillips, 1998; Perotti, Todd, and Norman, 1996). In texture-and-motion informative stimuli, texture and motion cues to the shape of a cylinder were provided. Circular texture elements were mapped to a cylinder's surface, and these elements moved horizontally along the cylinder's surface. A more detailed discussion of the visual stimuli, experimental procedure, and experimental results can be found in Jacobs (1999).

The subjects' depth judgments are compared to those of an ideal observer, a computational model whose judgments are optimal according to Bayesian statistical criteria. The optimal estimate of depth given motion and texture cues is the depth, denoted d, that maximizes the probability $p(d|m,t)$ where m and t denote the motion and texture cues. Using Bayes' rule, this probability may be written as

$$p(d|m,t) \propto p(m,t|d)\, p(d). \tag{3.1}$$

If we assume that the motion and texture cues are conditionally independent given the depth, and if we assume that the prior probability distributions of the depth, $p(d)$, of the motion cue, $p(m)$, and of the texture cue, $p(t)$, are uniform, then the posterior distribution of the depth may be expressed as

$$p(d|m,t) \propto p(d|m)\, p(d|t). \tag{3.2}$$

The posterior probability of depth d factors into the product of the probability of d given the motion cue and the probability of d given the texture cue. We assume that these two distributions are Normal distributions. Let d_m^* denote the optimal estimate of depth given the motion cue [$d_m^* = \mathrm{argmax}_d\, p(d|m)$], and let d_t^* denote the optimal estimate of depth given the texture cue [$d_t^* = \mathrm{argmax}_d\, p(d|t)$]. If $d_m^* \approx d_t^*$, then Yuille and Bülthoff (1996) showed that the optimal estimate of depth based on both cues, denoted d^*, is given by

$$d^* = w_m d_m^* + w_t d_t^* \tag{3.3}$$

where

$$w_m = \frac{\sigma_m^{-2}}{\sigma_m^{-2} + \sigma_t^{-2}} \quad \text{and} \quad w_t = \frac{\sigma_t^{-2}}{\sigma_m^{-2} + \sigma_t^{-2}} \tag{3.4}$$

and σ_m^2 and σ_t^2 are the variances of the distributions $p(d|m)$ and $p(d|t)$ respectively. This solution has several appealing properties. The optimal estimate of depth based on both cues is a linear combination of the optimal estimates based on the individual cues in which the linear coefficients, the weights w_m and w_t, are non-negative and sum to one. In addition, the weight on a cue, such as the motion weight w_m, is large when that cue is relatively reliable (the variance σ_m^2 is smaller than the variance σ_t^2), and small when the cue is relatively unreliable (σ_m^2 is larger than σ_t^2).

In general, Bayesian models may lie anywhere on the continuum between weak and strong fusion models depending on the statistical assumptions that underlie the model (Yuille and Bülthoff, 1996). Due to the particular assumptions described above, the ideal observer (Equations 3.3 and 3.4) is a linear cue combination rule and, thus, is an instance of a weak fusion model. Readers familiar with adaptive filter theory will recognize that the ideal observer is also an instance of a Kalman filter. A derivation of this ideal observer from a Kalman filter perspective is given in Luo and Kay (1992).

We now present the subjects' responses in the depth-matching experiment, and then compare these responses to the depth judgments of the ideal observer. The mean squared error (MSE) of a subject's response at depth d is defined as

$$\mathrm{mse}(d) = \; < (\hat{d} - d)^2 > \tag{3.5}$$

where $\hat{d}$ is a subject's depth estimate when shown a stimulus depicting a cylinder whose true depth was d, and the brackets $< >$ denote an average. It is easy to show that this error can be expressed as the sum of two terms (Casella and Berger, 1990):

$$\mathrm{mse}(d) = (<\hat{d}> - d)^2 + <(\hat{d} - <\hat{d}>)^2 > . \tag{3.6}$$

The first term is the square of the bias of a subject's response at depth d where the bias is equal to the difference between the average of a subject's depth estimate and the true depth (i.e. bias(d) $=< \hat{d} > -d$). The bias is positive if the subject tended to overestimate the true depth of a cylinder, and negative if the subject tended to underestimate this depth. The second term is the variance of a subject's response at depth d (i.e. variance(d) $=< (\hat{d}- < \hat{d} >)^2 >$).

Figure 3.2 shows the results of the depth-matching experiment for three subjects. Each column corresponds to a different subject. The horizontal axis of each graph gives the depth of a cylinder in pixels. The vertical axes of the graphs in the top row give the bias of a subject's response on the test trials for each depth; the standard deviation of a subject's response is given in the graphs in the middle row; the root mean squared error (RMSE) of a subject's response is given in the graphs in the bottom row. The dotted line in each graph is for responses to motion-informative stimuli; the dashed line is for responses to texture-informative stimuli; the solid line is for responses to texture-and-motion informative stimuli. Using Equation 3.6, the square of the data in the top row (the square of the biases) plus the square of the data in the middle row (the square of the standard deviations is the variances) equals the square of the data in the bottom row (the square of the RMSEs is the MSEs).

The data in Figure 3.2 reveal many features of subjects' responses. The biases in subjects' responses tended to be positive when subjects were viewing cylinders that are less deep than wide, and negative when they were viewing cylinders that are more deep than wide. This trend is most evident for subjects JC and JH, and appears to be strongest when these subjects were viewing stimuli that contained only a single cue to a cylinder's shape. This observation suggests that when subjects were viewing stimuli that contained only one informative cue, they tended to assume that the cylinders were roughly circular. However, when viewing stimuli that contained both cues, they either did not make this assumption or else they made it less strongly. Overall, subjects' responses tended to be less variable when they were viewing stimuli that contained both texture and motion cues compared to when they were viewing stimuli that contained only a texture cue or only a motion cue. Consistent with these observations regarding biases and variances, it was also the case that subjects' depth judgments had a smaller error when viewing multiple-cue stimuli than when viewing single-cue stimuli.

We compared the subjects' responses on test trials using the texture-and-motion informative stimuli to those predicted by the ideal observer defined above. The parameter values of the ideal observer were set based on subjects' responses on trials when only one cue was informative. Let optimal(d) denote the ideal observer's response; this is the predicted average response of a subject to a texture-and-motion stimulus depicting a cylinder of depth d. Let $< \hat{d}_m >$ and $< \hat{d}_t >$ denote a subject's average responses to motion-informative and texture-informative stimuli depicting a cylinder of depth d. The optimal response is equal to

$$\text{optimal}(d) = w_m < \hat{d}_m > + w_t < \hat{d}_t > \tag{3.7}$$

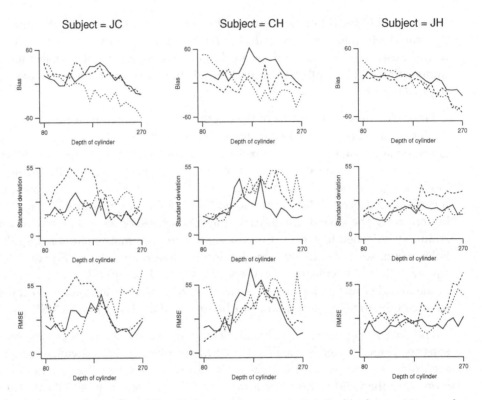

Figure 3.2: The results of the depth-matching experiment. Each column corresponds to a different subject. The horizontal axis of each graph gives the depth of a cylinder in pixels. The vertical axes of the graphs in the top row give the bias of a subject's response on the test trials for each depth; the standard deviation of a subject's response is given in the graphs in the middle row; the root mean squared error (RMSE) of a subject's response is given in the graphs in the bottom row. The dotted line in each graph is for responses to motion-informative stimuli; the dashed line is for responses to texture-informative stimuli; the solid line is for responses to texture-and-motion informative stimuli.

where the linear coefficients w_m and w_t were computed based on the variances of a subject's responses to motion-informative stimuli and texture-informative stimuli according to Equation 3.4. For subject JC, the coefficients w_m and w_t equal 0.58 and 0.42; for subject CH, $w_m = 0.45$ and $w_t = 0.55$; for subject JH, $w_m = 0.72$ and $w_t = 0.28$. Thus, the motion cue was mildly more reliable than the texture cue for subject JC (i.e. depth estimates based on the motion cue were less variable than estimates based on the texture cue); for subject CH, the texture cue was mildly more reliable; for subject JH, the motion cue was strongly more reliable.

The optimal responses of the ideal observer are compared to the subjects' responses in Figure 3.3. The horizontal axis of each graph gives the values of optimal(d), the predicted average responses to texture-and-motion informative stimuli depicting

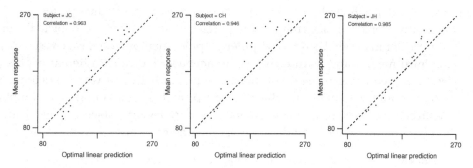

Figure 3.3: A comparison of the ideal observer's depth judgments with the subjects' actual depth judgments. The horizontal axis of each graph gives the values of optimal(d) in pixels, the predicted average responses to texture-and-motion informative stimuli depicting cylinders of depth d for each of the twenty possible values of d; the vertical axis gives a subject's actual average responses.

cylinders of depth d for each of the twenty possible values of d; the vertical axis gives a subject's actual average responses (the dashed diagonal line indicates where the data would lie if the predicted and actual responses are identical). The correlation between the optimal responses and the actual responses for subject JC is 0.96; the correlation for subject CH is 0.95; the correlation for subject JH is 0.99.

Based on these data, it seems that subjects combined the visual depth information provided by texture and motion cues in a statistically optimal manner. Consequently, the ideal observer is a good model of subjects' cue combination strategies. This is a surprising result because the ideal observer is strongly constrained (it is linear) and it does not have any free parameters. We conclude that observers' cue combination strategies are indeed optimal, at least under the conditions studied here.

Experience-Dependent Adaptation

This section examines the role that visual learning may play in cue integration. We address the question of whether or not observers' cue integration strategies for visual depth are adaptable in an experience-dependent manner. If the weight assigned to a depth judgment based on a particular cue reflects the estimated reliability of that cue, and if observers' cue integration strategies are adaptable, then it ought to be the case that changes in the reliability of a visual cue should result in changes in observers' cue weights.

We conducted an experiment in which the relative reliabilities of visual cues changed during the course of training. In each trial of the experiment, subjects monocularly viewed two sequentially presented stimuli where each stimulus depicted an elliptical cylinder defined by texture and motion cues. Subjects then performed a two-alternative forced-choice comparison, judging which of the two depicted cylinders was greater in depth. Using a computer graphics manipulation, we created displays in which motion and texture cues simultaneously indicated different depths (subjects reported being unaware of this manipulation). Thus it was possible for us to design training conditions in which one cue provided useful information for making depth comparisons, whereas the other cue was irrelevant. Subjects received auditory feedback on training trials indicating whether their response was correct or incorrect.

Unbeknownst to the subjects, the experiment used two types of training conditions. Under motion relevant conditions, the motion cue in one display of a trial indicated a cylinder that was deeper than the cylinder indicated by the motion cue in the other display, whereas the texture cue in each display indicated cylinders with identical depths. Therefore, only the motion cue was useful for performing the experimental task under these conditions. Under texture relevant training conditions, the situation was reversed. The texture cue distinguished the depths of the cylinders depicted in the two displays, whereas the motion cue was identical in the displays. That is, only the texture cue was useful for discriminating the cylinders' depths under texture relevant conditions. Subjects initially received training in which one cue (e.g., motion) was informative and the other cue (e.g., texture) was irrelevant. Each subject's relative weighting of motion and texture cues was then estimated. Then subjects were re-trained under new experimental conditions; in these new conditions, the previously informative cue was irrelevant, and the previously irrelevant cue was informative. Subjects' relative weighting of motion and texture cues was again estimated. A more detailed discussion of the visual stimuli, experimental procedure, and experimental results can be found in Jacobs and Fine (1999).

Subjects' motion and texture weights were estimated on the basis of their responses on test trials. Similar to training trials, subjects viewed two displays of cylinders and judged which cylinder was greater in depth. In one display of a test trial (display M), the motion cue indicated one of seven possible depths, whereas the texture cue indicated that the cylinder was equally deep as wide. In the other display (display T), the texture cue indicated one of seven possible depths, whereas the motion cue indicated that the cylinder was equally deep as wide. That is, whereas the texture cue of display M and the motion cue of display T indicated cylinders with identical depths, the motion cue of display M and the texture cue of display T indicated cylinders of different depths. In this way it was possible to evaluate how much each subject used the motion cue versus the texture cue.

Each subject's pattern of responses on the test trials was modeled using a logistic function. Let $d^M(m, t)$ denote a subject's depth percept based on display M, and let $d^T(m, t)$ denote his depth percept based on display T. Assuming a linear cue combination rule, these quantities can be written as

$$d^M(m, t) = w_m d^M(m) + w_t d^M(t) \tag{3.8}$$

$$d^T(m,t) = w_m d^T(m) + w_t d^T(t) \qquad (3.9)$$

where $d^M(m)$ and $d^M(t)$ are the depths indicated by the motion and texture cues in display M, $d^T(m)$ and $d^T(t)$ are the depths indicated by the motion and texture cues in display T, w_m and w_t are the motion and texture weights, and w_m and w_t are constrained to be non-negative and to sum to one. The probability that the subject selected display M as depicting the deeper cylinder is approximated with a logistic function:

$$P(\text{response} = M) = \frac{1}{1 + \exp\{-[d^M(m,t) - d^T(m,t)]/\tau\}} \qquad (3.10)$$

where τ is a temperature parameter. The model has two free parameters: the motion weight w_m (recall that $w_t = 1 - w_m$) and the temperature τ. The values of these parameters were estimated using a maximum likelihood estimation procedure based on a Bernoulli likelihood function:

$$P(\mathcal{X}|w_m,\tau) = \prod_{i=1}^{I} P(r_i = M)^{r_i} [1 - P(r_i = M)]^{1-r_i} \qquad (3.11)$$

where $\mathcal{X}$ is the subject's responses on the test trials, $P(r_i = M)$ is the probability that the subject selected display M on trial i according to the logistic function (Equation 3.10), r_i is a binary variable indicating whether the subject selected display M ($r_i = 1$) or display T ($r_i = 0$) on trial i, and I is the number of test trials. Equations 10 and 11 are justified as follows. Recall that subjects are performing a two-alternative forced choice task; they are choosing either display M or display T as depicting the deeper cylinder. Consequently, subjects' data are instances of a class often referred to as binary response data. Binary response data can frequently be modeled by a Bernoulli probability model. When doing so, it is convenient to use the logistic function to map the covariate variables (e.g., the depths indicated by motion and texture cues in displays M and T) to the response variable (e.g., the probability of selecting display M as depicting the deeper cylinder). Indeed, the inverse of the logistic function is known as the canonical link function for a Bernoulli probability model (McCullagh and Nelder, 1989).

The response data of one subject, subject DA, on the test trials are shown in Figure 3.4. This figure contains four graphs. The axis labeled 'motion shape' gives the cylinder shape indicated by the motion cue in display M; the axis labeled 'texture shape' gives the cylinder shape indicated by the texture cue in display T (recall that seven shapes were used: 1 is the shape with the smallest depth, 7 is the shape with the greatest depth). The values of the texture cue in display M and the motion cue in display T are not shown because they were constant (they always indicated a cylinder whose horizontal cross-section was circular). The axis labeled '$P(\text{response} = M)$' gives the probability that a subject judged display M as depicting the deeper cylin-

After motion relevant training

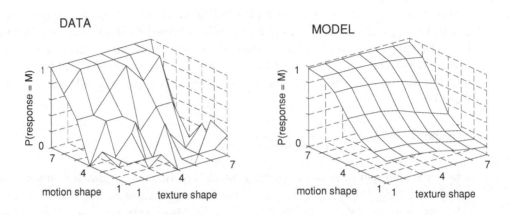

After texture relevant training

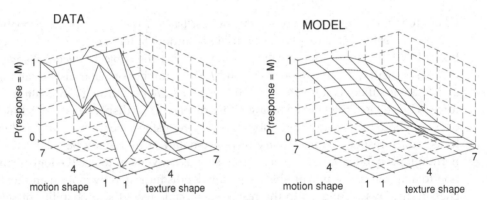

Figure 3.4: The response data of subject DA on test trials following motion relevant training (top-left graph) and texture relevant training (bottom-left graph). The logistic model was used to fit surfaces to these two datasets. These surfaces are shown in the top-right and bottom-right graphs, respectively.

der. The top-left graph gives the subject's response data on the test trials following motion relevant training; the top-right graph shows the surface that was fit to the subject's data by the logistic model. The shape of the data is sensible. As the motion cue in display M indicated a deeper cylinder (that is, as the value along the motion shape axis increased), the probability that the subject judged display M as depicting a deeper cylinder increased. Similarly, as the texture cue in display T indicated a deeper cylinder (as the value along the texture shape axis increased), the probability that the subject judged display M as depicting a deeper cylinder decreased. Analogous graphs for the response data on test trials following texture relevant training are shown in the bottom row. The bottom-left graph shows the subject's response data; the bottom-right graph shows the surface that was fit to the subject's data by the logistic model.

A comparison of the graphs in the top and bottom rows of Figure 3.4 reveals that the subject responded to the same set of test trials in different ways following training under motion relevant and texture relevant conditions. We conclude that the subject showed experience-dependent adaptation of her cue combination rule for depth, and that this adaptation occurred in a logical way. Following motion relevant training, the subject was highly sensitive to the motion cue and relatively insensitive to the texture cue. This is evidenced by the fact that the graph of the subject's data rises sharply along the motion shape axis, but declines gradually along the texture shape axis (this is most easily seen in the top-right graph of Figure 3.4). Comparing the subject's responses after texture relevant training with her responses after motion relevant training, the subject was relatively less sensitive to the motion cue and more sensitive to the texture cue. The graph of the data rises less steeply along the motion shape axis following texture relevant training, and rises more steeply along the texture shape axis.

The graph on the left of Figure 3.5 gives the estimated values of the motion weight w_m following motion relevant training and following texture relevant training for four subjects. All four subjects had larger motion weights following motion relevant training than following texture relevant training. Define the motion weight *difference* to be the estimate of a subject's motion weight following motion relevant training minus the value of this estimate following texture relevant training. The graph on the right side of Figure 3.5 gives the motion weight differences for the four subjects. The rightmost bar in the graph is the average motion weight difference; the error bar gives the standard error of the mean. Using a one-tailed t-test, the average motion weight difference is significantly greater than zero ($t = 2.357$, $p < 0.05$). Because subjects had larger motion weights after motion relevant training than after texture relevant training, we conclude that observers' cue combination strategies are adaptable as a function of experience; subjects adjusted their cue combination rules to more heavily use a cue when that cue was informative on a given task versus when the cue was irrelevant.

Summary and Conclusions

In summary, this chapter has addressed two important aspects of visual cue integration for depth perception. First, we addressed the question of whether or not observers' cue integration strategies can be characterized as "optimal" where the optimality criteria are based on Bayesian statistics. An experiment was reported in which

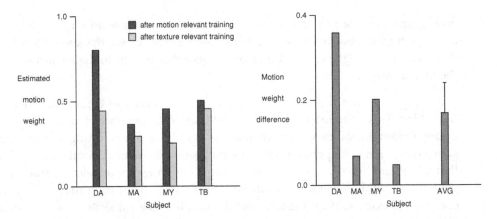

Figure 3.5: The graph on the left shows the estimated values of the motion weights w_m following motion relevant training and following texture relevant training for four subjects. The graph on the right shows the motion weight differences for the subjects.

it was found that subjects integrated the depth information provided by texture and motion cues in a statistically optimal manner. Second, we addressed the question of whether or not observers' cue integration strategies for visual depth are adaptable in an experience-dependent manner. We reported an experiment in which it was found that subjects adapted their weightings of depth-from-texture and depth-from-motion information as a function of training experience. Subjects adjusted their cue combination rules to use a cue more heavily after training in which that cue was reliable versus after training in which the cue was unreliable.

This work raises a number of questions. In regard to optimal cue integration, we would like to know if it is always the case that observers' depth percepts are closely approximated by a Bayesian model with a non-informative prior distribution, or are there circumstances in which observers' percepts are biased such that their responses can only be approximated with a model that is also suitably biased? If the latter, then what are the circumstances in which observers' depth percepts are biased, and what are those biases? Interesting findings regarding observers' biases are reported in Chapter 1 by Mamassian, Landy, and Maloney. In regard to experience-dependent adaptation of cue integration strategies, we would like to know what factors influence the amount of adaptation, and under what conditions is the degree of adaptation maximal? Do such conditions naturally occur during the everyday course of observers' lives? These questions are the focus of our future research.

Acknowledgement

I thank R. Aslin and I. Fine for many interesting conversations on this topic, and E. Bero, L. O'Brien, A. Pauls, and M. Saran for help in conducting the experiments. This work was supported by NIH grant R29-MH54770.

References

[1] Backus, B.T. and Banks, M.S. (1999) Estimator reliability and distance scaling in stereoscopic slant perception. *Perception*, 28, 217-242.

[2] Bruno, N. and Cutting, J.E. (1988) Minimodularity and the perception of layout. *Journal of Experimental Psychology*, 117, 161-170.

[3] Bülthoff, H.H. and Mallot, H.A. (1988) Integration of depth modules: Stereo and shading. *Journal of the Optical Society of America*, 5, 1749-1758.

[4] Casella, G. and Berger, R.L. (1990) *Statistical Inference*. Belmont, CA: Wadsworth.

[5] Clark, J. and Yuille, A.L. (1990) *Data Fusion for Sensory Information Processing Systems*. Norwell, MA: Kluwer.

[6] Cutting, J.E. and Vishton, P.M. (1995) Perceiving layout and knowing distances: The integration, relative potency, and contextual use of different information about depth. In W. Epstein and S. Rogers (Eds.), *Perception of Space and Motion*. San Diego: Academic Press.

[7] Dosher, B.A., Sperling, G. and Wurst, S. (1986) Tradeoffs between stereopsis and proximity luminance covariance as determinants of perceived 3D structure. *Vision Research*, 26, 973-990.

[8] Hearn, D. and Baker, M.P. (1997) *Computer Graphics (C Version)*. Upper Saddle River, NJ: Prentice Hall.

[9] Jacobs, R.A. (1999) Optimal integration of texture and motion cues to depth. *Vision Research*, 39, 3621-3629.

[10] Jacobs, R.A. and Fine, I. (1999) Experience-dependent integration of texture and motion cues to depth. *Vision Research*, 39, 4062-4075.

[11] Johnston, E.B., Cumming, B.G., and Landy, M.S. (1994) Integration of motion and stereopsis cues. *Vision Research*, 34, 2259-2275.

[12] Knill, D.C. (1998) Ideal observer perturbation analysis reveals human strategies for inferring surface orientation from texture. *Vision Research*, 38, 2635-2656.

[13] Landy, M.S., Maloney, L.T., Johnston, E.B., and Young, M. (1995) Measurement and modeling of depth cue combination: In defense of weak fusion. *Vision Research*, 35, 389-412.

[14] Landy, M.S., Maloney, L.T., and Young, M. (1991) Psychophysical estimation of the human depth combination rule. In P.S. Schenker (Ed.), *Sensor Fusion III: 3-D Perception and Recognition, Proceedings of the SPIE*, 1383, 247-254.

[15] Luo, R.C. and Kay, M.G. (1992) Data fusion and sensor integration: State-of-the-art 1990s. In M.A. Abidi and R.C. Gonzalez (Eds.), *Data Fusion In Robotics and Machine Intelligence*. San Diego: Academic Press.

[16] Maloney, L.T. and Landy, M.S. (1989) A statistical framework for robust fusion of depth information. *Visual Communications and Image Processing IV: Proceedings of the SPIE*, 1199, 1154-1163.

[17] Marroquin, J.L., Mitter, S.K., and Poggio, T. (1987) Probabilistic solution of ill-posed problems in computational vision. *Journal of the American Statistical Association*, 82, 76-89.

[18] McCullagh, P. and Nelder, J.A. (1989) *Generalized Linear Models*. London: Chapman and Hall.

[19] Nawrot, M. and Blake, R. (1989) Neural integration of information specifying structure from stereopsis and motion. *Science*, 244, 716-718.

[20] Nawrot, M. and Blake, R. (1991) The interplay between stereopsis and structure from motion. *Perception and Psychophysics*, 49, 230-244.

[21] Nawrot, M. and Blake, R. (1993) On the perceptual identity of dynamic stereopsis and kinetic depth. *Vision Research*, 33, 1561-1571.

[22] Perotti, V.J., Todd, J.T., Lappin, J.S., and Phillips, F. (1998) The perception of surface curvature from optical motion. *Perception and Psychophysics*, 60, 377-388.

[23] Perotti, V.J., Todd, J.T., and Norman, J.F. (1996) The visual perception of rigid motion from constant flow fields. *Perception and Psychophysics*, 58, 666-679.

[24] Rogers, B.J. and Collett, T.S. (1989) The appearance of surfaces specified by motion parallax and binocular disparity. *Quarterly Journal of Experimental Psychology*, 41, 697-717.

[25] Young, M.J., Landy, M.S., and Maloney, L.T. (1993) A perturbation analysis of depth perception from combinations of texture and motion cues. *Vision Research*, 33, 2685-2696.

[26] Yuille, A.L. and Bülthoff, H.H. (1996) Bayesian decision theory and psychophysics. In D.C. Knill and W. Richards (Eds.), *Perception as Bayesian Inference*. New York: Cambridge University Press.

4 Velocity Likelihoods in Biological and Machine Vision

Yair Weiss and David J. Fleet

Introduction

What computations occur in early motion analysis in biological and machine vision? One common hypothesis is that visual motion analysis proceeds by first computing local 2d velocities, and then by combining these local estimates to compute the global motion of an object. A well-known problem with this approach is that local motion information is often ambiguous, a situation often referred to as the "aperture problem" [13, 6, 2, 8]. Consider the scene depicted in Figure 4.1. A local analyzer that sees only the vertical edge of a square can only determine the horizontal component of the motion. Whether the square translates horizontally to the right, diagonally up and to the right, or diagonally down and to the right, the motion of the vertical edge will appear the same within the aperture. The family of velocities consistent with the motion of the edge can be depicted as a line in "velocity space", where any velocity is represented as a vector from the origin whose length is proportional to speed and whose angle corresponds to the direction of motion. Geometrically, the aperture problem is equivalent to saying that the family of motions consistent with the information at an edge maps to a straight line in velocity space, rather than a single point.

Because of ambiguities due to the aperture problem, as well as noise in the image observations, it would make sense that a system would represent the *uncertainty* in the local estimate as well as the best estimate. This would enable subsequent processing to combine the local estimates while taking their uncertainties into account. Accordingly, it has been argued that the goal of early motion analysis should be the extraction of local *likelihoods* (probability distributions over velocity), rather than a single estimate [10]. In a Bayesian approach to motion analysis, these local likelihoods would be combined with the observer's prior assumptions about the world, to estimate the motion of objects.

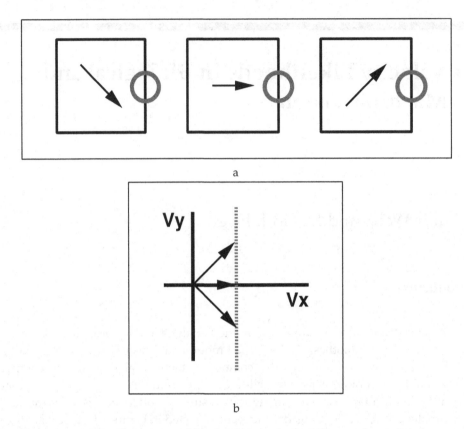

Figure 4.1: a. The "aperture problem" refers to the inability to determine the two dimensional motion of a signal containing a single orientation. For example, a local analyzer that sees only the vertical edge of a square can only determine the horizontal component of the motion. Whether the square translates horizontally to the right, diagonally up and to the right, or diagonally down and to the right, the motion of the vertical edge will be the same. **b.** The family of motions consistent with the motion of the edge can be depicted as a line in "velocity space", where any velocity is represented as a vector from the origin whose length is proportional to speed and whose angle corresponds to direction of motion. Graphically, the aperture problem is equivalent to saying that the family of motions consistent with the edge maps to a straight line in velocity space, rather than a single point.

In this paper, we assume that early motion analysis does indeed extract velocity likelihoods, and we address a number of questions raised by this assumption:

- What is the form of the likelihood? Can it be derived from first principles?
- What is the relationship between the local likelihood calculation and other models of early motion analysis?
- Can these likelihoods be represented by known physiology?

Motivation - Motion Analysis as Bayesian Inference

In the Bayesian approach to motion analysis, the goal is to calculate the posterior probability of a velocity given the image data. This posterior is related to the likelihoods and prior probabilities by Bayes' rule. Denoting by $I(x, t)$ the spatiotemporal brightness observation (measurement) at location x and time t, and by v the 2d image motion of the object, then

$$P(v \,|\, I(x,t))) \,=\, \alpha\, P(v)\, P(I(x,t)\,|\,v)\,, \tag{4.1}$$

where α is a normalization constant that is independent of v.

Bayes' rule represents a normative prescription for combining uncertain information. Assuming that the image observations at different positions and times are conditionally indpendent, given v, it is straightforward to show that this simplifies into:

$$P(v \,|\, I(x,t)) \,=\, \alpha\, P(v) \prod_{i,j} P(I(x_i,t_j)\,|\,v))\,, \tag{4.2}$$

where the product is taken over all positions x_i and times t_j. The important quantity to calculate at every image location is the *likelihood* of a velocity, $P(I(x_i,t_j)\,|\,v)$.

Interestingly, there is growing evidence that the human visual system can be described in terms of computations like these. For example, in [15, 5] it was shown that a large number of visual illusions are explained by a model that maximizes Equation 4.2 when $P(v)$ is taken to be a prior distribution that favors slow speeds. Figure 4.2 shows an example from [15]. Each stimulus consisted of a translating rhombus whose endpoints are occluded. When the rhombus is "fat", it is indeed perceived as moving horizontally. But when the rhombus is "narrow" the percevied motion is illusory — subjects perceive it as moving diagonally rather than horizontally.

Why do humans misperceive the motion of a narrow rhombus but not a fat one? To address this question, let us first consider models that do not represent uncertainty about local motion measurements. In the case of the fat rhombus, the perceived motion can be explained by an intersection-of-constraints (IOC) model [2]. According to this model, each local analyzer extracts the constraint line corresponding to the local moving contour. Subsequent processing then finds the intersection of these two constraint lines. This procedure will always give the veridical motion for a translating 2D figure, so it can explain the motion of the fat rhombus.

But, this IOC model does not account for the motion percept with the narrow one. As an alternative model, if each local analyzer were to extract the normal velocity of the contour followed by a *vector average* of these normal velocities, this would predict

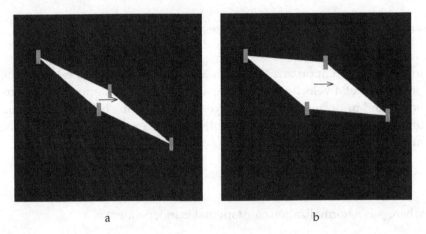

Figure 4.2: a. A "narrow" rhombus whose endpoints are occluded appears to move diagonally (consistent with VA). **b.** A "fat" rhombus whose endpoints are occluded appears to move horizontally

the diagonal motion for the narrow rhombus [16]. But, this vector average model does not explain the percept of the fat rhombus.

Figures 4.3–4.4 show how both percepts can be accounted for by Equation 4.2. Here, each local analyzer extracts a likelihood from the local contour motion. As shown in the figures these likelihoods are fuzzy constraint lines, indicating that velocities on the constraint lines have highest likelihoods, and the likelihood decreases gradually with increasing distance from the constraint line. When these likelihoods are multiplied together with the prior, as dictated by Equation 4.2, the predicted motion is horizontal for fat rhombuses and diagonal for narrow rhombuses.

These results and others in [15] suggest that a Bayesian model with a prior favoring slow speeds can explain a range of percepts in human vision. But our original question concerning the right likelihood function remains.

What Is the Likelihood Function for Image Velocity?

Previous approaches

In order to compute image velocity, one must first decide which property of the image to track from one time to the next. One common, successful approach in machine vision is based on the assumption that the light reflected from a object surface remains constant through time, in which case one can track points of constant

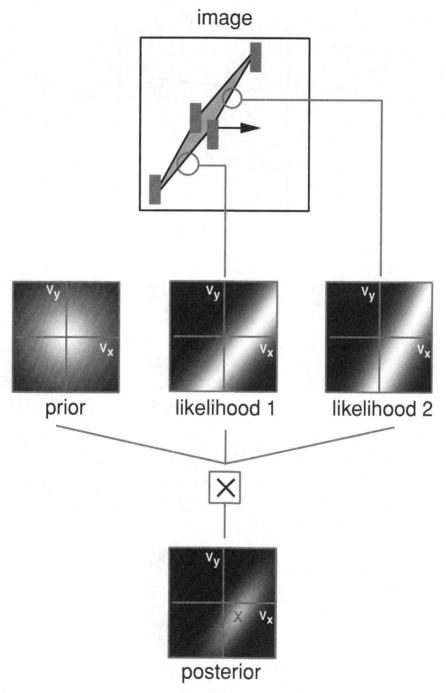

Figure 4.3: The response of the Bayesian estimator to a narrow rhombus (replotted from Weiss and Adelson 98).

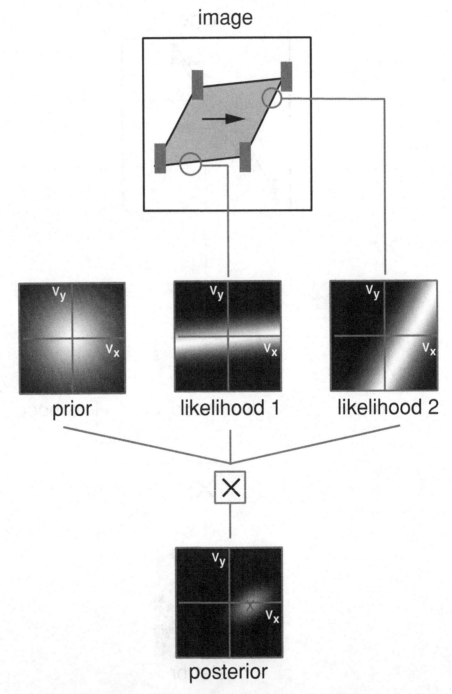

Figure 4.4: The response of the Bayesian estimator to a fat rhombus (replotted from Weiss and Adelson 98).

image intensity (e.g., [3, 6, 7]). Mathematically, this can be expressed in terms of a path, $x(t)$, along which the image, $I(x(t), t)$, remains constant: i.e.,

$$I(x(t), t) = C,\qquad(4.3)$$

where C is a constant. Taking the temporal derivative of both sides of Equation 4.3, and assuming that the path $x(t)$ is sufficiently smooth to be differentiable, with $v \equiv (v_x, v_y) = (\frac{dx}{dt}, \frac{dy}{dt})$, provides us with the constraint

$$\frac{\partial I}{\partial x}v_x + \frac{\partial I}{\partial x}v_y + \frac{\partial I}{\partial t} = 0 \qquad(4.4)$$

This is often refered to as the gradient constraint equation. When the exact solutions to Equation 4.4 are plotted in velocity space, one obtains a constraint line. This line represents all of the different 2d velocities that are consistent with the image derivative measurements, as given by Equation 4.4.

In estimating image velocity, it is the likelihood function that expresses our belief that certain velocities are consisten with the image measurements. Uncertainty in belief arises because the derivative measurements in Equation 4.4 only constrain velocity to somewhere along a line. Further uncertainty in belief arises because the partial derivative measurements are noisy. According to reasoning of this sort, most likelihood functions that have been proposed fall into one of two categories: "fuzzy constraint lines" (as in Figure 4.5c) and "fuzzy bowties" (as in Figure 4.5d). Examples of the two categories appeared in [10].

The first one defines the likelihood to be

$$P(I \mid v) = \alpha \exp\left(-\frac{1}{2\sigma^2} \int \left(\frac{\partial I}{\partial x}v_x + \frac{\partial I}{\partial y}v_y + \frac{\partial I}{\partial t}\right)^2 dx\, dt\right) \qquad(4.5)$$

This likelihood function is often derived by assuming that the temporal derivative measurement is contaminated with mean-zero Gaussian noise, but the spatial derivative measurements are noise-free [11]. Figure 4.5c shows an example of the likelihood for the image sequence shown in Figure 4.5a. For this image, that contains only a single orientation, this looks like a fuzzy constraint line.

The second category of likelihood function is defined to be:

$$P(I \mid v) = \alpha \exp\left(-\frac{1}{2\sigma^2} \int \frac{(\frac{\partial I}{\partial x}v_x + \frac{\partial I}{\partial y}v_y + \frac{\partial I}{\partial t})^2}{1 + v_x^2 + v_y^2} dx\, dt\right) \qquad(4.6)$$

This likelihood function has been shown to result from an assumption that mean-zero Gaussian noise is added to each of the spatial and temporal derivative measurements [9]. While this likelihood function has only recently been derived, the velocity at

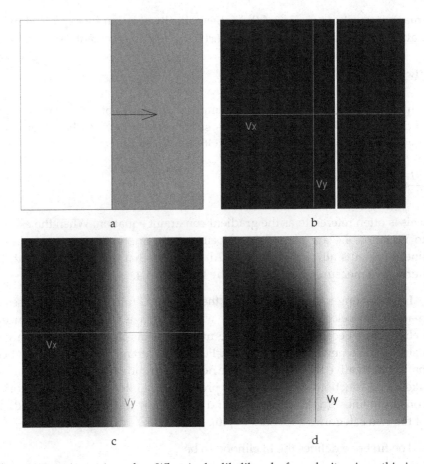

Figure 4.5: a: A moving edge. What is the likelihood of a velocity given this image sequence? **b.** The constraint line in velocity space. In the absence of noise, all velocities along the constraint line are consistent with the data. **c-d.** Likelihood functions in velocity space. White pixels correspond to high likelihood. Assuming only the temporal derivatives are noisy gives a fuzzy constraint line (as in b) but assuming all derivatives are equally noisy gives a fuzzy bowtie (as in c). What is the right likelihood to use?

which it is maximal corresponds to what has been usually called the total-least-squares velocity estimate [14]. Figure 4.5d shows the picture in velocity space. For a sequence that contains only a single orientation, this looks like a fuzzy bowtie. Given the assumption of noise in both spatial and temporal derivatices, the fuzzy bowtie seems slightly more attractive — why should one direction of differentiation behave differently than another?

The fuzzy constraint line has other desirable qualities however. One nice property can be illustrated in Figure 4.5. Obviously a vertical edge moving with velocity v is indistinguishable from a vertical edge moving with velocity $(v_x, v_y) + \alpha(0, 1)^T$. Thus if our image sequence contains only vertical edges, we might like the likelihood function to be invariant to an addition of a vertical component $P(I \,|\, (v_x, v_y)) = P(I \,|\, (v_x, v_y) + \alpha(0, 1)^T)$. This means that curve of equal likelihood should be lines that are parallel to the constraint line, a property that fuzzy lines have but fuzzy bowties do not.

Surprisingly, after many years of research into local motion analysis, there remains a lack of consensus regarding which likelihood to use, as these two and others have been suggested. To illustrate this, consider the recent paper of Fernmuller et al. [4] who have suggested yet another local likelihood function. It assumes that the noise in the spatial and temporal derivatives may be correlated. Specifically the noise in the two spatial derivatives is uncorrelated but the noise in the spatial and temporal derivatives is correlated with a correlation coefficient that depends on the sign of the derivatives, $E(I_x I_t) = -\sigma_{xt} sgn(I_x I_t)$. For $\sigma_{xt} = 0$ this reduces to the total-least-squares likelihood or the fuzzy bowtie. But when σ_{xt} is nonzero, they find that the likelihood is biased. That is, even if the noise is zero, the ML estimator using their likelihood function does not give the true velocity.

The problem with deriving these likelihoods from Equation 4.4 is that there is no generative model. The preceding discussion tries to derive noise models in the derivative domain rather than basing the noise assumptions in the imaging domain (where presumably we have better intuitions about what constitutes a reasonable noise model).

Generative model

In what follows we derive a likelihood function from a generative model of images. It is a natural extension of intensity conservation to a noisy imaging situation (see Figure 4.6). For notational simplicity we consider the generation of 1d images. The extension to 2d images is straightforward.

Let us assume that an unknown scene function $s(x)$ is first generated with probability $P(s)$. It is then translated with velocity v:

$$S(x, t) = s(x - vt) \tag{4.7}$$

In what follows we use capital $S(x, t)$ to denote the ideal, noiseless image sequence and $s(x) = S(x, 0)$ to denote a single image from that sequence.

Finally, to model the process of image formation, we assume that the observed image is equal to the translating scene plus imaging noise:

$$I(x, t) = S(x, t) + \sigma \eta \tag{4.8}$$

where η denotes zero mean Gaussian noise with variance 1 that is independent across

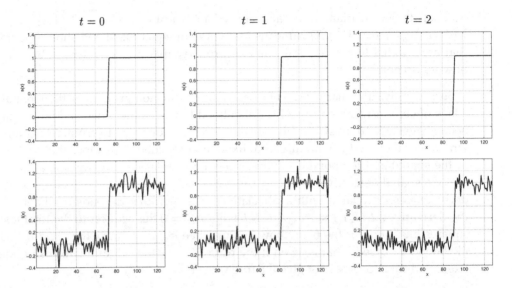

Figure 4.6: The generative model that we use to derive the likelihood function. The signal function (top panels) translates and conserves brightness. The image (bottom panels) equals signal plus imaging noise.

time and space, and independent of S. We assume that we observe $I(x, t)$ for a fixed time interval $|t| < t_m$ and for all x. Also, we will use the notation $\|f\|^2$ to denote the energy in the signal f; that is,

$$\|f\|^2 = \int_{|t|<t_m,x} f^2(x, t)\, dx\, dt \tag{4.9}$$

Claim 1: Assuming a uniform prior over scene functions ($P(s)$ is independent of s) then

$$P(I \mid v) = \alpha \exp\left(-\frac{1}{2\sigma^2}\|I - \hat{S}_v\|^2\right) \tag{4.10}$$

with

$$\hat{S}_v(x, t) = \hat{s}(x - vt), \tag{4.11}$$

and

$$\hat{s}_v(x, t) = \frac{1}{2t_m}\int_{-t_m}^{t_m} I(x + vt, t)\, dt \tag{4.12}$$

Figure 4.7 illustrates this calculation. For each velocity we calculate the predicted intensity assuming a scene function moving at that velocity (shown in the left col-

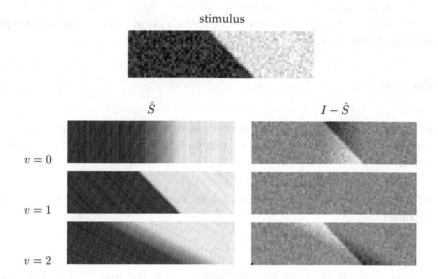

Figure 4.7: Top: A space versus time (xt) plot of an edge moving to the right. **Bottom:** Calculations of the log likelihood for different velocities. For each velocity we calculate the predicted intensity assuming a scene function moving at that velocity (shown in the left column). The residual intensity (shown in the right column) is explained as noise: the less energy in the residual the more likely the velocity.

umn). The residual intensity (shown in the right column) is explained as noise: the less energy in the residual the more likely the velocity.

Proof: A proof of claim 1 is obtained by first formulating the likelihood, $P(I|v)$, as the marginalization of the joint distribution over both I and the unknown scene function s, conditioned on v. More formally,

$$P(I \mid v) = \int_s P(s, I \mid v) \tag{4.13}$$

$$= \int_s P(s \mid v) P(I \mid s, v) \tag{4.14}$$

$$= \int_s \alpha \exp\left(-\frac{1}{2\sigma^2} \int (I(x,t) - s(x - vt))^2 dx\, dt\right) \tag{4.15}$$

$$= \max_s \alpha \exp\left(-\frac{1}{2\sigma^2} \int (I(x,t) - s(x - vt))^2 dx\, dt\right) \tag{4.16}$$

$$= \alpha \exp\left(-\frac{1}{2\sigma^2} \int (I(x,t) - \hat{s}(x,t))^2 dx\, dt\right) \tag{4.17}$$

where we have used the fact that $P(s|v)$ is independent of s and of v, and that for jointly Gaussian random variables, marginalization can be replaced with maximization: $\int_z P(x,z)dz = \alpha/\sqrt{V(z|x)} \max_z P(x,z)$ where $V(z|x)$ denotes the conditional variance of z given x. The maximization over s turns into a separate maximization over $s(x)$ for each x and it is easy to see that $s(x)$ is most likely when it is equal to the mean of $I(x + vt)$ over t. $\square$

Extensions

Of course the derivation given above makes several assumptions, many of which are somewhat restrictive. However, many of them can be relaxed in straightforward ways:

- Colored noise: If the noise is not white, then it can be shown that the likelihood becomes:

$$P(I \mid v) = \alpha \exp \left(-\frac{1}{2\sigma^2} \| I - \hat{S}_v \|_W^2 \right) \tag{4.18}$$

That is, rather than calculating the energy of the residual, we calculate a weighted energy; the weight of an energy band is inversely proportional to the expected noise variance in that band.

- Non-uniform prior over scene functions: Above we assumed that all scene functions are equiprobable. However, if we have some prior probability over the scene function, it can be shown that Equation 4.10 still holds but $\hat{S}_v$ is different. The estimated scene function is the one that is most probable given the prior scene probability and the observed data (unlike the present case where just the observed data determine the estimated scene function)

Connection to other models of early motion analysis

Sum of squared differences (SSD): In many computer vision applications motion is estimated using only two frames $I_1(x) = I(x, t_1)$ and $I_2(x) = I(x, t_2)$. Velocity is chosen by minimizing:

$$SSD(v) = \int (I_1(x) - I_2(x + v))^2 dx \tag{4.19}$$

It is straightforward to show that if we only observe $I(x, t)$ at two distinct times t_1, t_2 then:

$$P(I_1, I_2 \mid v) = \alpha \, exp(-SSD(v)/4\sigma^2) \tag{4.20}$$

so that minimizing $SSD(v)$ is equivalent to maximizing the likelihood (Figure 4.8).

stimulus: $I(x,t)$

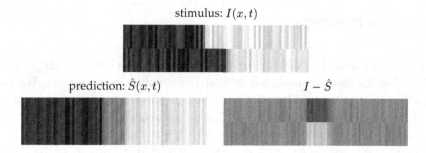

prediction: $\hat{S}(x,t)$ $I - \hat{S}$

Figure 4.8: When the image is sampled temporally to yield two frames. The likelihood of Equation 4.10 is monotonically related to the sum of squared difference (SSD) criterion.

stimulus $I(x,t)$

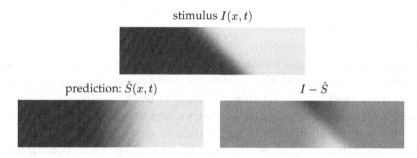

prediction: $\hat{S}(x,t)$ $I - \hat{S}$

Figure 4.9: When the image sequence is perfectly described by its linear Taylor series approximation, the likelihood of Equation 4.10 is a function of the gradient constraint.

The gradient constraint: A popular computer vision algorithm for estimating local velocities [7] is to find the vector v that minimizes:

$$J_{LK}(v) = \int_x \left(\frac{\partial I}{\partial x}v + \frac{\partial I}{\partial t} \right)^2 \tag{4.21}$$

It can be shown (Figure 4.9) that when $I(x,v)$ is well approximated by its Taylor series, i.e. $I(x + vt, t) = I(x, 0) + vt\frac{\partial I}{\partial x} + t\frac{\partial I}{\partial t}$ then:

$$P(I \,|\, v) = \alpha \exp \left(-\frac{1}{2\sigma^2} \frac{2t_m^3}{3} J_{LK}(v) \right) \tag{4.22}$$

This derivation is based on the assumption that $I(x,t)$ is perfectly approximated by its Taylor series, an assumption that will never hold with white noise, nor exactly in practice. In most situations, thus, Equation 4.22 will only be a rough approximation to Equation 4.10. Equation 4.22 is also based on the assumption that the image is observed for $|t| < t_m$ and for all x. When the image is observed within a spatial window of finite extent, then the likelihood changes.

Connection to Physiology

The most popular model for early motion calculations in primate visual cortex is based on the idea that motion is related to orientation in space-time. Accordingly, velocity tuned cells could be used to extract "motion energy" by applying space-time oriented filters to the spatiotemporal image sequence, followed by a squaring nonlinearity [1, 12]. The term "motion energy" refers to the fact that summing the squared output of oriented filters in all spatiotemporal bands is equivalent (by Parseval's theorem) to calculating the energy in an oriented hyperplane in the frequency domain.

To formalize this notion, we define the motion energy of a stimulus f as the energy of that stimulus convolved with an ideal oriented filter; i.e.,

$$ME(v; f) = \|f * \delta(x - vt)\|^2 \tag{4.23}$$

Equation 4.23 can also be interperted in the Fourier domain, where convolving f and $\delta(x - vt)$ are equivalent to multiplying their Fourier transforms $\hat{f}$ and $\delta(\omega_t + v\omega_x)$. Thus if we used infinite windows to analyze the stimulus, motion energy can be thought of as the total power of spatiotemporal frequencies that lie along the plane $\omega_t + v\omega_x = 0$. Recall, however, that our definition of energy integrates $(f * \delta(x - vt))^2$ over the window $|t| < t_m$, so that we also include spatiotemporal frequencies that are close to the plane $\omega_t + v\omega_x = 0$ but lie off it.

Claim 2: Let $P(I \mid v)$ be as defined in Equation 4.10. Then:

$$P(I \mid v) = \alpha \exp\left(\frac{ME(v; f)}{8\sigma^2 t_m^2}\right) \tag{4.24}$$

with $f = I(x, t)$ for $|t| < t_m$ and zero otherwise.

Claim 2 follows from the fact that the residual, $I - \hat{S}$, and the predicted signal $\hat{S}$ are *orthogonal* signals (see Figure 4.10):

$$\|I - \hat{S}_v\|^2 = \|I\|^2 - \|\hat{S}_v\|^2 \tag{4.25}$$

Equation 4.25 can be derived by performing the integration along lines of constant $x - vt$. Along such lines $\hat{S}_v$ is equal to the mean of I so that cross terms of the form $(I - \hat{S})\hat{S}$ cancel out. Using the fact that $\|I\|^2$ is independent of v and $\|\hat{S}_v\|^2 = \frac{ME(f; v)}{4t_m^2}$ gives Equation 4.24.

This shows that the likelihood of a velocity v can be computed as follows:

- compute the responses of a band of filters that are oriented in space-time with orientation dependent on v. The filters are shifted copies of $f(x, t) = \delta(x - vt)$.

$$\|residual\|^2 =$$

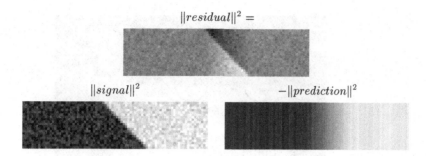

$$\|signal\|^2 \qquad\qquad -\|prediction\|^2$$

Figure 4.10: The energy of the residual is equal to the energy of the sequence minus that of the predicted sequence. This means that the likelihood of Equation 4.10 is montonically related to the motion energy of the sequence.

- square the output of the filters.
- pool the squared output over space.
- pass the pooled response through a pointwise nonlinearity.

If the input signal is band-limited we can replace $\delta(x - vt)$ with a sufficiently skinny oriented Gaussian. Thus the log likelihood can be calculated exactly by summing the squared response of space-time oriented filters.

The main difference between this calculation and the Adelson and Bergen [1] model is that the oriented filters are not band-pass. That is, the idealized filters $\delta(x - vt)$ respond to oriented structure in any spatiotemporal frequency band. The oriented filters in Adelson and Bergen as well as in Simoncelli and Heeger [12] respond to orientation only in a band of spatiotemporal frequencies. Note that the squared response to an all-pass oriented filter can be computed by adding the squared responses to band-pass oriented filters (assuming the band-pass filters are orthogonal). It would be interesting to find conditions under which the likelihood calculation requires band-pass oriented filters.

Examples of Likelihoods on Specific Stimuli

In the derivation so far, we have assumed that the sequence is observed for infinite space and finite time. Any calculation on real images, of course, will have to work with finite spatial windows. Finite spatial windows present the problem of window boundary effects. The predicted scene function at a point is the mean of all samples of this point in the window, but for finite sized windows, different velocities will have a different number of independent samples. This introduces a bias in favor of fast velocities.

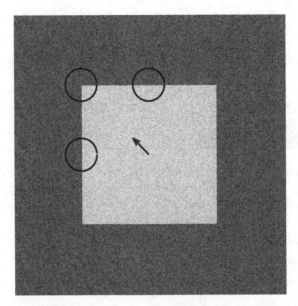

Figure 4.11: A single frame from the simple stimulus on which we calculated local likelihoods. The likelihoods were calculated at three locations: at the corner, side edge, and top edge. The image sequence was constructed by moving a square with velocity $(2, 2)$ and adding Gaussian noise with standard deviation 10% of the square contrast.

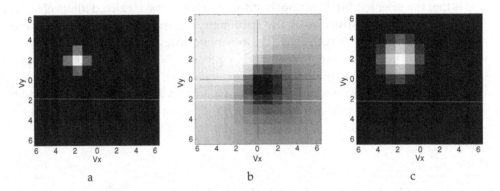

a   b   c

Figure 4.12: The likelihoods at the corner of the square calcuated using three equations. (a) The generative model likelihood (Eqn. 4.10) (b) the bowtie equation (Eqn. 4.6) (c) the fuzzy line equation (Eqn. 4.5).

To get an unbiased estimate as possible, we use windows whose spatial extent is much larger than the temporal extent. For these simulations we used rectangular windows of size $64 \times 64 \times 5$ pixels. The data for each window was obtained by zooming in on the moving square sequence shown in Figure 4.11.

Figures 4.12–4.15 show the results. We compare the likelihood from the genera-

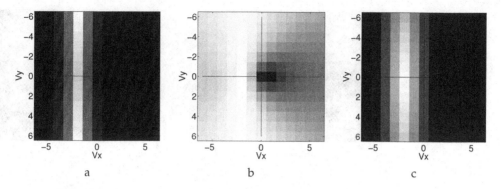

Figure 4.13: The likelihoods at the side edge of the square calcuated using three equations. (a) The generative model likelihood (Eqn. 4.10) (b) the bowtie equation (Eqn. 4.6) (c) the fuzzy line equation (Eqn. 4.5).

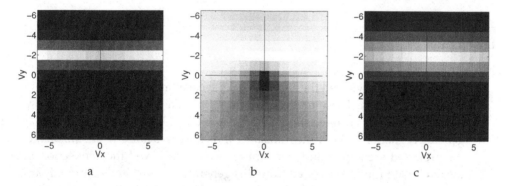

Figure 4.14: The likelihoods at the top edge of the square calcuated using three equations. (a) The generative model likelihood (Eqn. 4.10) (b) the bowtie equation (Eqn. 4.6) (c) the fuzzy line equation (Eqn. 4.5).

tive model (Equation 4.10) to the likelihood from the bowtie equation (4.6) and the likelihood from the fuzzy line equation (4.5). Gradients for the fuzzy bowties and fuzzy line equations were estimated by convolving the signal with derivatives of Gaussians. It can be seen that for edge locations the generative model likelihood is approximately a fuzzy line and for corner locations it is a fuzzy blob centered on the correct velocity. When contrast is decreased the likelihood becomes more fuzzy; uncertainty increases.

The fuzzy line likelihood gives qualitatively similar likelihood functions while the fuzzy bowtie equations give a very poor approximation.

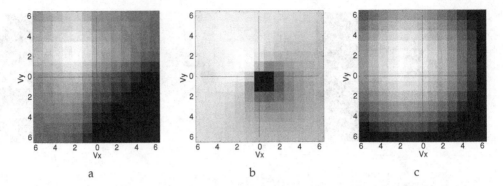

Figure 4.15: The likelihoods at the corner of the square calcuated using three equations. Here the contrast of the square was reduced by a factor of four and noise stays the same. Note that the likelihood becomes more fuzzy: uncertainty increases. (a) The generative model likelihood (Eqn. 4.10) (b) the bowtie equation (Eqn. 4.6) (c) the fuzzy line equation (Eqn. 4.5).

Discussion

We have briefly reviewed the successes of Bayesian models in accounting for human motion perception. These models require a formula for the likelihood of a velocity given image data. We have shown that such a formula can be derived from a simple generative model — the scene translates and conserves noise while the image equals the projected scene plus independent noise. We reviewed the connection between the likelihood function derived from this generative model and commonly used cost functions in computer vision. We also showed that the likelihood function can be calculated by summing the squared outputs of spatiotemporal oriented filters.

There are intriguing similarities between the calculation implied by the ideal likelihood function and common models for motion analysis in striate cortex. To a first approximation, complex cells in V1 can be modeled as squared outputs of spatiotemporal oriented filters. Again to first approximation, MT pattern cells can be modelled as pooling these squared responses over space [12]. This is consistent with the idea that a population of velocity tuned cells in area MT represent the likelihood of a velocity.

Acknowledgements

YW is supported by MURI-ARO-DAAH04-96-1-0341. DJF, on leave from Queen's University, is supported in part by an Alfred P. Sloan Research Fellowship.

References

[1] E. H. Adelson and J. R. Bergen. The extraction of spatio-temporal energy in human and machine vision. In *Proceedings of the Workshop on Motion: Representation and Analysis*, pages 151–155, Charleston, SC, 1986.

[2] E.H. Adelson and J.A. Movshon. Phenomenal coherence of moving visual patterns. *Nature*, 300:523–525, 1982.

[3] J.L. Barron, D.J. Fleet, and S.S. Beauchemin. Performance of optical flow techniques. *International Journal of Computer Vision*, 12:43–77, 1994.

[4] C. Fernmuller, R. Pless, and Y. Aloimoinos. The statistics of visual correspondence: Insights into the visual system. In *Proceedings of SCTV 99*. 1999. http://www.cis.ohio-state.edu/ szhu/workshop/Aloimonos.html.

[5] D. J. Heeger and E. P. Simoncelli. Model of visual motion sensing. In L. Harris and M. Jenkin, editors, *Spatial Vision in Humans and Robots*. Cambridge University Press, 1991.

[6] B. K. P. Horn and B. G. Schunck. Determining optical flow. *Artificial Intelligence*, 17(1–3):185–203, 1981.

[7] B. Lucas and T. Kanade. An iterative image registration technique with an application to stereo vision. In *Proc. DARPA Image Understanding Workshop*, pages 121–130, 1981.

[8] D. Marr and S. Ullman. Directional selectivity and its use in early visual processing. *Proceedings of the Royal Society of London B*, 211:151–180, 1981.

[9] O. Nestares, D.J. Fleet, and D.J. Heeger. Likelihood functions and confidence bounds for total-least-squares problems. In *Proc. IEEE Conference on Computer Vision and Pattern Recognition*, Hilton Head, Vol. II, pp. 760-767, 2000.

[10] E. P. Simoncelli. *Distributed Representation and Analysis of Visual Motion*. PhD thesis, Department of Electrical Engineering and Computer Science, Massachusetts of Technology, Cambridge, January 1993.

[11] E.P. Simoncelli, E.H. Adelson, and D.J. Heeger. Probability distributions of optical flow. In *Proc. IEEE Conf. Comput. Vision Pattern Recog.*, pages 310–315, 1991.

[12] E.P. Simoncelli and D.J. Heeger. A model of neuronal responses in visual area MT. *Vision Research*, 38(5):743–761, 1998.

[13] H. Wallach. Ueber visuell whargenommene bewegungrichtung. *Psychologische Forschung*, 20:325–380, 1935.

[14] J. Weber and J. Malik. Robust computation of optical flow in a multi-scale differential framework. *International Journal of Computer Vision*, 14:67–81, 1995.

[15] Y. Weiss and Edward H. Adelson. Slow and smooth: a Bayesian theory for the combination of local motion signals in human vision. Technical Report 1624,

MIT AI lab, 1998.

[16] C. Yo and H.R. Wilson. Perceived direction of moving two-dimensional patterns depends on duration, contrast, and eccentricity. *Vision Research*, 32(1):135–147, 1992.

5 Learning Motion Analysis

William T. Freeman, John Haddon, and Egon C. Pasztor

Introduction

The fundamental task of computer vision is the interpretation of images—what can we deduce about the world given one or more images of it? This understanding can be either at a high level—recognizing Albert Einstein, or identifying a chair— or at a low level—interpreting line drawings, estimating motion, or extrapolating resolution. The input is *image* data, which can be either a single image, or a collection of images over time. From that, for low-level vision problems, we want to estimate an underlying *scene*, which could be 3-dimensional shape, optical flow, reflectances, or high resolution detail. We will focus on low-level scene representations like these that are mapped over space. Reliable solutions to these vision tasks would have many applications in searching, editing, and interpreting images. Machine solutions might even give insight into biological mechanisms.

Much research has addressed these problems, providing important foundations. Because the problems are under-determined, regularization and statistical estimation theory are cornerstones (for example, [21, 26, 43, 34, 37, 28]). Unfortunately, solutions to these problems are often intractable; at best, they can be unreliable or slow. Often, the prior statistical models used are made up or tweaked by hand. Various image interpretation problems have defied generalization from initial simplified solutions [38, 2, 36].

In part to address the need for stronger models, researchers have analyzed the statistical properties of the visual world. Several groups derived V1-like receptive fields from ensembles of images [30, 4]; Simoncelli and Schwartz [35] accounted for contrast normalization effects by redundancy reduction. Li and Atick [1] explained retinal color coding by information processing arguments. Researchers have developed powerful methods to analyze and synthesize realistic textures by studying the response statistics of V1-like multi-scale, oriented receptive fields [18, 10, 43, 34]. These methods may help us understand the early stages of image representation and processing in the brain.

Unfortunately, they don't address how a visual system might *interpret* images. To do that, it is necessary to collect statistics relating images with their underlying scene interpretations. For natural scenes, this data is difficult to collect, since it involves gathering ground truth data of the scene attributes to be estimated, which is often not readily available in real-world situations.

A useful alternative is to use computer graphics to generate and render *synthetic* worlds, where every attribute is known, and record statistics from those. Several researchers have done so: Kersten and Knill studied linear shading and other problems [25, 24]; Hurlbert and Poggio trained a linear color constancy estimator [20]. Unfortunately, the simplified (usually linear) models which were used to obtain tractable results limited the usefulness of these methods.

Our approach is to use general statistical models, but to make the method tractable by restricting ourselves to *local* regions of images and scenes. We follow a learning-based approach, and use Markov networks to form models of image rendering and the underlying scene structure.

We believe that a visual system can correctly interpret a visual scene if it models (1) the probability that any local scene patch generated the local image patch, and (2) the probability that any local scene patch is the neighbor to any other. The first probabilities allow making scene estimates from local image data, and the second allow these local estimates to propagate. This approach leads to a Bayesian method for low level vision problems, constrained by Markov assumptions. We have applied this method to a number of problems, including that of extrapolating high-resolution from low-resolution images [12]. (This is the same problem as that addressed in the chapter by Papageorgiou, Girosi, and Poggio in this book, using a different approach). Here, we focus on the problem of optical flow estimation—given a pair of images from a moving scene, infer the projected velocities of the objects moving in the image.

Markov Network

We place the image and scene data in a Markov network [31, 15]. We break the images and scenes into localized patches where image patches connect with underlying scene patches; scene patches also connect with neighboring scene patches (see Fig. 5.1). (In general, the neighbor relationship can be with regard to position, scale, orientation, etc. Here, we consider neighbors in position and scale). This forms a network of scene nodes, each of which may have an associated observation.

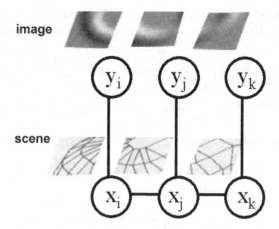

Figure 5.1: *Markov network for vision problems. Observations, y, have underlying scene explanations, x. Connections between nodes of the graphical model indicate statistical dependencies.*

Referring to Fig. 5.1, the Markov assumption asserts that complete knowledge of node x_j makes nodes x_i and x_k independent, *i.e.* $P(x_i, x_k | x_j) = P(x_i | x_j) P(x_k | x_j)$. We say x_i and x_k are conditionally independent given x_j.[1] The Markov assumption also implies that $P(x_i | x_j, x_k) = P(x_i | x_j)$. This lets us model a complicated spatial probability by a network of (tractable) probabilities governing local relationships.

To apply a Markov network to vision problems, we need to first *learn* the parameters of the network from a collection of training examples. Then, given new image data, we *infer* the corresponding scene.

Belief Propagation Derivation

Inference in networks without loops

For networks without loops, the Markov assumption leads to simple "message-passing" rules for computing the Maximum A Posteriori (MAP) and Minimum Mean Squared Error (MMSE) estimates [31, 40, 22]. To derive these rules, we first write the

---

1. Note that, in general, the random variables x and y may be vector-valued; for notational convenience, we drop the vector symbol.

MAP and MMSE estimates for x_j at node j by marginalizing (MMSE) or taking the maximum (MAP) over the other variables in the posterior probability:

$$\hat{x}_j^{\text{MMSE}} = \int_{x_j} x_j dx_j \int_{\text{all } x_i, i \neq j} P(x,y)\, dx \tag{5.1}$$

$$\hat{x}_j^{\text{MAP}} = \arg \max_{x_j} \max_{\text{all } x_i, i \neq j} P(x,y) \tag{5.2}$$

y is the observed image data.

For a Markov random field, the joint probability over the scenes x and images y can be written as [5, 15, 14]:

$$P(x,y) = \prod_{\text{neighboring } i,j} \Psi(x_i, x_j) \prod_k \Phi(x_k, y_k), \tag{5.3}$$

where we have introduced pairwise compatibility functions, Ψ and Φ, described below. The factorized structure of Eq. (5.3) allows the marginalization and maximization operators of Eqs. (5.1) and (5.2) to pass through compatibility function factors with unrelated arguments. For the example network in Fig. 5.1, we have

$$
\begin{aligned}
\hat{x}_1^{\text{MAP}} &= \arg \max_{x_1} \max_{x_2} \max_{x_3} P(x_1, x_2, x_3, y_1, y_2, y_3) \\
&= \arg \max_{x_1} \max_{x_2} \max_{x_3} \\
&\quad \Phi(x_1, y_1)\Phi(x_2, y_2)\Phi(x_3, y_3)\Psi(x_1, x_2)\Psi(x_2, x_3) \\
&= \arg \max_{x_1} \Phi(x_1, y_1) \\
&\quad \max_{x_2} \Psi(x_1, x_2)\Phi(x_2, y_2) \\
&\quad \max_{x_3} \Phi(x_3, y_3)\Psi(x_2, x_3)
\end{aligned} \tag{5.4}
$$

Each line of Eq. (5.4) is a local computation involving only one node and its neighbors. The analogous expressions for $\hat{x}_2^{\text{MAP}}$ and $\hat{x}_3^{\text{MAP}}$ use similar local calculations. Iterating those calculations lets each node j compute $\hat{x}_j^{\text{MAP}}$ from the messages passed between nodes.

Assuming a general network without loops, Eqs. (5.1) and (5.2) can be computed by iterating the following steps [31, 40, 22]. The MAP estimate at node j is

$$\hat{x}_j^{\text{MAP}} = \arg \max_{x_j} \Phi(x_j, y_j) \prod_k M_j^k \tag{5.5}$$

where k runs over all scene node neighbors of node j. M_j^k is the message sent from node k to node j. We calculate M_j^k from:

$$M_j^k = \max_{x_k} \Psi(x_k, x_j) \Phi(x_k, y_k) \prod_{l \neq j} \tilde{M}_k^l \qquad (5.6)$$

where $\tilde{M}_k^l$ is M_k^l from the previous iteration. The initial $\tilde{M}_k^l$s are vectors of all 1's. After at most one iteration of Eq. (5.6) per scene node variable, Eq. (5.5) gives the desired optimal estimate, $\hat{x}_j^{\text{MAP}}$. The MMSE estimate, Eq. (5.2), has analogous formulae, with the $\max_{x_k}$ of Eq. (5.6) replaced by $\int_{x_k}$, and $\arg\max_{x_j}$ of Eq. (5.5) replaced by $\int_{x_j} x_j$. For linear topologies, these propagation rules are equivalent to standard Bayesian inference methods, such as the Kalman filter and the forward-backward algorithm for hidden Markov models [31, 28, 39, 22, 13]. Weiss showed the advantage of belief propagation over regularization methods for several 1-d problems [39]; with the expectation of similar benefits, we apply belief propagation to our 2-d problems.

Networks with loops

Markov networks may also contain loops where messages can pass from node to node and return to the original node (e.g. Figure 5.3). This unfortunately means that the message passing algorithm presented above is not exactly correct.

Some theoretical justifications exist for using the message passing algorithm for networks with loops, however. In [41], it is shown that the MMSE rules give the correct means, but underestimate the variance for Gaussian distributions. For MAP rules, for arbitrary distributions, if the algorithm converges, it must converge to at least a local maximum of the posterior. [42] shows that the MMSE belief propagation equations are equivalent to the stationarity conditions for the Bethe approximation to the "free energy" of the network. This suggests that it might be acceptable to use message passing, ignoring the fact that there are loops present; and indeed, experiments give good results using this approach [27, 40].

Belief propagation algorithm	Network topology	
	no loops	*arbitrary topology*
MMSE rules	MMSE, correct posterior marginal probs.	For Gaussians, correct means, wrong covs.
MAP rules	MAP	Local max. of posterior, even for non-Gaussians.

Table 5.1: Summary of results from [41] regarding belief propagation after convergence.

Motion

The image analysis problem which we focus on here is that of estimating the optical flow between a pair of images. There are many existing techniques for computing optical flow from the differences between the two frames (e.g. [19, 6, 28]). We applied our method for learning low-level vision to this problem to show results on a well-studied problem. There have been many related applications of Markov networks to vision, in the form of Markov random fields [15, 32, 14, 24, 6, 28, 26, 33]. For other learning or constraint propagation approaches in motion analysis, see [28, 29, 23].

We examined two classes of scene—first, a "blobs world", in which planar blobs translate in the plane; and then, more realistic images generated using a 3D rendering package. In both cases, the "image" consists of two concatenated image frames from sequential times. The "scene" is the corresponding projected velocities of the moving objects in the world.

Blobs world

In the blobs world, the training images were randomly generated moving, irregularly shaped blobs, as typified by Fig. 5.2 (a). The background was a random shade of gray, which yielded a range of contrasts with the blobs. Each blob was moving in a randomized direction, at some speed between 0 and 2 pixels per frame.

We represented both the images and the velocities in 4-level Gaussian pyramids [8], to efficiently communicate across space. Each scene patch then additionally connects with the patches at neighboring resolution levels. Figure 5.2 shows the multiresolution representation (at one time frame) for images and scenes.[2] Figure 5.3 shows the corresponding Markov network for the scene nodes. (Each scene node connects to an observation node, not shown, at the corresponding scale and position). Luettgen et al [28] use a related multi-resolution Markov model to analyze motion, with exact inference. We use approximate inference, but use a more general model, allowing non-Gaussian statistics and Markov network connections between nodes at the same resolution level, which avoids discontinuities at quad-tree pyramid boundaries.

We applied the training method and propagation rules to motion estimation, using a vector code representation [16] for both images and scenes. We wrote a tree-structured vector quantizer, to code 4 by 4 pixel by 2 frame blocks of image data for each pyramid level into one of 300 codes for each level. We also coded scene patches

---

2. To maintain the desired conditional independence relationships, we appended the image data to the scenes. This provided the scene elements with image contrast information, which they would otherwise lack.

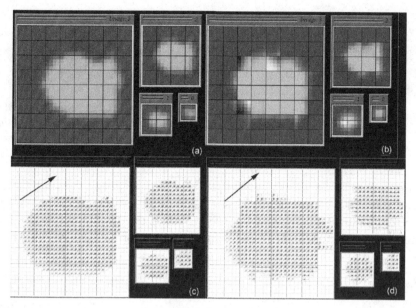

Figure 5.2: *(a) First of two frames of typical image data (in Gaussian pyramid). We observe the image at four different spatial scales. The blob is undergoing uniform translation in a random direction. (b) We represent the input frames by a collection of vector quantized pairs of image patches. (c) The true optical flow scene information that we hope to recover. (d) The system can only describe the estimated scene by a set of vector quantized patches of optical flow. Large arrow added to show small vectors' orientation. The goal is to estimate (c) from (a), viewed over two time steps. In our vector quantized representation, the best we can do is to estimate (d) from (b), viewed over two time frames. Figure 5.6 shows the velocity field estimated by our algorithm.*

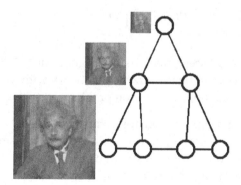

Figure 5.3: *Schematic illustration of multi-scale representation used for motion analysis problem. The image data is presented to the Markov network at multiple resolutions. Each scene node (representing the a patch of velocity data at some resolution and position) connects with its neighbors both in space and across scale. Each scene node also has connections (not shown) with a patch of image observations at the corresponding position and scale.*

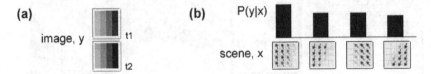

Figure 5.4: *The local likelihood information for motion problem, in a vector quantized representation. Conditional probabilities for the image data y (pair of image patches), given the scene x (projected velocities over a patch) are derived from co-occurence histograms. For a given image data sample, (a), the four scene elements with the highest likelihood of generating the image data are shown in (b).*

into one of 300 codes. Figure 5.2 shows an input test image, (a) before and (b) after vector quantization. The true underlying scene, the desired output, is also shown in figure 5.2, (c) before and (d) after vector quantization.

Learning

For the blobs world problem, we used a different factorization of the posterior probability than Eq. (5.3), based on repeated applications of the rule $P(a,b) = P(a|b)P(b)$. This factorization, described in [11, 12], yields very similar belief propagation rules as Eq. (5.6), using compatibility functions learned from image-scene and scene-scene co-occurance statistics. The update and estimation rules are:

$$M_j^k = \max_{x_k} P(x_k|x_j)P(y_k|x_k) \prod_{l \neq j} \tilde{M}_k^l, \tag{5.7}$$

$$x_{j\,MAP} = \text{argmax}_{x_j} P(x_j)P(y_j|x_j) \prod_k M_j^k. \tag{5.8}$$

where k runs over all scene node neighbors of node j. While the expression for the joint probability does not generalize to a network with loops, we nonetheless found good results for the motion estimation problem using these update rules.

During learning, we presented approximately 200,000 examples of different moving blobs, some overlapping, of a contrast with the background randomized to one of 4 values. Using co-occurence histograms, we measured the statistical relationships that embody the algorithm: $P(x)$, $P(y|x)$, and $P(x_n|x)$, for scene x_n neighboring scene x. Figures 5.4 and 5.5 show examples of these measurements.

Inference

Given a new image to analyze, we first break it into local patches of image data (image pairs). For each image pair patch, we collect a set of candidate scene interpreta-

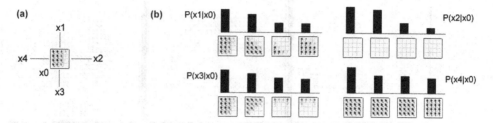

Figure 5.5: *Some scene conditional probabilities, for the motion problem. For the given scene element, (a), the four most likely nodes from four different neighboring scene elements are shown. For example, the top left plot of (b) shows the four motion patches most likely to appear at position $x1$, above the given patch of velocity data, and similarly for the three other positions relative to $x0$. Scene elements also connect to patches at other scales, not shown in this figure.*

tions from the training database. The belief propagation algorithm updates a set of probability assignments for each candidate scene interpretation, based initially only on the local image data at that patch, then taking into account more and more image data as the algorithm iterates.

Figure 5.6 shows six iterations of the inference algorithm as it converges to a good estimate for the underlying scene velocities. The local probabilities we learned ($P(x)$, $P(y|x)$, and $P(x_n|x)$) lead to figure/ground segmentation, aperture problem[3] constraint propagation, and filling-in (see caption). The resulting inferred velocities are correct up to the accuracy of the vector quantized representation.

Extension to more realistic images

The blob world discussed above is a very simple model of motion in real images. In order to apply the Markov network formalism to more realistic images, we generated a number of scenes using 3D Studio Max, release 2.5, a 3D modelling and rendering program. Distorted cubes in various orientations and positions were rendered from a camera directly overhead, and then from a slighly rotated and translated camera to generate a second frame (examples of overhead images may be seen in figures 5.7(a) and 5.8(a)).

For the blobs problem, we used a simple approach of storing (through our training observations) all possible local patches we would observe, and all possible scene observations for each one of those. In applying this approach to these more realistic images, we ran into a number of problems, related to the complexity of more realistic

---

3. The aperture problem refers to the fact that when you observe only a small piece of edge, you can only determine the component of its velocity across the edge, but not the component in the direction of the edge.

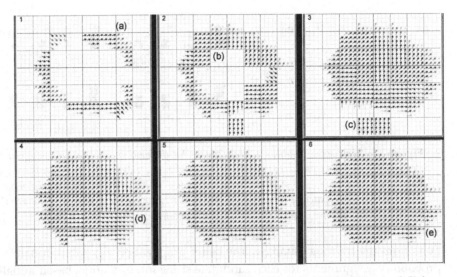

Figure 5.6: *The most probable scene code for Fig. 5.2b at first 6 iterations of Bayesian belief propagation. (a) Note initial motion estimates occur only at edges. Due to the "aperture problem", initial estimates do not agree. (b) Filling-in of motion estimate occurs. Cues for figure/ground determination may include edge curvature, and information from lower resolution levels. Both are included implicitly in the learned probabilities. (c) Figure/ground still undetermined in this region of low edge curvature. (d) Velocities have filled-in, but do not yet all agree. (e) Velocities have filled-in, and agree with each other and with the correct velocity direction, shown in Fig. 5.2.*

images. There are two major reasons why the blob world is easier to deal with than realistic images:

- *The background is stationary.* A stationary background means that if we observe a moving edge in an image patch, we know that one side of the edge is stationary, and we know the component of the velocity of the foreground in the direction perpendicular to the edge. Thus, the possible scene patches (optical flow) at an edge consist of a pair of one-dimensional spaces (the velocity parallel to the edge is the continuous dimension, and either side of the edge can be the foreground).

For real images, the background may also be moving, and unless it has significant texture, it is difficult to tell which direction it is moving in. In the absence of other (global) information, the possible motions at a patch are a pair of three-dimensional spaces (we have two extra dimensions because the background can be moving at any velocity). It is more difficult both to learn and to do inference in this higher-dimensional space.

- *The blobs are untextured.* Because the blobs have no surface texture, there are relatively few possible image patches. Consider an image patch in the interior of a blob: every such patch will look identical, and we only need to describe the different possible scene motions.

But real surfaces do have texture. To sample from all possible input data we need to sample from all possible patch textures combined with all possible motions that the patches could undergo.

Inference

If we were to use the same approach as we did with the blobs world, of choosing a set of image/scene pairs for each node, the number of candidates would have to be very large. There are many possible image patches in real images; we found that in order to ensure including the correct scene among the candidates, we needed to maintain a very long list of candidates.

Instead, we used the brightness constraint equation (BCE) common in optical flow work in computer vision [19], and generated a list of candidate scene explanations on the fly for each image patch of the test image. The BCE assumes that an object that moves from frame to frame will have the same brightness in each frame, possibly appearing at different points in the image.

Suppose that the pixel at point (x, y) at time t has moved to point $(x + dx, y + dy)$ at time $t + dt$. Then we have

$$I(x, y, t) = I(x + dx, y + dy, t + dt)$$

If we take a Taylor series on the right to first order,

$$I(x, y, t) = I(x, y, t) + \frac{\partial I}{\partial x} dx + \frac{\partial I}{\partial y} dy + \frac{\partial I}{\partial t} dt$$

In other words,

$$\nabla I \cdot v = -\frac{\partial I}{\partial t}$$

For real images, the equality will not be exact, and so it is standard practice to take a least squares estimate. Using this equation, we can evaluate the likelihood of different optical flow vectors at any pixel. (See the chapter by Weiss and Fleet for a complete discussion of likelihood functions for motion analysis). Of course, the aperture problem arises if we just consider a single pixel (we will only be able to determine one component of the velocity), but taking the sum over several pixels generally avoids this issue.

This raises the question of which pixels to sum over. Because of the difficulty mentioned above with edges in environments with nonstationary backgrounds, we assume that the optical flow is constant over a patch. This assumption is used in regularization approaches to the optical flow problem [19, 7] in which motion is smoothed across discontinuities. By making the optical flow constant over a patch, we are essentially ignoring the presence of object boundaries, but we gain significantly in that we no longer need to represent all possible optical flow vectors on either side of the boundary.

Due to the large numbers of samples that we would otherwise need to observe in training, instead of learning the statistics of neighbouring patches, we adopted a heuristic which gives us a measure of the correspondence between adjacent patches. Adjacent patches overlap by one pixel; then the compatibility of two adjacent patches can be estimated by the agreement that the two patches have on their common pixels. If the two patches have very different beliefs about the values of the pixels they share, those patches cannot be side by side.

Specifically, let k and j be two neighboring scene patches. Let d^l_{jk} be a vector of the pixels of the lth possible candidate for scene patch x_k which lie in the overlap region with patch j. Likewise, let d^m_{kj} be the values of the pixels (in correspondence with those of d^l_{jk}) of the mth candidate for patch x_j which overlap patch k. We say that scene candidates x^l_k (candidate l at node k) and x^m_j are compatible with each other if the pixels in their regions of overlap agree. We assume that the scene training samples differ from the "ideal" training samples by Gaussian noise of covariance σ_s. Those covariance values are parameters of the algorithm. We then define the compatibility matrix between scene nodes k and j as

$$\Psi(x^l_k, x^m_j) = \exp^{-|d^l_{jk} - d^m_{kj}|^2 / 2\sigma_s^2} \tag{5.9}$$

The rows and columns of the compatibility matrix $\Psi(x^l_k, x^m_j)$ are indexed by l and m, the scene candidates at each node, at nodes j and k. We evaluate $\Phi(x_k, y_k)$ in an analogous fashion [12].

In using this heuristic, we are no longer *learning* the statistics of adjacent patches. Since for these images, we constrain our velocity samples to be uniform over each patch, the method of evaluating $\Psi(x_k, x_j)$ is equivalent to a smoothness constraint on the reconstructed motion. This is similar to other motion smoothness constraints (e.g. [19]), although enforced by Bayesian belief propagation.

Initially, we chose our optical flow vectors by sampling from the distribution of velocities consistent with the BCE. But we found that at some nodes in the network, there would be a number of adjacent patches which all had very similar samples, not because of similar structure, but simply because of the randomness of sampling. Because these samples agreed with their neighbours, and other samples may not have had such good agreement, these nodes would end up with a strong belief, based on no evidence, which was often contradictory to the correct answer.

Thus, we chose to select candidates by choosing optical flow vectors on a uniform grid, and to keep all of the candidates for each node. This solved any problems with random agreement with neighbours, since each neighbour also had the complete candidate list, so no candidate had more agreement than any other.

Results

In figures 5.7 and 5.8, we show two examples of the optical flow algorithm working on our realistic images. Observe that initially, the optical flow vectors are mostly zero (we display the average vector for each patch, weighted by its belief) except at edges, where we have a good estimate of the perpendicular velocity. After one iteration, the information at the edges begins to be propagated, and after a few iterations, the solution is close to the correct answer.

In some cases, the final solution deviates from the correct answer, especially at the image boundary. This is partially due to the fact that in this model, there is no way for a node at the boundary to have a greater magnitude than its neighbours. If the images are from a camera rotating about its optical axis, we observe the centre of the vector field rotating, and we expect the boundary of the image to be rotating more. Similarly, if the camera is moving towards the scene, we see expansion in the middle of the image, and we expect that effect to be exaggerated towards the boundary, even in the absence of any confirming evidence. But with a Markov network, if there is no information present at the boundary of an image, the nodes there will likely share the belief of the nearest nodes with good information. Since those nodes are closer to the centre of the image, the optical flow vectors will tend to have smaller magnitude, and the optical flow on the boundary will be underestimated.

Figure 5.9 shows a frame from the Yosemite image sequence [17], and the resulting optical flow from our algorithm. The clouds are correctly identified as moving to the right, and there is a focus of expansion somewhat to the right of the center of the image as we fly towards that point. A few scene patches in the clouds still have some error; the lack of texture in that part of the image makes accurate optical flow estimation there exceedingly difficult.

Summary

We have presented an algorithm for motion analysis which uses belief propagation in a Markov network to estimate the optical flow between a pair of images by communicating local information across space. The algorithm has been applied to a simple 2D blob world, as well as more realistic images generated in a 3D rendering package. The local probabilistic descriptions have power and flexibility. For the

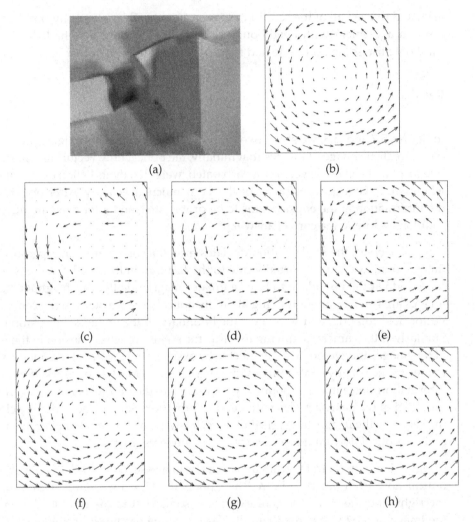

Figure 5.7: *Example of optical flow solution using belief propagation. (a) one frame of the two-frame input image pair. (b) The true rotational (synthetically generated) optical flow for this image. (c) The initial estimate of optical flow, with no information from a scene node's neighbors. (d)–(h) Reconstructed optical flow after 1–5 iterations of belief propagation. The initial iterations show little motion in regions where there is little image contrast perpendicular to the direction of motion, such as the right hand side, and upper left hand corner. The spatial continuity of the motion, enforced by the belief propagation, fills in the motion smoothly.*

motion problem, they lead to filling-in motion estimates in a direction perpendicular to object contours and resolution of the aperture problem (Fig. 5.6).

The algorithm uses simple notions, which can apply to other vision problems: form hypotheses from local data, and propagate these across space. Of course, these are well-known principles in computational vision [38, 9, 2, 3]; what we propose is simple machinery to implement these principles. We have shown elsewhere the

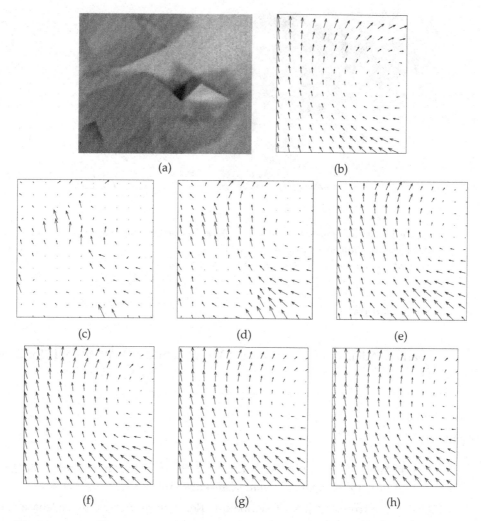

(a) (b)

(c) (d) (e)

(f) (g) (h)

Figure 5.8: *Another example of optical flow solution using belief propagation. See caption to figure 5.7.*

usefulness of this method for the problems of super-resolution and discriminating shading from paint [12]. From a synthetically generated world, we learn a training set of local examples of image (image pairs) and scene (projected image velocities) data. Using the machinery of Bayesian belief propagation applied to Markov networks with loops, we quickly find approximate solutions for the scene explanation which maximizes the posterior probability.

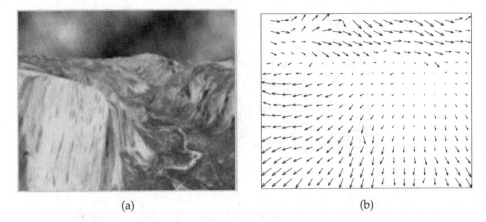

(a)   (b)

Figure 5.9: *Results of motion estimation on Yosemite sequence. (a) Single frame from sequence. (b) estimated optical flow, based on that frame and the subsequent one. The clouds are flowing to the right, and the land underneath is expanding as we fly into the valley.*

Acknowledgements

We thank E. Adelson, O. Carmichael, J. Tenenbaum, and Y. Weiss for helpful discussions.

References

[1] J. J. Atick, Z. Li, and A. N. Redlich. Understanding retinal color coding from first principles. *Neural Computation*, 4:559–572, 1992.

[2] H. G. Barrow and J. M. Tenenbaum. Recovering intrinsic scene characteristics from images. In A. R. Hanson and E. M. Riseman, editors, *Computer Vision Systems*, pages 3–26. Academic Press, New York, 1978.

[3] H. G. Barrow and J. M. Tenenbaum. Computational vision. *Proc. IEEE*, 69(5):572–595, 1981.

[4] A. J. Bell and T. J. Sejnowski. The independent components of natural scenes are edge filters. *Vision Research*, 37(23):3327–3338, 1997.

[5] J. Besag. Spatial interaction and the statistical analysis of lattice systems (with discussion). *J. Royal Statist. Soc. B*, 36:192–326, 1974.

[6] M. J. Black and P. Anandan. A framework for the robust estimation of optical flow. In *Proc. 4th Intl. Conf. Computer Vision*, pages 231–236. IEEE, 1993.

[7] M. J. Black and P. Anandan. The robust estimation of multiple motions: Parametric and piecewise-smooth flow fields. *Computer Vision and Image Understanding*, 63(1), 1996.

[8] P. J. Burt and E. H. Adelson. The Laplacian pyramid as a compact image code. *IEEE Trans. Comm.*, 31(4):532–540, 1983.

[9] M. B. Clowes. On seeing things. *Artificial Intelligence*, 2:79–116, 1971.

[10] J. S. DeBonet and P. Viola. Texture recognition using a non-parametric multi-scale statistical model. In *Proc. IEEE Computer Vision and Pattern Recognition*, 1998.

[11] W. T. Freeman and E. C. Pasztor. Learning to estimate scenes from images. In M. S. Kearns, S. A. Solla, and D. A. Cohn, editors, *Adv. Neural Information Processing Systems*, volume 11, Cambridge, MA, 1999. MIT Press. See also http://www.merl.com/reports/TR99-05/.

[12] W. T. Freeman, E. C. Pasztor, and O. T. Carmichael. Learning low-level vision. *Intl. J. Computer Vision*, 2000. In press. See also http://www.merl.com/reports/TR2000-05/.

[13] B. J. Frey. *Graphical Models for Machine Learning and Digital Communication*. MIT Press, 1998.

[14] D. Geiger and F. Girosi. Parallel and deterministic algorithms from MRF's: surface reconstruction. *IEEE Pattern Analysis and Machine Intelligence*, 13(5):401–412, May 1991.

[15] S. Geman and D. Geman. Stochastic relaxation, Gibbs distribution, and the Bayesian restoration of images. *IEEE Pattern Analysis and Machine Intelligence*, 6:721–741, 1984.

[16] R. M. Gray, P. C. Cosman, and K. L. Oehler. Incorporating visual factors into vector quantizers for image compression. In A. B. Watson, editor, *Digital images and human vision*. MIT Press, 1993.

[17] D. Heeger. Yosemite fly-by sequence. ftp://csd.uwo.ca/pub/vision/TESTDATA/.

[18] D. J. Heeger and J. R. Bergen. Pyramid-based texture analysis/synthesis. In *ACM SIGGRAPH*, pages 229–236, 1995. In *Computer Graphics* Proceedings, Annual Conference Series.

[19] B. K. P. Horn and B. G. Schunk. Determining optical flow. *Artificial Intelligence*, 17:185–203, 1981.

[20] A. C. Hurlbert and T. A. Poggio. Synthesizing a color algorithm from examples. *Science*, 239:482–485, 1988.

[21] M. Isard and A. Blake. Contour tracking by stochastic propagation of conditional density. In *Proc. European Conf. on Computer Vision*, pages 343–356, 1996.

[22] M. I. Jordan, editor. *Learning in graphical models*. MIT Press, 1998.

[23] S. Ju, M. J. Black, and A. D. Jepson. Skin and bones: Multi-layer, locally affine, optical flow and regularization with transparency. In *Proc. IEEE Computer Vision and Pattern Recognition*, pages 307–314, 1996.

[24] D. Kersten. Transparancy and the cooperative computation of scene attributes.

In M. S. Landy and J. A. Movshon, editors, *Computational Models of Visual Processing*, chapter 15. MIT Press, Cambridge, MA, 1991.

[25] D. Kersten, A. J. O'Toole, M. E. Sereno, D. C. Knill, and J. A. Anderson. Associative learning of scene parameters from images. *Applied Optics*, 26(23):4999–5006, 1987.

[26] D. Knill and W. Richards, editors. *Perception as Bayesian inference*. Cambridge Univ. Press, 1996.

[27] F. R. Kschischang and B. J. Frey. Iterative decoding of compound codes by probability propagation in graphical models. *IEEE Journal on Selected Areas in Communication*, 16(2):219–230, 1998.

[28] M. R. Luettgen, W. C. Karl, and A. S. Willsky. Efficient multiscale regularization with applications to the computation of optical flow. *IEEE Trans. Image Processing*, 3(1):41–64, 1994.

[29] S. Nowlan and T. J. Sejnowski. A selection model for motion processing in area MT of primates. *J. Neuroscience*, 15:1195–1214, 1995.

[30] B. A. Olshausen and D. J. Field. Emergence of simple-cell receptive field properties by learning a sparse code for natural images. *Nature*, 381:607–609, 1996.

[31] J. Pearl. *Probabilistic reasoning in intelligent systems: networks of plausible inference*. Morgan Kaufmann, 1988.

[32] T. Poggio, V. Torre, and C. Koch. Computational vision and regularization theory. *Nature*, 317(26):314–139, 1985.

[33] E. Saund. Perceptual organization of occluding contours of opaque surfaces. In *CVPR '98 Workshop on Perceptual Organization*, Santa Barbara, CA, 1998.

[34] E. P. Simoncelli. Statistical models for images: Compression, restoration and synthesis. In *31st Asilomar Conf. on Sig., Sys. and Computers*, Pacific Grove, CA, 1997.

[35] E. P. Simoncelli and O. Schwartz. Modeling surround suppression in V1 neurons with a statistically-derived normalization model. In *Adv. in Neural Information Processing Systems*, volume 11, 1999.

[36] P. Sinha and E. H. Adelson. Recovering reflectance and illumination in a world of painted polyhedra. In *Proc. 4th Intl. Conf. Comp. Vis.*, pages 156–163. IEEE, 1993.

[37] R. Szeliski. *Bayesian Modeling of Uncertainty in Low-level Vision*. Kluwer Academic Publishers, Boston, 1989.

[38] D. Waltz. Generating semantic descriptions from drawings of scenes with shadows. In P. Winston, editor, *The psychology of computer vision*, pages 19–92. McGraw-Hill, New York, 1975.

[39] Y. Weiss. Interpreting images by propagating Bayesian beliefs. In *Adv. in Neural Information Processing Systems*, volume 9, pages 908–915, 1997.

[40] Y. Weiss. Belief propagation and revision in networks with loops. Technical Report 1616, AI Lab Memo, MIT, Cambridge, MA 02139, 1998.

[41] Y. Weiss and W. T. Freeman. Correctness of belief propagation in Gaussian graphical models of arbitrary topology. Technical Report UCB.CSD-99-1046, Berkeley Computer Science Dept., 1999. www.cs.berkeley.edu/~yweiss/gaussTR.ps.gz.

[42] J. S. Yedidia, W. T. Freeman, and Y. Weiss. Generalized belief propagation. Technical Report 2000–26, MERL, Mitsubishi Electric Research Labs., www.merl.com, 2000.

[43] S. C. Zhu and D. Mumford. Prior learning and Gibbs reaction-diffusion. *IEEE Pattern Analysis and Machine Intelligence*, 19(11), 1997.

6 Information Theoretic Approach to Neural Coding and Parameter Estimation: A Perspective

Jean-Pierre Nadal

Introduction

The idea that Shannon's Information Theory (Shannon and Weaver, 1949; Blahut 1988) is relevant for studying neural coding goes back to Attneave, 1954, and Barlow, 1960. Despite some very important early works (e.g. Stein, 1967; Laughlin, 1981), it has received considerable attention only since the late 80's (after the works of, e.g., Linsker, 1988; Barlow et al 1989; Bialek et al, 1991; Atick, 1992; van Hateren, 1992, and with many other works since then). The relevance of Information Theory to the field of parameter estimation has been acknowledged much more recently. On the one hand it has been shown that, in the Bayesian framework, the Bayes cumulative risk is precisely equal to the mutual information between parameters and data (see e.g. Clarke and Barron 1990; Haussler and Opper, 1995; and references therein). On the other hand, a simple relationship between the *Fisher Information*, a basic quantity in Estimation Theory, and the (Shannon) mutual information between parameters and data has been shown to exist only very recently (Clarke and Barron, 1990; Rissanen, 1996; Brunel and Nadal 1998). At the same time, the fact that neural coding and parameter estimation are intimately related subjects has been realized. In particular, a duality has been shown between neural architectures which allows one to translate a learning (or parameter estimation) task into a sensory coding problem (Nadal and Parga, 1994a).

In the next section, I introduce the general information theoretic framework which allows us to discuss both parameter estimation (from the Bayesian point of view) and neural (especially sensory) coding. Then, I present the generic behaviour of the mutual information between parameters and data (equivalently between stimuli and neural code), putting into perspective results published in the literature in both fields.

In the last section, I describe current and possible lines of research for going beyond the feedforward sensory coding problem.

General Framework

Neural coding

One possible approach to the problem of neural representations, or "neural codes", is illustrated on Figure 6.1. The environment is assumed to produce, at each instant of time, a new stimulus Θ with some probability distribution $\rho(.)$. Depending on the particular problem considered, Θ might be, say, the orientation of a bar presented in the visual field, or the multidimensional pattern elicited at the input of the neural system (e.g., the activities of the photoreceptors). The "neural code" is given by the activities $D = \{d^1, ..., d^p\}$ of p neurons. The activation rule is given by some probability distribution $P(D|\Theta)$, which depends on some set of parameters W (e.g. the set of synaptic efficacies).

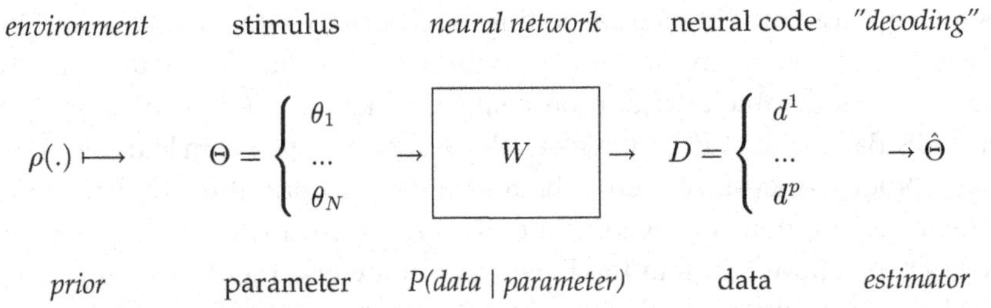

| *environment* | stimulus | *neural network* | neural code | *"decoding"* |

$$\rho(.) \longmapsto \quad \Theta = \left\{ \begin{array}{l} \theta_1 \\ ... \\ \theta_N \end{array} \right. \quad \rightarrow \boxed{\quad W \quad} \rightarrow \quad D = \left\{ \begin{array}{l} d^1 \\ ... \\ d^p \end{array} \right. \quad \rightarrow \hat{\Theta}$$

| *prior* | parameter | *P(data | parameter)* | data | *estimator* |

Figure 6.1: A single framework for neural coding and parameter estimation (see text).

The neural representation D is further processed by the neural system, and it may be the case - though not necessarily always - that there is *reconstruction* of the stimulus, that is, an *estimation* $\hat{\Theta}$ is produced as a result of the processing of D. One should note that the use of the name *code* in this context of neural modelling is generally not accepted by information-theorists for whom a code is *defined* as a *deterministic* mapping. The point of view taken in this paper is that a neural representation, or neural code, is the appropriate concept which generalises the engineer's deterministic code to the case of intrinsically noisy systems.

Parameter estimation

To study a parameter estimation task, one can make use of the very same formalism. Here the quantities D, p and Θ will be given a different interpretation as explained below.

In the context of parameter estimation, one has some data D, a set of p observations $D = \{d^1, ..., d^p\}$. In the simplest setting, one assumes that the probability distribution from which the data have been generated is known, except for some (possibly multi-dimensional) parameter Θ which is thus the parameter to be estimated from the data. In the general case, the probability distribution $P(D|\Theta)$ may depend on additional parameters W, called *hyper-parameters* if they are considered as additional degrees of freedom useful for modelling the unknown distribution, or *nuisance* parameters if they correspond to parameters of the true model in which one is not interested. In the standard Bayes framework, one considers that the unknown parameter Θ has been chosen by Nature according to some *prior* distribution $\rho(.)$, so that Figure 6.1 illustrates the Bayes framework when the goal is to compute a parameter estimate $\hat{\Theta}$ (another important Bayesian task is to *predict* the next datum, d^{p+1}, but we will here mainly focus on the parameter estimation task). In practice, the prior $\rho(.)$ is typically taken as the maximum entropy distribution taking into account all known constraints on the parameter. The neural coding framework presented here can thus be considered as a particular case of Bayesian modelling, where there is a *true* parameter (the actual stimulus) and a *true* prior distribution (the environment distribution).

Other related points of view

The general setting $\rho(.) \longmapsto \Theta \to D$ introduced here corresponds also to recognition and generative models in data analysis. In a recognition model, the data Θ are presented to a network (more generally a learning machine) which produces, say, the independent components (hence in that case Θ plays the role of data, and D the role of independent components). In a generative approach, the data D is considered as having been produced by some random variables, Θ. The framework applies as well to signal processing, Θ being the signal and D the filtered signal.

In this general framework, our interest is in the characterisation of typical and optimal performances making use of information theoretic concepts (for an introduction to Information Theory see Blahut 1988 and Cover and Thomas 1991). This information theoretic approach, and related information theoretic criteria (*infomax, redundancy reduction*), are introduced in the next section. Before that, let us consider some specific examples of models.

Specific examples

In this section, several specific examples are briefly presented. Each model is introduced by giving the particular definitions of N, Θ, p and D which make the model fit into the framework presented in Figure 6.1.

First some neural coding models:

(1) early visual system: infomax and redundancy reduction approaches to neural coding in the early visual system (Linsker 1988 and 1993, van Hateren 1992, Atick 1992, Li and Atick 1994a, Li 1995) assume $p \sim N$ large. Here, Θ is the set of activities of the photoreceptors, and D the resulting activities of the ganglion cells or of V1 cells.

(2) early visual system: with a *sparse coding* hypothesis for V1, one takes $p > N$, and a code is built such that the number of active output cells for any given input is small (Field 1987, Olshausen and Field 1997, and this book, chapter by Olshausen).

(3) Independent Component Analysis (ICA; for general references on ICA see Jutten and Herault 1991, Comon 1994, and the web site ICA Central, http://sig.enst.fr/~cardoso/icacentral/). ICA can be formulated in various ways, we give here the recognition and generative approaches. Recognition model: Θ is the signal, W the network parameters to be adapted in order to have $\{d^1, ..., d^p\}$ as estimates of the independent components (see Nadal and Parga 1994, Bell and Sejnowski 1995 for the *infomax* approach). In a generative approach, Θ is the set of IC's, and D the observed signal (this corresponds to the maximum likelihood approach to ICA, see Cardoso 1997). Both points of view can be put together if one consider Θ as the set of IC's, D the observed signal, and $\hat{\Theta}$ as the estimate of Θ.

(4) *population coding*: Θ is a low dimensional field, e.g. an angle, $N = 1$, and the number p of coding cells is very large, each cell responding with a specific *tuning curve* centred at some particular value of the stimulus; in the simplest models, the cells' activities are given by Poisson processes. In (Seung and Sompolinsky 1993), population coding is for the first time approached with a parameter estimation point of view (the neural activities D being the data from which the system must extract an estimate $\hat{\Theta}$ of the stimulus). Their analysis is based on the *Fisher information*, whereas the present (Shannon) information theoretic approach is developed in (Brunel and Nadal 1998) (see below). For other approaches and references on population coding, see the chapter by Zemel and Pillow in this book.

Let us now consider three specific examples in the parameter estimation context:

(1) We are given a data set $D = \{d^k, k = 1, ..., p\}$, the d^ks being real numbers i.i.d., drawn from a Gaussian distribution with zero mean and unknown variance Θ which we want to estimate.

(2) Supervised classification task to be performed by a simple perceptron: the data are $d^k = \{\xi^k, v^k\}, k = 1, ..., p$, with ξ^k an N-dimensional pattern, randomly picked with say, some Gaussian distribution, and $v^k = \pm 1$ are the binary targets. Θ is the N-dimensional perceptron coupling vector which has generated the data; for a deterministic rule, $v^k = \text{sgn} \sum_{j=1}^{N} \Theta_j \xi_j^k$.

(3) Unsupervised learning task: the goal is to estimate an N-dimensional direction Θ from the observations of p N-dimensional vectors, $D = \{d^k = \xi^k, k = 1, ..., p\}$, independently drawn from some probability distribution that depends on the parameter only through the scalar product of Θ with the pattern: $P(d^k|\Theta) = p(\lambda^k \equiv \sum_{j=1}^{N} \Theta_j \xi_j^k)$.

The models (2) and (3) have been intensively studied (see in particular Biehl and Mietzner 1993, Watkin and Nadal 1994, Reimann and Van den Broeck 1996, Van den Broeck 1998, Buhot and Gordon 1998).

In the following, I will make equivalent use of the terminologies associated with either the parameter estimation or the neural coding contexts: thus, I will call the output D either the "data" or the "neural code", and the input Θ either the "parameter" or the "stimulus" (or the "signal").

Information Theoretic Framework

The Mutual Information between data and parameter

In all the cases mentioned above (neural coding, parameter estimation...), the main quantity of interest is the *Mutual Information* $I[\Theta; D]$ between the two random variables, the input Θ and the output D. This Shannon information quantity is defined as the Kullback divergence between the joint and the product distributions of $\{\Theta, D\}$, and can be written as (see e.g. Blahut 1988):

$$I[\Theta; D] = \int d\Theta \rho(\Theta) \int dD P(D|\Theta) \ln \frac{P(D|\Theta)}{P(D)} \tag{6.1}$$

where $P(D)$ is the marginal probability distribution of D,

$$P(D) = \int d\Theta \rho(\Theta) \, P(D|\Theta). \tag{6.2}$$

The mutual information $I[\Theta; D]$ measures the number of bits (if we take base 2 logarithms in 6.1) conveyed by D about Θ. This is an a priori relevant quantity for both neural coding and parameter estimation: intuitively, it measures all the information actually available in the data to be used for estimating the parameters. Without specifying in advance any particular estimator, the best possible performance that can ever be achieved in this estimation task is controlled by the mutual information. Indeed, the basic but fundamental information processing theorem tells us that processing cannot increase information (see e.g. Blahut 1988), that is, whatever the estimator (the algorithm for computing $\hat{\Theta}$ from D) may be,

$$I[\Theta; \hat{\Theta}] \leq I[\Theta; D]. \tag{6.3}$$

The mutual information $I[\Theta; D]$ can also be understood as the Bayes risk in the probability estimation task (for the prediction of d^{p+1}), that is, the cumulative entropy loss assuming that the true parameter has been generated by Nature according to $\rho(.)$ (see Haussler and Opper 1997).

The *information channel capacity*, or simply the *capacity*, $C = C(W)$ is defined as the supremum of the mutual information over all possible choices of input distributions $\rho(.)$, the parameters W of the channel being fixed:

$$C = \max_{\rho} I[\Theta; D] \tag{6.4}$$

In the neural coding context, it is the maximal amount of information that the network can convey, whatever the statistics of the environment.

For parameter estimation, it gives the *minimax risk*, that is, the smallest possible worst case risk in the Bayesian framework (see Haussler and Opper 1997 and references therein). It is related to Vapnik's growth function (Vapnik 1995) considered in computational learning theory. To see this, consider the simplest case of a supervised binary classification task by a perceptron (example (2) above). The choice of couplings Θ is equivalent to a choice of a particular dichotomy. The total number Δ of realizable dichotomies is a function of p and N alone - not of the set of patterns to be classified. The mutual information is then upper bounded by the logarithm of the number of possible classifications, that is, by $\ln \Delta$ (which is the growth function for the perceptron). The maximum of the mutual information is reached for ρ giving the same weight to all possible classifications, hence

$$C(\text{perceptron}) = \ln \Delta(N, p) \tag{6.5}$$

(for more details, see Nadal and Parga 1993 and 1994a, Opper and Kinzel 1995).

Infomax, Redundancy and ICA

One specificity of neural coding is the adaptation of the system to a *given* environment $\rho(.)$. A possible criterion for efficient coding is then the maximisation of mutual information over the choice of system (network) parameters W - a criterion called *infomax* after Linsker, 1988:

$$\text{(Infomax)} \quad I_{\max}[\rho] = \max_W I[\Theta; D] \tag{6.6}$$

Optimal coding according to this criterion has been studied by various authors, see in particular (Stein 1967, Laughlin 1981, Linsker 1988, van Hateren 1992, Nadal and Parga 1993, Stemmler and Koch 1998).

An alternative is the *minimisation of redundancy* based on the original ideas of F. Attneave (1954) and H. Barlow (1960). The redundancy considered here is the redundancy R in the neural code, that is, the mutual information between the p output units. It is thus defined as the Kullback divergence between the joint probability distribution of the code D and the factorial distribution of its components $d^1, ..., d^p$:

$$R = \int \prod_{k=1}^{p} dd^k P(D) \ln \frac{P(D)}{\prod_{k=1}^{p} P_k(d^k)} \tag{6.7}$$

with $P_k(d^k)$ the marginal probability distribution of d^k. The redundancy is zero iff the probability distribution $P(D)$ is equal to the product of the marginals (except possibly on a set of zero measure),

$$P(D) = \prod_{k=1}^{p} P_k(d^k) \tag{6.8}$$

in which case one speaks of a *factorial code*. If such a code is achieved, each coding cell is carrying some information statistically independent of the one conveyed by the other cells. In the signal processing language, this is equivalent to stating that the system is performing an Independent Component Analysis (ICA) of the input signal. Barlow's proposal is thus that the efficient coding scheme (again for a given environment ρ) corresponds to adapting the parameters W in order to minimise the redundancy:

$$\text{(Barlow's principle)} \quad \min_W R \tag{6.9}$$

Minimisation of redundancy has been considered in the modelling of the early visual system (Atick and coworkers 1992, Redlich 1993, Li and Atick 1994a and 1994b).

The fact that (6.7) is an appropriate cost function for performing ICA has been also recognised in the signal processing context (Comon, 1994).

In many cases, the output distribution *given the input* is factorised:

$$P(D|\Theta) = \prod_{k=1}^{p} P_k(d^k|\Theta) \tag{6.10}$$

This is so for the most studied case in parameter estimation, where one considers the data to be statistically independent realizations of the same law ($P_k(.|\Theta)$ is in addition independent of k); this is also the case for multilayer feedforward neural networks, where each output d^k is a (possibly stochastic) function of Θ alone (see the examples given above). Whenever this conditional factorisation (6.10) holds, one has

$$R = \sum_{k=1}^{p} I_k[\Theta; d^k] - I[\Theta; D] \tag{6.11}$$

where $I_k[\Theta; d^k]$ is the mutual information between the kth output unit alone and the input Θ. Since $R \geq 0$, one has then

$$I[\Theta; D] \leq \sum_{k=1}^{p} I_k[\Theta; d^k]. \tag{6.12}$$

Remark: conversely (6.11) implies (6.10) a.s.; it is not difficult to construct examples where (6.10) does not hold, and with the r.h.s. of (6.11) strictly negative.

As the above relations (6.11) and (6.12) suggest, maximisation of the mutual information (infomax) leads to redundancy reduction, and hence to ICA (Nadal and Parga 1994b, Nadal et al 1998). Sufficient conditions for this result to hold are: vanishing input noise, and infomax done over the choice of both synaptic couplings and transfer functions. In the particular case where the input is a linear mixture of IC's, and the network a simple nonlinear feedforward network (no hidden units), the infomax criterion is also equivalent to the maximum likelihood approach to ICA (Cardoso 1997). Specific algorithms based on these information theoretic cost functions have been proposed (see e.g. Pham et al 1992, Comon 1994, Bell and Sejnowski 1995).

Remark: Throughout this paper, I am considering memoryless channels: the output D at some time t is a function of a single input Θ. Generalisation to systems with memory, that is, where $D(t)$ depends on $\{\Theta(t - \tau), 0 \leq \tau \leq T\}$ for some possibly infinite T, can be done - and in some cases has been done, see e.g. Li 1995 (case of early visual system) and Pham 1996 (case of ICA). In particular, the relevant mutual information to be considered in such cases is $I[D(t); \{\Theta(t - \tau), 0 \leq \tau < T\}]$ for finite T and the limit when $T \rightarrow \infty$.

Typical Behaviour of the Mutual Information

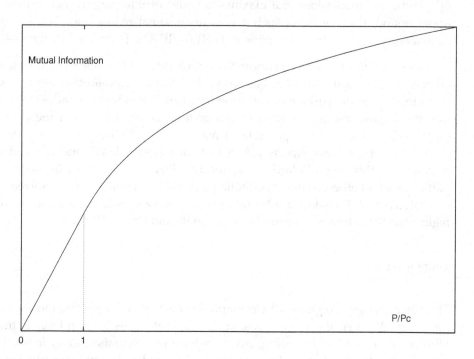

Figure 6.2: Typical behaviour of the mutual information I between input and output, as a function of the number of coding cells P scaled to the critical value, P_c. For $P \leq P_c$, I is (at best) proportional to P. For $P \gg P_c$, I has a logarithmic behaviour.

The typical behaviour of the amount of information conveyed by the (neural) system about the stimulus/parameter, as function of the number of coding cells (the number of observations) p, is shown on Figure 6.2, for the case of a real valued N-dimensional parameter. One can show (Herschkowitz and Nadal 1999) that for any p, the mutual information is upper bounded by a quantity linear in p: this is simply because, at best, every datum conveys some information statistically independent of what is conveyed by the others, in which case the information will be essentially proportional to p. However, it is not always possible to saturate this linear behaviour, and in general, for large p, the mutual information has a logarithmic behaviour in p. I discuss now, in more detail, these two regimes of particular interest: the small p ($p < N$), and large p ($p \gg N$) regimes.

Small p regime

At small values of p (typically $p < N$, or more generally $p \leq p_c \sim d_{VC}$ where d_{VC} is the VC dimension), the maximal amount of information may saturate the upper bound, linear in p. In such a regime, maximal redundancy is achieved or, equivalently, Independent Component Analysis (ICA) is performed by the system.

In the context of learning/parameter estimation, such a linear regime may be observed and is related to what has been called *retarded classification*: in this regime, no estimation of the parameter can be made. This may appear paradoxical: on one side the largest possible amount of information is extracted from the data, and on the other side it is not possible to make any prediction concerning the next observation. These two aspects are in fact intimately related, and we will come back later to this point. Retarded classification has been exhibited in models with particular symmetries, in the asymptotic limit $N \to \infty$ with $\alpha = \frac{p}{N}$ kept fixed (Biehl and Mietzner 1993, Watkin and Nadal 1994). A rigorous proof of the existence of this regime has been derived recently (Herschkowitz and Opper, 1999).

Large p regime

The other important regime is the asymptotic one, that is, for $p \to \infty$, more precisely for $p >> N$ when the VC dimension d_{VC} is finite. This large p limit is the one of interest for population coding, over-complete representations, and in particular, sparse codes. It is the standard asymptotic limit considered in statistics (the limit of a large number of available data).

In this regime, the mutual information grows logarithmically in p:

$$\lim_{p >> N} I[\Theta; D] \sim K \, N \ln \frac{p}{N} \tag{6.13}$$

where the prefactor K depends on the smoothness of the statistical relationship between observations (activities of neural cells) and parameter (stimulus). This logarithmic behaviour is very related to the one obtained for the growth function discussed in Vapnik's framework. Indeed, as mentioned in the previous section, in the case of a binary classification by a perceptron, the growth function is an upper bound on the mutual information. One should note however that in (6.13), N is the dimension of the parameter (more exactly the number of independent degrees of freedom), and *not* the VC dimension of the system.

For a smooth enough distribution, the leading behaviour is always $\frac{N}{2} \log \frac{p}{N}$. In such a smooth case, one has in fact a simple exact expression for the mutual information in the asymptotic regime: it is found that it is given in terms of the *Fisher information*, that is (restricting here for simplicity to the scalar case, $N = 1$)

$$I[D; \Theta] = - \int d\theta \rho(\theta) \ln \rho(\theta) + \int d\theta \rho(\theta) \frac{1}{2} \ln \left(\frac{F(\theta)}{2\pi e} \right) \tag{6.14}$$

where the Fisher information $F(\Theta)$ is defined by:

$$F(\Theta) = \left\langle -\frac{\partial^2 \ln P(D|\Theta)}{\partial \Theta^2} \right\rangle_\Theta \tag{6.15}$$

in which $\langle \, . \, \rangle_\Theta$ denotes the integration over D *given* Θ with the p.d.f. $P(D|\Theta)$. Fisher information is related through the Cramer-Rao bound to the smallest possible variance of an estimator (Blahut 1988): the largest the Fisher information, the smallest the variance.

It is quite remarkable that the existence of a direct relationship between a Shannon information and the Fisher information has been known for less than ten years. Indeed, this relation (6.14) (and its generalisation to arbitrary N) was first derived by Clarke and Barron, 1990, in the case of i.i.d. data; with weaker hypothesis, it appears as a side result in the 1996 Rissanen's paper on the Minimum Description Length (MDL) principle. A direct derivation in the context of neural coding and information processing (including cases of correlated data) is given in Brunel and Nadal 1998.

One should insist that it is only in this asymptotic limit that one has a direct relationship between number of bits and quadratic errors. In particular, for $p \sim N$ and/or with spiking neurons optimisation of the neural code at short times will be different whether the goal is optimal reconstruction or information preservation (Ruderman 1994, Brunel and Nadal 1998).

In the case of non smooth distribution, that is, when the Fisher information is infinite, there is no known general expression for the asymptotic behaviour of the mutual information. However, recent results suggest (Haussler and Opper 1997) that the prefactor - the numerical constant K in (6.13) - can take only a small number of possible values. Specific models have been studied (Nadal and Parga 1993, Opper and Kinzel 1995) and general bounds derived (Haussler and Opper 1997, Herschkowitz and Nadal 1999), showing that one always has a log behaviour with a rational prefactor. In the particular case of a binary classification by a perceptron, the prefactor is 1 (indeed $\ln \Delta(N, p) \sim N \log \frac{p}{N}$ for large p). This means that when the probability distribution of the data D given the parameter Θ has a discontinuity, the mutual information is asymptotically twice as large than for a smooth distribution.

The optimal performance in the estimation task, in the asymptotic limit of large p, is directly related to the behaviour of the mutual information: the typical discrepancy between the (best possible) estimator and the true parameter will go to zero as an inverse power law in p, with an exponent which depends on the prefactor K (for more details, see Opper and Kinzel 1995, Haussler and Opper 1997, Herschkowitz and Nadal 1999). One interesting qualitative aspect is the fact that good performance is obtained in the regime where the mutual information has the slowest (*log*) growth, in contrast with the poorest performance obtained in the linear regime. Indeed, if after learning p examples, one has a good prediction for the next one, d^{p+1}, this means that when the new datum d^{p+1} is actually given, one is only partly "surprised" by its value - precisely because one had already a good idea of what it would be. Hence, the new information (the part not already contained in the first p examples) conveyed by this new datum is small: the information growth has to be sublinear. Conversely, a linear growth means that d^{p+1} conveys some totally new information, hence that no prediction at all was possible based on the first p examples.

In the context of neural coding, the asymptotic (*log*) regime gives a highly redundant code: indeed, the fact that it is possible to have a good prediction of the activity d^{p+1} of the $p+1$th cell, given the activities of the first p cells, means that the amount of information conveyed by the $p+1$th cell is not independent of the information conveyed by the other cells. As we have seen, this redundancy cannot be avoided: for a given number N of inputs (sensory receptors), the marginal gain of information obtained by adding a new coding cell becomes smaller and smaller as p increases. However, such redundancy may be useful for various reasons - e.g. noise robustness, or in order to satisfy other constraints such as sparseness (see chapter by Olshausen in this book).

Finally, one should add that the log behaviour is obtained whenever one has a real valued parameter belonging to a finite dimensional space. For a parameter with discrete components, the mutual information is upper bounded by the finite entropy of the parameter; this bound is saturated for large p, either at a finite value of p or asymptotically with an exponential convergence rate (Haussler and Opper 1995). When the parameter is a function (which means in particular $N = \infty$), one may find a power law behaviour (Opper, 1999) with an exponent smaller than one - in agreement with the fact that the growth must be sublinear.

Beyond Sensory Coding

I have presented some common and generic properties of information processing in the dual context of neural coding and parameter estimation. To conclude, I would like to make some comments on possible further developments, and on the limitations, of the approach illustrated on Figure 6.1. I will propose several possible lines of research which still make use of the information theoretic framework but try to address computing aspects not necessarily obviously related to efficient coding.

First, one should say that information theoretic criteria may not be, or not always be, the appropriate ones: as put forward by Z. Li (Li 1998), one may have to contrast optimal coding versus computation. An example of this is already presented in the previous section: for p small, optimal coding (via infomax, that is, maximisation of information preservation) is not equivalent to optimal reconstruction (minimisation of quadratic error); however, for large p the two criteria become identical. More generally, one can say, as we have seen, that the mutual information is the relevant quantity for parameter estimation - if the cost is taken as an entropic loss, and not the quadratic error.

As already said for neural coding, it is not always the case that one has to compute an estimate of Θ. It might be also that one is interested in some function $F(\Theta)$, so that the final output is not $\hat{\Theta}$ but the estimate $\widehat{F(\Theta)}$. If the desired computation task is known, that is, if $F(.)$ is known, then one is interested in $I[D; F]$ instead of $I[D; \Theta]$. One can note that the input Θ can be considered as a "noisy" representation of $F(\Theta)$ if $\Theta \rightarrow F(\Theta)$ is not invertible.

A different but similar approach would be the one followed in Communication Theory (see e.g. Blahut 1988), when a cost for decoding errors is prescribed in advance. For instance, suppose the task is to minimise the quadratic error, $E =< (\hat{\Theta} - \Theta)^2 >$. Then, one may ask for the *minimisation* of the mutual information with the constraint that E is smaller than some prescribed level: one is then building a code which conveys just the information directly needed for this particular task.

Another line of research is one followed by Phillips (Phillips, 1995, Phillips and Singer, 1997): one considers the N inputs to be composed of the external stimulus and of what defines the task or context (other external stimuli and/or internal states of the system); an *infomax* cost function is then built which distinguishes the two types of inputs.

Another important aspect is the search for codes preserving topological or geometrical properties (Victorri and Derome 1984, Rao and Ruderman 1999). It is not obvious whether the building of a code showing invariance through particular transformations should be the result of ad-hoc constraints imposed in addition to a coding criterion (see e.g. the approach in Li and Atick, 1994b, where translational and scale invariance is a constraint added to redundancy reduction), or whether such properties must appear as a consequence of efficient coding. I would expect the second hypothesis to be correct, as suggested by work on natural image analysis (Field 1987, Ruderman and Bialek 1994, Turiel and Parga 2000, chapter in this book by Piepenbrock).

One should note also that the framework illustrated on Figure 6.1 applies as well to time dependent activities. Particular cases are very briefly mentioned in this chapter. To give an example, one can consider a single spiking cell responding to a particular stimulus. In our framework, p is then the time during which one collects the number of spikes emitted by the cell. The behaviour of the mutual information between the cell activity and the stimulus as a function of time (of p) is the one discussed in this chapter - linear at short times, logarithmic at long times - (Stein 1967, Bialek et al 1991, Brunel and Nadal 1998). The information content of more complex time dependent codes have yet to be studied (for various approaches to the modelling of spiking neural cells, see this book, Part II: Neural Function).

A last remark is that the framework illustrated on Figure 6.1 seems to imply a purely feedforward system, where each output d^k is a function of the input Θ. This is not the case. Indeed, our basic tool is the mutual information, which is a symmetric quantity with respect to the two random variables Θ and D (it does not distinguish an "input" from an "output"): it is well defined whenever one can write the joint probability distribution $P(\Theta, D)$. Hence, most of what has been said above applies as well for motor coding (D being the internal motor representation and Θ the motor action), and population coding is indeed studied for both sensory and motor representations. The framework also applies regardless of the complexity of the network, including with correlated outputs: in particular, D might be the activities of an attractor network whose initial state has been, directly or indirectly, imposed by the stimulus Θ. One should note also that mutual information is a relevant tool for characterising the neural code, even when optimal information preservation is not the chosen criterion: for example, it would be interesting to study the information content of sparse codes.

The comments in the previous paragraph lead to one of the most interesting problems for which the general framework in Figure 6.1 may not be fully appropriate: the building of neural codes *via* the sensori-motor loop. One would like the system to build its internal representations through *active perception*, which implies that the source distribution, ρ, is not externally given by the environment: the sequence of successive inputs depends on the past history - the past sequence of {stimuli,actions}. I would suggest that one can stay within the same framework, using the following point of view: a joint sensori-motor representation may be built by considering the mutual information between the neural code D and the pair $\{perception(t), action(t+1)\}$; the decision to make a particular action can be considered as trying to choose a particular stimulus, the one which would be the most efficient in the learning process leading to the neural code. This is then the same as *learning by queries* in statistical learning theory (Kinzel and Rujan 1990), a learning strategy in which at each step, one picks the training example which provides the largest possible amount of information. The result is then a learning (adaptation) process which can be efficient in terms of convergence rate towards the optimal solution - but it does not affect the nature of the optimal solution (the optimal code).

Acknowledgements

This contribution is based on work done mainly with Nestor Parga, Nicolas Brunel and Didier Herschkowitz. I thank Zhaoping Li, Alexandre Pouget, Sophie Denève, Anthony Bell and Manfred Opper for stimulating discussions during the NIPS meeting. This work has been partly supported by the French grant DGA 96 2557A/DSP.

References

[1] Atick J. J., Could information theory provide an ecological theory of sensory processing. *NETWORK*, 3:213–251, 1992.

[2] Attneave F., Informational aspects of visual perception. *Psychological Review*, 61:183–193, 1954.

[3] Barlow H. B., The coding of sensory messages. In W. H. Thorpe and O. L. Zangwill, editors, *Current Problems in Animal Behaviour*, pages 331–360. Cambridge University Press, 1960.

[4] Barlow H. B., Kaushal T. P., and Mitchison G. J., Finding minimum entropy codes. *Neural Comp.*, 1:412–423, 1989.

[5] Bell A. and Sejnowski T., An information-maximisation approach to blind separation and blind deconvolution *Neural Computation* 7:1129–1159, 1995.

[6] Bialek W., Rieke F., de Ruyter, van Steveninck R., and Warland D., Reading a neural code. *Science*, 252:1854–57, 1991.

[7] Biehl M. and Mietzner A., Statistical Mechanics of Unsupervised Learning, *Europhys. Lett.* 24:421, 1993;

[8] Blahut R. E., *Principles and Practice of Information Theory*, Addison-Wesley, Cambridge MA, 1988.

[9] Buhot A. and Gordon M., Phase transitions in optimal unsupervised learning. *Phys. Rev. E*, 57(3):3326–3333, 1998.

[10] Brunel N. and Nadal J.-P., Mutual information, Fisher information and population coding. *Neural Computation*, 10:1731–1757, 1998.

[11] Cardoso J.-F., Infomax and maximum likelihood for blind separation *IEEE Signal Processing Letters* 4:112-114, 1997.

[12] Clarke B. S. and Barron A. R., Information-theoretic asymptotics of bayes methods. *IEEE Trans. on Information Theory*, 36(3):453–471, 1990.

[13] Comon P., Independent component analysis, a new concept ? *Signal Processing*, 36:287–314, 1994.

[14] Cover, T. M. and Thomas, J. A., *Information Theory*, John Wiley, 1991.

[15]   Field D., Relations between the statistics of natural images and the response properties of cortical cells. *J. Opt. Soc. Am.*, 4:2379, 1987.

[16]   van Hateren J.H., Theoretical predictions of spatiotemporal receptive fields of fly LMCs, and experimental validation. *J. Comp. Physiology A*, 171:157-170, 1992.

[17]   Haussler D. and Opper M., General bounds on the mutual information between a parameter and n conditionally independent observations. In *VIIIth Ann. Workshop on Computational Learning Theory (COLT95)*, pages 402–411, Santa Cruz, 1995 (ACM, New-York).

[18]   Herschkowitz D. and Nadal J.-P., Unsupervised and supervised learning: the mutual information between parameters and observations *Phys. Rev. E,* 59(3):3344-3360, 1999

[19]   Herschkowitz D. and Opper M., Retarded Learning in High Dimensional Data Spaces, *in preparation*, 1999.

[20]   Jutten C. and Herault J., Blind separation of sources, Part I: An adaptive algorithm based on neuromimetic architecture, *Signal Proc.*, 24:1–10, 1991.

[21]   Kinzel W. and Rujan P., Learning by queries, *Europhys. Lett.* 13:473, 1990.

[22]   Laughlin S. B., A simple coding procedure enhances a neuron's information capacity. *Z. Naturf.*, C 36:910–2, 1981.

[23]   Li Z., A theory of the visual motion coding in the primary visual cortex *Neural Computation* 8(4):705-30, 1995.

[24]   Li Z., *This Workshop*, and: A neural model of contour integration in the primary visual cortex *Neural Computation* 10:903-940, 1998

[25]   Li Z. and Atick J. J., Towards a theory of the striate cortex. *Neural Comp.*, 6:127–146, 1994.

[26]   Li Z. and Atick J. J., Efficient stereo coding in the multiscale representation. *Network: Computation in Neural Systems*, 5(2):157-174, 1994.

[27]   Linsker R., Self-organization in a perceptual network. *Computer*, 21:105–17, 1988.

[28]   Linsker R., Deriving receptive fields using an optimal encoding criterion. In Hanson S. J., Cowan J. D., and Lee Giles C., editors, *Neural Information Processing Systems 5*, pages 953–60. Morgan Kaufmann, San Mateo, 1993.

[29]   Nadal J.-P., Brunel N. and Parga N., Nonlinear feedforward networks with stochastic ouputs: infomax implies redundancy reduction *Network: Computation in Neural Systems* 9(2):207-217, 1998.

[30]   Nadal J.-P. and Parga N., Information processing by a perceptron in an unsupervised learning task. *NETWORK*, 4:295–312, 1993.

[31]   Nadal J.-P. and Parga N., Duality between learning machines: a bridge between supervised and unsupervised learning. *Neural Computation*, 6:489–506, 1994.

[32]   Nadal J.-P. and Parga N., Nonlinear neurons in the low noise limit: a factorial

code maximizes information transfer *Network: Computation in Neural Systems* 5:565-581, 1994.

[33] Olshausen B. A. and Field D. J., Sparse coding with an overcomplete basis set: A strategy employed by V1? *Vision Research*, 37:3311-3325, 1997.

[34] Opper M. and Haussler D., Bounds for predictive errors in the statistical mechanics of supervised learning, *Phys. Rev. Lett.*, 75:3772-3775, 1995.

[35] Opper M. and Kinzel W., Statistical mechanics of generalization. In E. Domany J.L. van Hemmen and K. Schulten, editors, *Physics of Neural Networks*, p. 151, Springer, 1995.

[36] Pham D.-T., Blind Separation of Instantaneous Mixture of Sources via an Independent Component Analysis *IEEE Trans. SP* 44(11):2768–2779, 1996.

[37] Pham D.-T., Garrat Ph. and Jutten Ch., Separation of a mixture of independent sources through a maximum likelihood approach in *Proc. EUSIPCO*, pp 771–774, 1992.

[38] Phillips W. A., Kay J. and Smyth D., The discovery of structure by multi-stream networks of local processors with contextual guidance *Network: Computation in neural systems* 6:225-246, 1995.

[39] Phillips W. A. and Singer W., In search of common foundations for cortical computation *Behavorial and Brain Sciences* 20(4):657-722, 1997.

[40] Rao R. P. N. and Ruderman D. L., Learning Lie Groups for Invariant Visual Perception, In *Advances in Neural Information Processing Systems 11* (proceedings of NIPS98), Ed. by M. S. Kearns, S. A. Solla and D. A. Cohen, p. 810-816, MIT Press, 1999.

[41] Redlich A. N., Redundancy reduction as a strategy for unsupervised learning. *Neural Comp.*, 5:289–304, 1993.

[42] Reimann P. and Van den Broeck C., Learning by examples from a non uniform distribution. *Phys. Rev. E*, 53 (4):3989–3998, 1996.

[43] Rissanen J., Fisher information and stochastic complexity. *IEEE Trans. on Information Theory*, 42 (1):40-47, 1996.

[44] Ruderman D., Designing receptive fields for highest fidelity. *NETWORK*, 5:147–155, 1994.

[45] Ruderman D. and Bialek W., Statistics of natural images: scaling in the woods. In Cowan J. D., Tesauro G., and Alspector J., editors, *Neural Information Processing Systems 6*, Morgan Kaufmann, San Mateo, 1994.

[46] Shannon C. E. and Weaver W., *The Mathematical Theory of Communication*. The University of Illinois Press, Urbana, 1949.

[47] Stein R., The information capacity of nerve cells using a frequency code *Biophys. Journal* **7** (1967) 797–826.

[48] Stemmler M. and Koch Ch., Information maximization in single neurons In *Advances in Neural Information Processing Systems 11*, Ed. by M. S. Kearns, S. A.

Solla and D. A. Cohen (The MIT Press 1999), p. 160.

[49]   Seung H. S. and Sompolinsky H., Simple models for reading neural population codes *P.N.A.S. USA* 90:10749–10753, 1993.

[50]   Turiel A. and Parga N., The multi-fractal structure of contrast changes in natural images: from sharp edges to textures, *Neural Computation*, 12:763–793, 2000.

[51]   Van den Broeck C., Unsupervised learning by examples: on-line versus off-line learning. In *proceedings of the TANC workshop* (Hong-Kong May 26-28), 1997.

[52]   Victorri B. and Derome J.-R., Mathematical model of visual perception, *J. Theor. Biol.* 108:227-260, 1984.

[53]   Watkin T. and Nadal J.-P., Optimal unsupervised learning. *J. Phys. A: Math. and Gen.*, 27:1899–1915, 1994.

7 From Generic to Specific: An Information Theoretic Perspective on the Value of High-Level Information

A.L. Yuille and James M. Coughlan

Introduction

What are the fundamental limits of vision? How much information can an ideal observer [11] extract from the light rays reaching his/her eyes? And, more importantly for this chapter, how much does this depend on the prior knowledge that the observer has about the world/domain?

It should be emphasized that we are concerned with decoding the input signal to extract useful information (as is presumably the function of the cortex) and not with efficiently encoding the signal for transmission (which may well be performed by the retina or LGN; see [2]). We are also not concerned with neural encoding. For a different information theoretic perspective on these issues, see the chapter by Nadal in this book.

To make our ideas more concrete, consider the relative difficulties of the three detection tasks in figure 7.1. Segmenting and locating the informational sign (left panel) is straightforward using low level cues such as edge detection (such signs are intended to be easily detectable) though high-level knowledge about signs is needed to interpret it. Finding the gila monster (central panel) is difficult (because the animal has evolved to blend into the background to increase its survival chances) and seems to require mid-level knowledge, combining texture and shapes cues like symmetry, even to segment it. Finally, detecting the Dalmatian dog (right panel) is very difficult and would seem to require high level knowledge about the shape and appearance of Dalmatians.

These examples have implications for theories of the human visual system. Many theories of vision are bottom-up – e.g. Marr [14] – where low level processing feeds

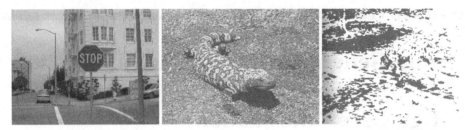

Figure 7.1: Left to right, three detection tasks of increasing degrees of difficulty. The stop sign (left) is easy to find. The gila monster (centre) is harder. The Dalmatian dog (right) is almost impossible.

forward without any feedback from higher levels. In other words, visual tasks such as segmentation are performed without using high-level knowledge about objects. Marr himself notes that such theories would have difficulty in detecting the Dalmatian dog and states that "our general view is that although some top-down information is sometimes necessary, it is only of secondary importance in early visual processing" (pp 100-101 in [14]).

On the other extreme, Mumford [15] has advocated a model of the visual system based on Grenander's pattern theory [9]. This approach proposes algorithms based on the principle of analysis through synthesis which, in its most extreme form, would involve synthesizing an image of a Dalmatian (presumably in V1) in order to segment and recognize it. Mumford has argued that such theories could be implemented using feedback loops to enable high-level models of objects to directly access the raw input images (in order to compare them to the synthesized images). These theories are certainly powerful enough in principle to detect the Dalmatian dog but would seem too slow for general image processing, given current pattern theory algorithms, particularly since it is claimed that humans can recognize objects in roughly 150 msec. Analysis through synthesis theories appear to be more computationally, and biologically, plausible for tracking objects over time [16] where only small changes in the object's appearance need to be synthesized. Alternatively, Ullman [19] has proposed a theory where bottom-up cues help activate top-down hypotheses, which may combine the best of both worlds.

What are the trade-offs between top-down and bottom-up strategies of vision? A top-down strategy is theoretically optimal given infinite computational resources. One simply stores high-level Bayesian models of everything one needs to detect (e.g. stop signs, gila monsters, Dalmatian dogs) – and applies each model to the image in order to detect whether the object is present or not [9]. In certain cases, this search can be performed very efficiently for individual objects (see, for example, Coughlan's Dynamic Programming algorithm for detecting a hand in an image [3]). Nevertheless, such an approach is computationally prohibitive, when one takes into account the enormous number of objects that one would like to detect, and seems far too slow. By contrast, a bottom-up approach which segments out objects based purely on low-level (i.e. object independent cues) is a lot faster (in principle), but it will sometimes fail – for example on the Dalmatian dog. (We assume, here, of course that recognizing the object is considerably easier once it has been detected and segmented).

To understand these trade-offs further, we seek to quantify when high-level knowledge is required for low-level processing. Clearly, one needs high-level knowledge of signs, gila monsters, and Dalmatians in order to recognize them. But when is high-level knowledge about them required to *segment them from the image*? We believe that quantifying the value of high-level information for visual tasks will help throw light on the bottom-up/top-down debate and will lead to more effective algorithms for segmentation and object recognition.

This chapter addresses these questions for the specific task of detecting a target in background clutter and assumes that visual perception is best posed as perceptual inference [12]. Our technical presentation follows the original material on this topic first described by Yuille and Coughlan in [22] for the analysis of the Geman and Jedynak model of road detection [8]. The concepts have later been developed and generalized by Wu and Zhu [20] and then by Yuille, Coughlan, Zhu and Wu [23].

Our approach, of course, lies entirely within the Bayesian framework for vision [12]. The chapter by Schrater and Kersten in this book gives a nice discussion of Bayes and its relationship to psychophysics. The chapters by Mamassian *et al.*, Jacobs, Weiss and Fleet, and Freeman *et al.* all describe interesting aspects of this approach.

The Detectability of Targets

How easy is it to detect a target such as a road in an aerial image? This question was addressed by Coughlan and Yuille [21, 5] when analyzing the theory proposed by Geman and Jedynak [8]. In this theory, the properties of the target and the background were characterized by probability distributions (see "Background and Previous Work" section). Coughlan and Yuille showed that the detectability of the target depended on a single parameter K, called the *order parameter*, which could be computed from the underlying probability distributions specifying the problem and which can be thought of as a generalized signal to noise ratio. The larger the value of K the easier the task. Moreover, if $K < 0$ then the task is impossible because it is impossible, with reasonable probability, to distinguish the target from the background (i.e. it becomes similar to looking for a needle in a haystack). These results will be summarized in the section entitled "Fundamental limits."

In this chapter, we use similar techniques to explore a related problem. How much harder do we make target detection by using a weaker *generic* model (i.e. a weaker prior probability distribution)? Or more positively, how much easier do we make the task by using more information about the target?

This relates to the bottom-up versus top-down distinction which we discussed in the previous section. More concretely, a recent system by Geiger and Liu [7] for detecting human figures uses low-level prior knowledge of edge smoothness, as implemented by snakes [10], to detect boundary segments of objects which are then grouped, using object specific knowledge, to locate specific objects. This system is effective and computationally efficient but it will break down if the background clutter is sufficiently complicated that the snake algorithms are unable to find the object boundaries. In such situations, however, it *may still be possible to detect the object if a high-level prior model is used.*

This chapter develops a theory to contrast bottom-up and top-down approaches for the specific problem of road tracking [8]. This is a domain which is simple enough to allow rigorous mathematical analysis. It also helps that the Geman and Jedynak theory for road tracking [8] is both theoretically elegant and also highly effective in practice. Very similar theories have been proposed for the related tasks of bounding contour detection (for example, [7, 3]).

More precisely, our approach characterizes the road detection task in terms of order-parameters for both the bottom-up and top-down strategies. It will be shown that in certain *regimes* of the order parameters, both strategies will be effective (in the sense of finding a close approximation to the true solution). In other regimes, the top-down strategy will work but the bottom-up strategy will not. In yet other regimes, the target detection problem becomes impossible to solve by any approach. Our results suggest that the bottom-up strategy can often be significantly quicker than the top-down strategy and it makes sense to use it, particularly if we are searching for one of several different types of road.

Background and Previous Work

Tracking curved objects in real images is an important practical problem in computer vision. We consider a specific formulation of the problem of road tracking from aerial images by Geman (D.) and Jedynak [8]. This approach assumes that both the intensity properties and the geometrical shapes of the target path (i.e. the edge contour) can be modelled statistically. This path can be considered to be a set of elementary path segments joined together. We first consider the intensity properties along the edge and then the geometric properties.

The image properties of segments lying on the path are assumed to differ, in a

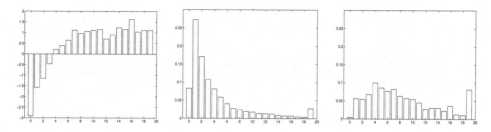

Figure 7.2: The log likelihood ratios (far left) of the off-edge probabilities $p_{off}(y)$ (center) and the on-edge probabilities $p_{on}(y)$(right), where $y = \left|\vec{\nabla} I\right|$. These distributions, and ratios, were very consistent for a range of images. The filter responses y, on the horizontal line, were quantized to take 20 values.

statistical sense, from those off the path. More precisely, we can design a filter $\phi(.)$ with output $\{y_x = \phi(I(x))\}$ for a segment at point x so that:

$$P(y_x) = P_{on}(y_x) \ \text{ if "x" lies on the true path}$$
$$P(y_x) = P_{off}(y_x) \ \text{ if "x" lies off the true path.}$$

For example, we can think of the $\{y_x\}$ as being values of the edge strength at point x and P_{on}, P_{off} as being the probability distributions of the response of $\phi(.)$ on and off an edge. Figure (7.2) provides examples of P_{on}, P_{off} expressed as histograms (see Konishi *et al.* [13] for examples of P_{on}, P_{off} evaluated on a large dataset of real images). The set of possible values of the random variable y_x is the *alphabet* with *alphabet size* M.

We now consider the geometry of the target contour. We require the path to be made up of connected segments $x_1, x_2, \ldots, x_N$ (see figure (7.3)). There will be a Markov probability distribution $P_g(x_{i+1}|x_i)$ which specifies prior probabilistic knowledge of the target. Each point x has a set of Q neighbours. Following terminology from graph theory, we refer to Q as the *branching factor*. We will assume that the distribution P_g depends only on the relative positions of x_{i+1} and x_i. In other words, $P_g(x_{i+1}|x_i) = P_{\Delta g}(x_{i+1} - x_i)$. An important special case is when the probability distribution is uniform for all branches (i.e. $P_{\Delta g}(\Delta x) = U(\Delta x) = 1/Q \ \forall \Delta x$).

By standard Bayesian analysis, the optimal (MAP estimate) path $X^* = \{x_1^*, \ldots, x_N^*\}$ maximizes the sum of the log posterior ratios:

$$R(X) = \sum_i \log \frac{P_{on}(y_{(x_i)})}{P_{off}(y_{(x_i)})} + \sum_i \log \frac{P_{\Delta g}(x_{i+1} - x_i)}{U(x_{i+1} - x_i)}, \tag{7.1}$$

where the sum i is taken over all points on the target. $U(x_{i+1} - x_i)$ is the uniform distribution and its presence merely changes the log posterior $R(X)$ by a constant

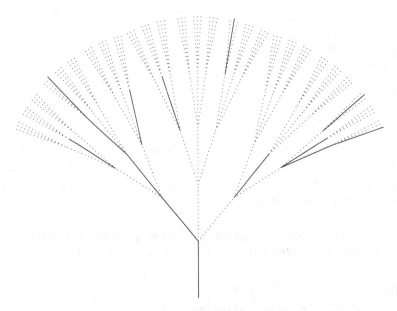

Figure 7.3: A simulated road tracking problem where dark lines indicate strong edge responses and dashed lines specify weak responses. The branching factor is three. The data was generated by stochastic sampling using a simplified version of the models analyzed in this paper. In this sample there is only one strong candidate for the best path (the continuous dark line) but chance fluctuations have created subpaths in the noise with strong edge responses.

value. It is included to make the form of the intensity and geometric terms similar, which simplifies our later analysis.

We will refer to $R(X)$ as the *reward* of the path X which is the sum of the *intensity rewards* $\log \frac{P_{on}(y_{(x_i)})}{P_{off}(y_{(x_i)})}$ and the *geometric rewards* $\log \frac{P_{\Delta g}(x_{i+1}-x_i)}{U(x_{i+1}-x_i)}$.

Intuitively, any path in the image has a reward which can be computed from equation (7.1). One path in the image corresponds to the true road path and we expect, or hope, that its reward will be higher than the rewards for all the other possible image paths. We refer to these non-road paths as *distractor* paths. If, with high probability, the reward of one of the distractor paths is higher than the reward for the true path then the task of detecting the true road path becomes impossible.

At a more abstract level, the road is represented by $X = x_1, ..., x_N$ and the Markov distribution $P_g(x_{i+1}|x_i)$ specifies a prior distribution $P(X) = \prod_{i=1}^{N-1} P_g(x_{i+1}|x_i)$ on the geometry of the road. The image measurements are represented by $Y = \{\phi(I(x)) : x \in D\}$ where D is the entire image. The likelihood function $P(Y|X)$ is given by:

$$P(Y|X) = \prod_{x \in D \cap X} P_{on}(y_x) \prod_{x \in D \cap X^c} P_{off}(y_x), \tag{7.2}$$

where $D \cap X$ is the set of image pixels which are on the road and $D \cap X^c$ are the set of pixels which are not. X^c is the complement of X in D (i.e. $X \cup X^c = D$ and $X \cap X^c = \phi$ where ϕ is the empty set).

The two distributions $P(Y|X)$ and $P(Y)$ determine the joint distribution $P(X, Y) = P(Y|X)P(X)$ which defines a probability distribution on the set of problem instances.

As we will show, this formulation can be extended to deal with second order and higher level priors (provided they are shift-invariant). (See figures (7.7,7.8,7.9, 7.10) for examples of first order models and figure (7.11) for examples of second order Markov models.) This allows our theory to apply to models such as snakes [10]. (It is straightforward to transform the standard energy function formulation of snakes into a Markov chain by discretizing and replacing the derivatives by differences. The smoothness constraints, such as membranes and thin plate terms, will transform into first and second order Markov chain connections respectively). Recent work by Zhu [25] shows that Markov chain models of this type can be learnt using Minimax Entropy Learning theory from a representative set of examples.

Fundamental limits

As described above, the Bayesian formulation of our problems *naturally gives rise to a probability distribution $P(X, Y)$ on the ensemble of problem instances*, which is called the *Bayesian Ensemble*.

Using the Bayesian Ensemble, Coughlan and Yuille showed [21] that the difficulty of detecting targets, such as roads, in images can be characterized in terms of an *order parameter K*. This order parameter was defined in terms of the statistical properties of the images and the target and was used to characterize both the *expected error* in the solution and the *expected convergence rate*. It was shown that the detection task had a phase transition at $K = 0$. For $K < 0$ it was impossible, on average, to detect the target by any algorithm – but for $K > 0$ detection is possible (see figure (7.4)). More precisely, the detection task is formulated as MAP estimation and is equivalent to maximizing an appropriate *reward function*. We proved that the expected number of *ghosts* (false paths caused by random alignments of off-road pixels) with higher reward than the *true path reward* decreases as 2^{-KN} where N is the length of the road. Moreover, the expected error rate and the algorithmic convergence time decrease exponentially with K. The size of K increases with the effectiveness of the edge detector and with the amount of prior knowledge available about the target. The results were obtained by mathematical proofs on the Bayesian ensemble of target detection problem instances using the formulation of road tracking by Geman and Jedynak [8].

The exact form of the order parameter depends the precise specification of the problem. In this case, we restrict ourselves to analyzing the chances that the rewards

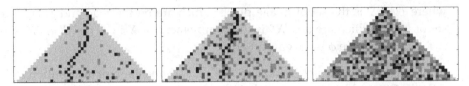

Figure 7.4: The difficulty of detecting a target path increases as the amount of background clutter increases. In this chapter, the difficulty of detection is quantified by a single parameter K, the order parameter, which is derived from the underlying probability distributions which characterize the domain. The larger K the easier the task and so K can be thought of as a generalized signal to noise measure. Left, an easy detection task with $K = 0.8647$. Middle, a harder detection task with $K = 0.2105$. Right, an impossible task with $K = -0.7272$.

of *any* of the distractor paths is higher than the *expected reward* of the true road path. (See [21] for a discussion of the different ways the problem can be specified and how this affects the exact form of the order parameter.) For the road tracking task (with the problem specification given above) the *order parameter* $K = D(P_{on}||P_{off}) + D(P_{\Delta G}||U) - H(U)$. (In other words, K is the sum of the Kullback-Leibler distances $D(P_{on}||P_{off}) = \log\{\sum_y P_{on}(y) \log\{P_{on}(y)/P_{off}(y)\}$ and $D(P_{\Delta G}||U)$ minus the entropy $H(U)$ of the uniform distribution.) The smaller these two distances the harder the problem becomes. Intuitively, the better the local edge cues – as evaluated by $D(P_{on}||P_{off})$ – and the more prior knowledge we have of the geometry – as measured by $D(P_{\Delta g}||U) - H(U)$, the easier it is to detect the true road path. For example, the easiest road to detect is one that is known to be perfectly straight (which makes $D(P_{\Delta g}||U) - H(U) = 0$) and for which the local edge cues are unambiguous (i.e. $D(P_{on}||P_{off}) \mapsto \infty$).

Technically, the proofs of Yuille and Coughlan [21] involve adapting techniques from information theory, such as Sanov's theorem, which were developed to bound the probability of rare events occurring [6]. For the road tracking problem, a rare event would be when a subpath in the background noise/clutter has greater reward than a subpath of the true road – i.e. looks more like a road. The proofs are fairly complicated [21] but we give some of the basic ingredients in the appendix. We note that related techniques are mentioned in the chapter by Nadal.

All these results, however, assumed that there was a fixed geometric prior model. What happens if we use a weaker *generic* prior for the reasons specified in the introduction? (I.e. we may not know the true prior and/or it may be easier to compute with the wrong prior). How badly do our results degrade? Suppose we have several types of roads and we do not know which one we should be looking for – can we get away with using a simple generic prior to detect these different types of road simultaneously? We now address these issues.

High-Level and Generic Models

Suppose we have a single high-level model for a road with a *high level* geometric prior $P_H(\Delta x)$. Let us assume a weaker *generic* prior $P_G(\Delta x)$. We can define two different rewards R_G and R_H:

$$R_G(\{x_i\}) = \sum_i \log \frac{P_{on}(y_{(x_i)})}{P_{off}(y_i)} + \sum_i \log \frac{P_G(\Delta x_i)}{U(\Delta x_i)},$$

$$R_H(\{x_i\}) = \sum_i \log \frac{P_{on}(y_{(x_i)})}{P_{off}(y_i)} + \sum_i \log \frac{P_H(\Delta x_i)}{U(\Delta x_i)}. \tag{7.3}$$

The optimal Bayesian strategy to search for the road would be to use the high level model and evaluate paths based on their rewards R_H. But this strategy ignores the computation time involved in using the prior P_H. For example, P_H might be a second or higher order model while P_G might be a first order Markov model (which would be easier to search over). Also, we might not know the exact form of P_H. Perhaps the most important situation, to be considered in a later section, is when we can use a single generic model to search for a target which may be one of several different models. Using a single generic model (provided it is powerful enough) to detect the road can be significantly faster than testing each possible road model in turn.

But how "weak" should the generic prior P_G be? One possibility is that P_G is an approximation to P_H. Such a situation will often arise when we do not know the true prior distribution of a target. If P_G is just a minor perturbation of P_H then standard analysis shows that the concavity of the Bayes risk means the system will be stable to such perturbations. A more important case arises when P_G *is a poor approximation to* P_H. In what regimes can we get away with using a poor approximation? We will give results for this case.

A more interesting form of "weakness" is when the generic prior P_G is a projection of the high-level prior P_H onto a simpler class of probability distributions. This allows us to formulate the idea of a hierarchy in which the priors for several high-level objects would all project onto the identical low-level prior (see figure (7.5)). For example, we might have a set of priors $\{P_{H_i} : i = 1, ..., M\}$ for different members of the cat family. There might then be a generic prior P_G onto which all the $\{P_{H_i}\}$ project and which is considered the embodiment of "cattiness".

In this chapter, for ease of exposition, we will restrict ourselves to the special case when the P_H are related to P_G by the *Amari condition*:

$$\sum_x P_H(x) \log P_G(x) = \sum_x P_G(x) \log P_G(x). \tag{7.4}$$

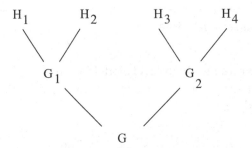

Figure 7.5: The Hierarchy. Two high-level models H_1, H_2 "project" onto a low-level generic model P_{G_1}. In situations with limited clutter, it will be possible to detect either H_1 or H_2 using the single generic model P_{G_1}. This idea can be extended to have hierarchies of projections. This is analogous to the superordinate, basic level, and subordinate levels of classification used in cognitive psychology.

This condition is important because it often arises in Amari's theory of information geometry [1] (though the same condition can arise in other completely unrelated situations). In information geometry, we consider families of probabilities distributions which are called *exponential distributions*. These distributions are specified by the values of *sufficient statistics* (the simplest examples are Gaussian distributions where the sufficient statistics correspond to the mean and variance of the distribution). The set of exponential distributions defined by a specified class of sufficient statistics form a sub-manifold in probability space (in the information geometry perspective) where points of the submanifold correspond to specific distributions indexed by particular values of the sufficient statistics (e.g. the set of Gaussian distributions forms a submanifold where each point corresponds to a particular Gaussian specified by its mean and variance). Within this geometrical framework one can approximate a given distribution by *projecting it down onto an exponential submanifold* (see figure (7.6)). This projection is governed by equation (7.4), where P_H is the original distribution and P_G is its best projection onto a specified submanifold.

In vision, an important example of this arises in the minimax entropy criterion used in the learning theory developed by Zhu, Wu, Mumford [24]. This can be interpreted in terms of information geometry and projections onto exponential submanifolds [4]. More precisely, Minimax Entropy learning naturally gives rise to a sequence of increasingly accurate Gibbs distributions (figure (7.6)) by pursuing additional features and statistics $p_0 = U, p_1, p_2, ..., p_k \rightarrow p_{\text{true}}$ where k is the number of features and statistics included in the model p_k. The sequence starts with p_0 being a uniform distribution U and approaches the true distribution p_{true} in the limit [24]. Each distribution p_i is an Amari projection of the distributions p_j for $j > i$. Moreover, there is a close connection between the goodness of a minimax entropy learning model and its corresponding order parameter (see [23]).

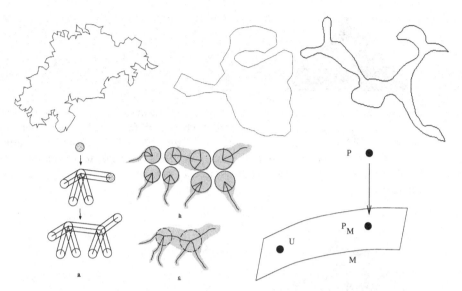

Figure 7.6: The *Amari projection* and a sequence of prior models for animate object shapes by minimax entropy using an increasing number of feature statistics. See text for interpretation.

The Order Parameters

We use the techniques outlined in the "Fundamental limits" section to calculate the order parameters. These calculations are variants of those used in [21] and are too lengthy to include here. (More details appear in [23]).

We assume the generic prior P_G is obtained from a high-level prior P_H by Amari projection. For reasons of space, we also use this example to illustrate what happens if we use a "poor" approximation to the true high-level model. We consider using the generic reward R_G and the high-level reward R_H. The criterion is to determine the probability that *a ghost* (a fluctuation of off-road pixels) will have higher reward than the *expected true path reward* under either of the two rewards. We obtain order parameters K_H^A, K_G^A for the high-level and generic rewards respectively (the superscript A refers to Amari):

$$K_H^A = D(P_{on}||P_{off}) + D(P_H||U) - \log Q,$$
$$K_G^A = D(P_{on}||P_{off}) + D(P_G||U) - \log Q. \tag{7.5}$$

It follows from the definition of Amari projection that $K_H^A - K_G^A = D(P_H||U) - D(P_G||U) = D(P_H||P_G)$ (where $D(P||Q) = \sum_y P(y)\log P(y)/Q(y)$ is the *Kullback-Leibler* divergence between distributions $P(y)$ and $Q(y)$). Therefore the high-level prior P_H has a bigger order parameter by an amount which depends on the dis-

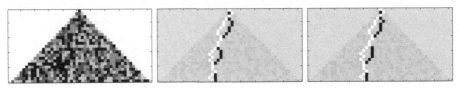

Figure 7.7: The Ultra Regime $K_H^G < K_G^A < 0$. Left, the input image. Centre, the true path is shown in white and the *errors* of the best path found using the Generic model are shown in black. Right, similarly for the High-Level model. Observe that although the best paths found are close to the true path there is comparatively little overlap. A dynamic programming algorithm was used to determine the best solution for either choice of reward.

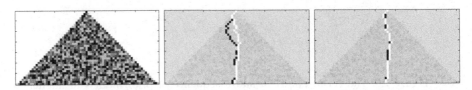

Figure 7.8: The Challenging Regime $K_G^A < 0 < K_H^A$. Same conventions as previous figure. Observe that the Generic models fails (centre) but the High-Level model succeeds (right).

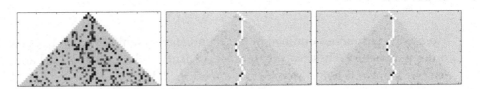

Figure 7.9: The Easy Regime $0 < K_G^A < K_H^A$. Same conventions as previous figure. In this regime both the Generic (centre) and High-Level (right) models succeed.

tance between it and P_G as measured by the Kullback-Leibler divergence $D(P_H \| P_G)$. Recall [21] that the target detection problem becomes insolvable (by any algorithm) when the order parameter is less than zero. Hence, there are three regimes: (I) The *Ultra Regime* (figure (7.7)) is when $K_G^A < K_H^A < 0$ (i.e. $D(P_H \| U) + D(P_{on} \| P_{off}) < \log Q$) and the problem cannot be solved (on average) by any model (or algorithm). (II) The *Challenging Regime* (figure (7.8)) where $K_G^A < 0 < K_H^A$ (i.e. $\log Q < D(P_H \| U) + D(P_{on} \| P_{off}) < \log Q + D(P_H \| P_G)$) within which the problem can be solved by the high-level model but not by the generic model. (III) The *Easy Regime* (figure (7.9)) where $K_H^A > K_G^A > 0$ and the problem can be solved by either the generic or the high-level model.

In our simulations (figures (7.7,7.8,7.9)), we *generate* the target true paths by *stochastic sampling from the high level model*. To *detect* the best path we apply a dynamic programming algorithm to optimize the high-level or generic reward functions applied to the generated data. Dynamic programming is guaranteed to find the solution with highest reward.

Multiple Hypotheses and Higher-Order Markov Models

We now apply our theory to deal with multiple (two or more) high-level models and with high-level models defined by second-order Markov chains.

The prototypical case for two, or more, high-level models is illustrated in figure (7.10). High-level model H_1 prefers roads which move to the right (see the white paths in the left hand panels of figure (7.10)) while high-level model H_2 likes roads moving to the left (see white paths in the right panels). Both models H_1 and H_2 *project to the same generic model G*, by Amari projection, and thus form part of a hierarchy (see figure (7.5)). Our theory again enables us to calculate order parameters and identify three regimes: (I) The Ultra Regime where none of the models (H_1, H_2 or G) can find the target. (II) The Challenging Regime where the high-level models H_1, H_2 can find targets generated by H_1 and H_2 *respectively* but the generic model G cannot find either. (III) The Easy Regime where all the models can locate the targets effectively. Once again, the best paths for the different rewards was found using dynamic programming (which is guaranteed to find the global solution).

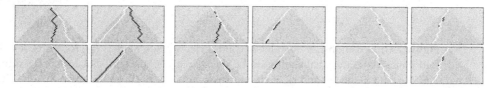

Figure 7.10: Two High-Level models H_1, H_2. Three sets of four panels for Ultra, Challenging, and Easy regimes (left to right). For each of the three sets, the data in the left and right columns is generated by H_1 and H_2 respectively. The upper rows gives the solutions found by the Generic model and the lower rows give the solutions found by the High-Level model (H_1 or H_2 as appropriate) with the true paths (white) and the errors of the best paths (black). Observe that all models give poor results in the Ultra regime (left panel). In the Challenging regime (centre panel) we get good results for the High-Level models and significantly poorer results for the Generic. The rightmost panel (same conventions) demonstrate the effectiveness of all models in the Easy regime.

In the Easy Regime, little is gained by using the two high-level models. It may indeed be more computationally efficient to use the generic model to detect the target. The target could then be classified as being H_1 or H_2 in a subsequent classification stage. We will discuss computational tradeoffs of these two approaches in the next section.

We now repeat this example using high-level models H_3, H_4 defined by second order Markov chains (see figure (7.11)). This second order property allows us to obtain more interesting models. For example, model H_3 generates very wiggly roads ("English" roads) (see left panel of figure (7.11)) while model H_4 generates roads that have long straight sections with occasional sharp changes in direction ("Roman" roads, see right hand panels). It is straightforward to compute order parameters for these models (the second-order Markov property requires slight modifications to the earlier calculations) and, as before, we get order parameters which specify the three standard Ultra, Challenging, and Easy regimes – see figure (7.11). In this figure, we point out a fluke where the high-level model H_4 correctly found the target even in the Ultra Regime. By our theory, this is possible though highly unlikely. Another unlikely outcome is shown in the bottom right panel where the H_4 model has detected the target to *one hundred percent accuracy*. This is reflected in the overall darkness of the panel because, with no black pixels to indicate errors, our graphics package has altered the brightness of the panel (compared to the other panels which do contain black errors). Dynamic programming is used to find the best solutions by global optimization.

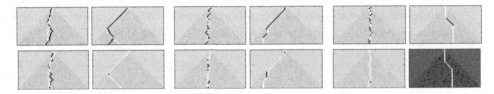

Figure 7.11: Two High-Level models second-order Markov models H_3, H_4. Three sets of four panels for Ultra, Challenging, and Easy regimes (left to right). For each of the three sets, the data in the left and right columns is generated by H_3 and H_4 respectively. The upper rows gives the solutions found by the Generic model and the lower rows give the solutions found by the High-Level model (H_3 or H_4 as appropriate) with the true paths (white) and the errors of the best paths (black). Observe that all models give poor results in the Ultra regime (left panel). In the Challenging regime (centre panel) we get good results for the High-Level models and significantly poorer results for the Generic. The rightmost panel (same conventions) demonstrate the effectiveness of all models in the Easy Regime.

Discussion and Conclusions

This chapter investigated how much prior knowledge is needed to detect a target road in the presence of clutter. We used the concept of order parameters to determine whether a target could be detected using a general purpose "generic" model or whether a more specific high level model was needed. At critical values of the order parameters the problem becomes unsolvable without the addition of extra prior knowledge. We discussed the implication of these results for bottom-up and top-down theories of vision. The analysis can also be extended to yield more precise performance measures which determine the accuracy of the solution [21] and the complexity of A* search algorithms for finding the solution [5].

The results of this chapter were obtained by analysis of the Bayesian ensemble of problem instances where the probability distributions are of the specific form required by Sanov's theorem [6]. More recently, however, more powerful techniques have been used [20], [23] to compute order parameters for other classes of probability distributions, including those learnt by Minimax Entropy learning theory for modelling textures [24]. Similar results on the value of high-level information can be obtained for such distributions [23].

Our work complements the theoretical analysis by Tsotsos on the complexity of visual search [18]. Tsotsos uses techniques from theoretical computer science to prove that certain search tasks can be performed in polynomial time while others are NP-complete (and so presumably have exponential complexity). Our approach differs by relying on probabilistic analysis which takes advantage of the Bayesian formulation of the problem. This naturally leads to a probability distribution on the set of problem instances which enables us to consider the behaviour of the algorithms on typical problem examples (i.e. those which occur with large probability) [5]. By contrast, theoretical computer science generally deals with worst case performance. Interestingly, recent work by Selman and Kirkpatrick [17] investigates the behaviour of algorithms for NP-complete problems, such as 3-SAT, by defining probability distributions on the set of problem instances. They demonstrate that the complexity of the problem changes, on average, as this probability distribution changes. In particular, there are phase transitions at critical values of the parameters which define the probability distributions. This analysis is performed by computer simulations aided by non-rigourous (but often highly effective) statistical physics techniques such as replica calculations. The relationships between this work and our own is a topic for further analysis.

Hopefully, analysis of the type performed in this chapter can help quantify when high-level knowledge is needed to perform visual tasks such as object detection. The key step is to model the problem in terms of Bayesian inference. This enables us to specify the difficulty of the task in terms of the statistics of the domain and the knowledge about the target known to the modeller. Our opinion is that in most real world situations, the full high-level model is not required in order to do segmentation – in other words, we are in the easy domain and simple bottom-up processing may often be sufficient to do tasks such as detection.

Acknowledgments

We want to acknowledge funding from NSF with award number IRI-9700446, from the Center for Imaging Sciences funded by ARO DAAH049510494,from the Smith-Kettlewell core grant, and the AFOSR grant F49620-98-1-0197 to ALY. We thank Mario Ferraro for asking interesting questions which inspired some of this work. Scott Konishi and Song Chun Zhu gave useful feedback.

Appendix

We now briefly sketch how our results are obtained (for more details, see [21] and other references below).

First, recall that we seek to find the path that maximizes the reward given by equation (7.1):

$$R(X) = \sum_i \log \frac{P_{on}(y_{(x_i)})}{P_{off}(y_{(x_i)})} + \sum_i \log \frac{P_{\Delta g}(x_{i+1} - x_i)}{U(x_{i+1} - x_i)}, \tag{7.6}$$

Now consider the *expected reward* for the true road. For this path the geometry X is generated by the distribution $P_G(X) = \prod_{i=1}^{N-1} P_{\Delta g}(x_{i+1} - x_i)$ and the measurements $\{y_{(x_i)}\}$ are generated by the distribution $P_{on}(y)$. Hence, the expected reward for the true path is given by:

$$< R(X) >_{true} = \sum_i \sum_{y_{(x_i)}} P_{on}(y_{(x_i)}) \log \frac{P_{on}(y_{(x_i)})}{P_{off}(y_{(x_i)})} +$$

$$+ \sum_i \sum_{x_{i+1}} P_{\Delta g}(x_{i+1} - x_i) \sum_i \log \frac{P_{\Delta g}(x_{i+1} - x_i)}{U(x_{i+1} - x_i)}$$

$$= ND(P_{on}||P_{off}) + (N-1)D(P_{\Delta g}||U). \tag{7.7}$$

Similarly, the distractor paths have geometry generated by U and observations generated by P_{off} and hence, the expected reward for a distractor path can be computed to be $-ND(P_{off}||P_{on}) - (N-1)D(U||P_{\Delta g})$ (where the minus signs arise because of the form form of the reward function).

Clearly, the expected reward for the true path, $ND(P_{on}||P_{off}) + (N-1)D(P_{\Delta g}||U)$, is larger than the expected reward for any distractor path $-ND(P_{off}||P_{on}) - (N-1)D(U||P_{\Delta g})$ (because Kullback-Leibler distances $D(P||Q)$ are always non-negative and, almost always, positive).

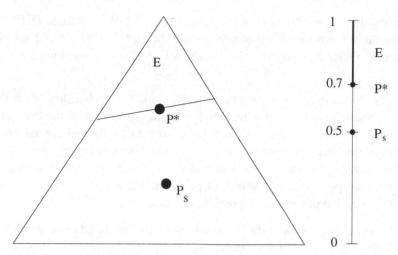

Figure 7.12: Left, Sanov's theorem. The triangle represents the set of probability distributions. P_s is the distribution which generates the samples. Sanov's theorem states that the probability that a type, or empirical distribution, lies within the subset E is chiefly determined by the distribution P^* in E which is closest to P_s. Right, Sanov's theorem for the coin tossing experiment. The set of probabilities is one-dimensional and is labelled by the probability $P_s(head)$ of tossing a head. The unbiased distribution P_s is at the centre, with $P_s(head) = 1/2$, and the closest element of the set E is P^* such that $P^*(head) = 0.7$.

But this analysis has ignored the fluctuations in the rewards. We need to estimate the probability than *any* of the many distractor paths has higher reward than the true road reward (even though each specific distractor path will almost certainly have lower reward). To analyze the effects of fluctuations, we need to appeal to large deviation theory [6] to determine bounds for fluctuations. For the problems considered in this chapter, there are tight bounds which are given by Sanov's theorem.

Sanov's Theorem. *Let $\theta_1, \theta_2, ..., \theta_N$ be i.i.d. from a distribution $Q(\theta)$ with alphabet size J and E be any closed set of probability distributions. Let $Pr(\vec{\phi} \in E)$ be the probability that the type of a sample sequence lies in the set E. Then:*

$$\frac{2^{-ND(\vec{\phi}^*||Q)}}{(N+1)^J} \leq Pr(\vec{\phi} \in E) \leq (N+1)^J 2^{-ND(\vec{\phi}^*||Q)}, \tag{7.8}$$

where $\vec{\phi}^* = \arg\min_{\vec{\phi} \in E} D(\vec{\phi}||Q)$ is the distribution in E that is closest to Q in terms of Kullback-Leibler divergence.

Sanov's theorem can be illustrated by a simple coin tossing example (figure (7.12)). Suppose we have a fair coin and want to estimate the probability of observing more than 700 heads in 1000 tosses. Then, set E is the set of probability distributions for which $P(head) \geq 0.7$ ($P(head) + P(tails) = 1$). The distribution generating the samples is $P_s(head) = P_s(tails) = 1/2$ because the coin is fair. The distribution in

E closest to P_s is $P^*(head) = 0.7, P^*(tails) = 0.3$. We calculate $D(P^*||P_s) = 0.119$. Substituting into Sanov's theorem, setting the alphabet size $J = 2$, we calculate that the probability of more than 700 heads in 1000 tosses is less than $2^{-119} \times (1001)^2 \leq 2^{-99}$.

Sanov's theorem can be applied to determine the probability of rare events, such as the chances that a distractor path has higher reward than the true path (see [21]). In other words, the subset E can be chosen to be the set for which this occurs. To determine the changes that *any* distractor path has higher reward than the true path we make use of Boole's inequality combined with Sanov's theorem. (Boole's inequality appears in any standard probability text book and puts a bound on the probability that one or many possible events occurs).

To apply Sanov's theorem to the case of High-Level and generic priors, we simply redefine our set E so that it corresponds to the appropriate choice of reward function (i.e. E could be chosen to be the set for which the generic reward for a distractor path is higher than the generic reward for the true path). Then, Sanov's theorem can be applied to determined probability bounds as before.

References

[1]   S. Amari. "Differential Geometry of curved exponential families – Curvature and information loss. Annals of Statistics, vol. 10, no. 2, pp 357-385. 1982.

[2]   J.J. Atick and A.N. Redlich. "What does the retina know about natural scenes?" *Neural Computation*, vol. 4: pp 196-210. 1992.

[3]   James M. Coughlan, A.L. Yuille, D. Snow and C. English. "Efficient Optimization of a Deformable Template Using Dynamic Programming". In *Proceedings Computer Vision and Pattern Recognition. CVPR'98. Santa Barbara. California.* 1998.

[4]   James M. Coughlan and A.L. Yuille. "A Phase Space Approach to Minimax Entropy Learning". In *Proceedings of NIPS98.* 1998.

[5]   James M. Coughlan and A.L. Yuille. "Bayesian A* tree search with expected O(N) convergence rates for road tracking". In *Proceedings EMMCVPR'99.* Springer-Verlag Lecture Notes in Computer Science 1654. 1999.

[6]   T.M. Cover and J.A. Thomas. *Elements of Information Theory.* Wiley Interscience Press. New York. 1991.

[7]   D. Geiger and T-L Liu. "Top-Down Recognition and Bottom-Up Integration for Recognizing Articulated Objects". In *EMMCVPR'97.* Ed. M. Pellilo and E. Hancock. Springer-Verlag. CS 1223. 1997.

[8]   D. Geman. and B. Jedynak. "An active testing model for tracking roads in satellite images". *IEEE Trans. Patt. Anal. and Machine Intel.* Vol. 18. No. 1, pp

1-14. January. 1996.

[9]   U. Grenander, *Lectures in Pattern Theory I, II, and III: Pattern Analysis, Pattern Synthesis and Regular Structures.* Springer-Verlag. Berlin. 1976.

[10] M. Kass, A. Witkin, and D. Terzopoulos. "Snakes: Active Contour models". In *Proc. 1st Int. Conf. on Computer Vision.* 259-268. 1987.

[11] D. Kersten. "Statistical Limits to Image Understanding". In *Computational Models of Visual Processing*, Eds. M. Landy and A. Movshon. MIT Press: Cambridge, MA. 1990.

[12] D.C. Knill and W. Richards. (Eds). *Perception as Bayesian Inference.* Cambridge University Press. 1996.

[13] S. M. Konishi, A.L. Yuille, J.M. Coughlan and Song Chun Zhu. "Fundamental Bounds on Edge Detection: An Information Theoretic Evaluation of Different Edge Cues." In *Proceedings Computer Vision and Pattern Recognition CVPR'99.* Fort Collins, Colorado. 1999.

[14] D. Marr. *Vision.* W.H. Freeman: San Francisco, CA. 1982.

[15] D. Mumford. "Neuronal Architecture for Pattern-theoretic Problems". In *Large-Scale Neuronal Theories of the Brain.* Eds. C. Koch and J.L. Davis. (2nd edition). A Bradford Book. The MIT Press: Cambridge, MA. 1995.

[16] R.P.N. Rao and D.H. Ballard. "Dynamic Model of Visual Recognition Predicts Neural Response Properties in the Visual Cortex." *Neural Computation.* Vol. 9. No. 4. pp 721-734. 1997.

[17] B. Selman and S. Kirkpatrick. "Critical Behaviour in the Computational Cost of Satisfiability Testing". Artificial Intelligence. 81(1-2); 273-295. 1996.

[18] J.K. Tsotsos. "Analyzing Vision at the Complexity Level". *Behavioural and Brain Sciences.* Vol. 13, No. 3. September. 1990.

[19] S. Ullman. "Sequence Seeking and Counterstreams: A Model for Bidirectional Information Flow in the Cortex". In *Large-Scale Neuronal Theories of the Brain.* Eds. C. Koch and J.L. Davis. (2nd edition). A Bradford Book. The MIT Press: Cambridge, MA. 1995.

[20] Y. Wu and S.C. Zhu. "Equivalence of Image Ensembles and Fundamental Bounds". International Journal of Computer Vision (Marr Prize special issue). To appear. 2000.

[21] A. L. Yuille and James M. Coughlan. "Fundamental Limits of Bayesian Inference: Order Parameters and Phase Transitions for Road Tracking." *IEEE Transactions on Pattern Analysis and Machine Intelligence* (PAMI). Vol. 22. No. 2. February. 2000.

[22] A.L. Yuille and James M. Coughlan. "High-Level and Generic Models for Visual Search: When does high level knowledge help?" In *Proceedings Computer Vision and Pattern Recognition CVPR'99.* Fort Collins, Colorado. 1999.

[23] A.L. Yuille, J.M. Coughlan, Y. Wu and S.C. Zhu. "Order Parameters for Mini-

max Entropy Distributions: When does high level knowledge help?". To appear in *Proceedings Computer Vision and Patern Recognition*. CVPR'2000. Hilton Head, South Carolina. June, 2000.

[24]   S-C Zhu, Y-N Wu and D. Mumford. FRAME: Filters, Random field And Maximum Entropy. Int'l Journal of Computer Vision 27(2) 1-20, March/April. 1998.

[25]   S.C.Zhu, "Embedding Gestalt Laws in Markov random fields". *IEEE Trans. on Pattern Analysis and Machine Intelligence*, PAMI. Vol. 21, No.11, pp 1170-1187, Nov, 1999.

8 Sparse Correlation Kernel Reconstruction and Superresolution

Constantine P. Papageorgiou, Federico Girosi, and Tomaso Poggio

Introduction

This chapter presents a new paradigm for signal reconstruction and compression that is based on the selection of a sparse set of bases from a large dictionary of class-specific basis functions. In our case, the basis functions we use are derived from the correlation functions of the class of images we are analyzing. The concept of sparsity enforces the requirement that, given a certain reconstruction error, we should choose the smallest subset of basis functions that yields a reconstruction with this error. The problem of signal reconstruction is formulated as one where we are given only a small, possibly unevenly sampled, subset of points in a signal where the goal is to accurately reconstruct the entire signal. We also investigate a closely related subject, lossy compression, that is, given an entire signal of N bits, we see how well we can represent the signal with only $M \ll N$ bits of information, using the same general technique. For an expanded version of this chapter that includes supplemental appendices, see Papageorgiou *et al.*, 1998 (available at ftp://publications.ai.mit.edu/ai-publications/1500-1999/AIM-1635.ps).

The signal approximation problem we present assumes that we have prior information about the class of signals we are reconstructing or compressing; this information is in the form of the correlation function of the class of signals to which this signal belongs, as defined by a representative set of signals from this class (Penev and Atick, 1996; Poggio and Girosi, 1998a; Poggio and Girosi, 1998b). For this chapter, the signals that we will be looking at are images of pedestrians (Papageorgiou, 1997; Oren *et al.*, 1997; Papageorgiou *et al.*, 1998). Using an initial set of pedestrian images, we compute the correlation function and use the pointwise-defined functions as the dictionary of basis functions from which we can reconstruct subsequent out-of-sample images of pedestrians. Our choice of using the correlation kernel can be motivated from a Bayesian point of view. We show that, if we assume a Gaussian noise process on our measurements, the kernel to use, in a Bayesian sense, is the correlation kernel.

To approximate or reconstruct an image, rather than using the entire set of correlation based basis functions comprising the dictionary – this would result in no compression whatsoever – we choose a small subset of the kernels via the criteria of sparsity. We obtain a sparse representation by approximating the signal using the Support Vector Machine (SVM) (Boser, Guyon, and Vapnik, 1992; Vapnik, 1995) formulation of the regression problem. Based on recently reported results (Girosi, 1997; Girosi, 1998), we note that this framework is equivalent to using a modified version of the Basis Pursuit De-Noising (BPDN) approach of Chen, Donoho, and Saunders (1995) to obtaining a sparse representation of a signal.

We push this paradigm further by investigating the use of dictionaries of multiscale basis functions that encode different levels of detail. To obtain a sparse, multiscale approximation of a signal, we use BPDN; this leads to improved reconstruction error and a more sparse representation. We also show that the empirical results highlight a drawback in using traditional formulations of sparsity.

The results presented in this chapter can be useful in low-bandwidth videoconferencing, image de-noising, reconstruction in the presence of occlusions, signal approximation from sparse data, as well as in superresolving images. It is important to note that the results are not particular to image analysis; this technique can also be seen as an alternative to traditional means of function approximation and signal reconstruction, such as Principal Components Analysis (PCA), for a wider class of signals.

The chapter is organized as follows: We first introduce generalized correlation kernels, followed by Bayesian motivation for our choice of kernels. We then describe the concept of sparsity and present both the SVM regression and BPDN formulations of this approach. We present results of several image reconstruction experiments using this technique for sparse approximations with the generalized correlation kernels and describe a superresolution reconstruction experiment. We also present results of image compression experiments and a comparison between SVM and BPDN on this task. We then show results of experiments that use a dictionary with basis functions at multiple scales to do lossy image compression using BPDN. We conclude by discussing the error norms that our different reconstruction techniques use and their psychophysical plausibility. The final section summarizes our results and presents several observations and open questions.

Generalized Correlation Kernels

To reconstruct or compress a function f, we use information about the class of point-wise mean-normalized signals that f is a part of, derived from a set of representative examples from that class. This information is in the form of the correlation function of the signals in the class:

$$R(\mathbf{x}, \mathbf{y}) = E[(f_\alpha(\mathbf{x}) - \mu(\mathbf{x}))(f_\alpha(\mathbf{y}) - \mu(\mathbf{y}))] \qquad (8.1)$$

where f_α are instances of the class of functions to which f belongs, $\mathbf{x}$ and $\mathbf{y}$ are coordinates in the 2-dimensional signal, and μ are the point means across the class of functions: $\mu(\mathbf{x}) = E[f_\alpha(\mathbf{x})]$.

We can also generate the eigen-decomposition of the symmetric, positive definite correlation matrix by solving

$$\int d\mathbf{x} R(\mathbf{x}, \mathbf{y}) \phi_n(\mathbf{x}) = \lambda_n \phi_n(\mathbf{y}) \qquad (8.2)$$

where ϕ_n are the eigenvectors and λ_n are the eigenvalues of the system[1]. After generating this decomposition, we can write R in the form,

$$R(\mathbf{x}, \mathbf{y}) = \sum_{n=1}^{M} \lambda_n \phi_n(\mathbf{x}) \phi_n(\mathbf{y}) \qquad (8.3)$$

where $M \leq \infty$; this result is due to the spectral theorem.

The set of functions ϕ_n are ordered with decreasing positive eigenvalue λ_n and are normalized to form an orthonormal basis for the correlation function of f_α. The classical Principal Component Analysis (PCA) approach approximates a function f as a linear combination of a finite number, M', of the basis functions ϕ_n:

$$f(\mathbf{x}) = \sum_{n=1}^{M'} b_n \phi_n(\mathbf{x}) \qquad (8.4)$$

where the coefficients b_i are determined so as to minimize the L_2 approximation error of f.

---

1. Estimating the correlation function is in general non-trivial; we ignore numerical issues here.

Poggio and Girosi (1998a) show that the correlation function R, which is positive definite, induces a Reproducing Kernel Hilbert Space (RKHS) that allows us to approximate the function f as:

$$f(\mathbf{x}) = \sum_{i=1}^{N} c_i R(\mathbf{x}, \mathbf{x}_i) \tag{8.5}$$

where i ranges over pixel locations in the image; R is the reproducing kernel in this space and the norm is:

$$\|f\|_R^2 = \sum_{n=1}^{M} \frac{c_n^2}{\lambda_n} \tag{8.6}$$

We can obtain a wider class of kernels spanning exactly the same space of functions as the correlation function in Equation 8.3 by varying the degree of λ_n, which in effect controls the prior information regarding the strength of each eigenfunction, an observation due to Penev and Atick (1996). We therefore define the *generalized correlation kernel* as:

$$R_d(\mathbf{x}, \mathbf{y}) = \sum_{n=1}^{M} (\lambda_n)^d \phi_n(\mathbf{x}) \phi_n(\mathbf{y}) \tag{8.7}$$

and notice that the parameter d controls the locality of the kernel; for small d, R_d approaches a delta function in the space of ϕ_n, and as d gets larger, R_d gets smoother[2].

Each of these correlation kernels is a function in four variables (x_1, x_2, y_1, y_2) so, to effectively visualize them, we hold the x_1 and x_2 positions constant and vary y_1 and y_2. Figure 8.1 shows several examples of the kernels generated with varying d, for a set of 924 grey-level 128×64 images of pedestrians that have been normalized to the same scale and position; this database has been used in Papageorgiou (1997), Oren *et al.* (1997), and Papageorgiou *et al.* (1998). Each column shows $R_d((x_1 = a, x_2 = b), \mathbf{y})$ for an image where, from the top to bottom rows, $d = 0.0$, $d = 0.5$, and $d = 1.0$; for example, the first column shows the kernels for $R_d((11, 10), \mathbf{y})$. The progressive delocalization of the kernels when d is varied from 0.0 to 1.0 is evident in these figures.

---

2. This particular parameterization is one of many possibilities.

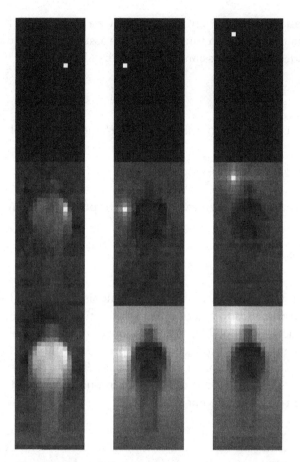

Figure 8.1: Examples of the correlation kernels we can compute. Each column shows the kernels, $R_d((x_1 = a, x_2 = b), \mathbf{y})$, for a specific (a, b) where $d = 0.0$, $d = 0.5$, and $d = 1.0$ in the top, middle, and bottom rows, respectively. These images demonstrate that $d = 1.0$ corresponds to a very smooth kernel, while $d = 0.0$ is highly localized.

Bayesian Motivation

Our choice of the correlation function, R, as the kernel can be motivated from a Bayesian perspective; see Wahba (1990) and Poggio and Girosi (1998a) for background material. Consider the general regularization problem:

$$\min_{f \in \mathcal{H}} H[f] = \sum_{i=1}^{N} (y_i - f(\mathbf{x}_i))^2 + \gamma \|f\|_K^2 \tag{8.8}$$

In a Bayesian interpretation, the data term is a model of the noise and the stabilizer is a prior on the regression function f. If we assume that the data, y_i, are affected by additive independent gaussian noise, then the likelihood has the following form:

$$P(\mathbf{y}|f) \propto e^{-\sum_{i=1}^{N}(y_i - f(\mathbf{x}_i))^2} \tag{8.9}$$

and, when we use the correlation kernel R, the prior probability is:

$$P(f) \propto e^{-\|f\|_R^2} \propto e^{-\sum_{n=1}^{M} \frac{c_n^2}{\lambda_n}} \tag{8.10}$$

where $M < \infty$. As shown earlier, this corresponds to a representation of the form:

$$f(\mathbf{x}) = \sum_{n=1}^{M} c_n \phi_n(\mathbf{x}) \tag{8.11}$$

Thus, the stabilizer measures the Mahalanobis distance of f from the mean signal. This also corresponds to a zero mean multivariate Gaussian density on the Hilbert space of functions defined by R and spanned by ϕ_n, e.g., the space spanned by the principal components introduced in the previous section. From a Bayesian point of view, under the assumption of gaussian noise, R is the right kernel to use, whenever it is available. It is important to note that in our SVM and BPDN formulations, we use gaussian priors but do not assume gaussian additive noise in the data.

Sparsity

The operational definition of a sparse representation in the context of regression that we will use is the smallest subset of elements from a large dictionary of features such that a linear superposition of these features can effectively reconstruct the original signal. In this chapter, we will focus on sparse representations using the correlation kernels introduced in the previous section:

$$f(\mathbf{x}) = \sum_{i=1}^{N'} c_i R(\mathbf{x}, \mathbf{x}_i) \tag{8.12}$$

where N' is smaller than the size of the signal.

Suppose that we have a large dictionary of core building blocks for a class of signals we are analyzing. Given a new signal of the same class, obtaining a sparse representation of this signal amounts to choosing the smallest subset of building blocks from the dictionary that will allow us to achieve a certain level of performance.

It is important to note that comparing representations for sparsity is only fair for a given performance criterion.

Here, we present a brief introduction to the concepts of Support Vector Machine regression and Basis Pursuit De-Noising as they apply to sparse representations; for a more in depth treatment of these subjects, the reader is referred to (Boser, Guyon, and Vapnik, 1992; Vapnik, 1995; Burges, 1998; Chen, Donoho, and Saunders, 1995; Girosi, 1997; Girosi, 1998).

Support vector machine regression

Given a kernel K that defines a RKHS and with the appropriate choice of the scalar product induced by K, the empirical risk minimization regularization theory framework suggests to minimize the following functional:

$$H[f] = \frac{1}{N} \sum_{i=1}^{N} \| z_i - f(\mathbf{x}_i) \|_{L_2}^2 + \gamma \|f\|_K^2 \tag{8.13}$$

where $\|f\|_K^2$ is as previously defined. This corresponds to minimizing the sum of the empirical error measured in L_2 and a smoothness functional. The Support Vector Machine regression formulation minimizes a similar functional, differing only in the norm on the data term; instead of using the L_2 norm, the following ϵ-insensitive error function, called the L_ϵ norm, is used:

$$|z_i - f(\mathbf{x}_i)|_\epsilon = \begin{cases} 0 & \text{if } |z_i - f(\mathbf{x}_i)| < \epsilon \\ |z_i - f(\mathbf{x}_i)| - \epsilon & otherwise \end{cases} \tag{8.14}$$

The functional that is minimized is therefore:

$$H[f] = \frac{1}{N} \sum_{i=1}^{N} |z_i - f(\mathbf{x}_i)|_\epsilon + \gamma \|f\|_K^2 \tag{8.15}$$

yielding a function of the form:

$$f(\mathbf{x}) = \sum_{i=1}^{N'} c_i R(\mathbf{x}, \mathbf{x}_i) \tag{8.16}$$

where the coefficients c are obtained by solving a quadratic programming problem (Vapnik, 1995; Osuna, Freund, and Girosi, 1997; Girosi, 1997). Depending on the value of the sparsity parameter γ, the number of c_i that differ from zero will be smaller than

N; the data points associated with the non-zero coefficients are called *support vectors* and it is these support vectors that comprise our sparse approximation.

Basis pursuit de-noising

The Basis Pursuit De-Noising approach of Chen, Donoho, and Saunders (1995) is a means of decomposing a signal into a small number of constituent dictionary elements. The functional that is minimized consists of an error term and a sparsity term and in the case of arbitrary basis functions, ϕ_i, is:

$$E[\mathbf{c}] = \|f(\mathbf{x}) - \sum_{i=1}^{N} c_i \phi_i(\mathbf{x}_i)\|_{L_2}^2 + \lambda\|\mathbf{c}\|_{L_1} \tag{8.17}$$

In our case, to sparsify Equation 8.12, the following functional must be minimized (Girosi, 1997; Girosi, 1998):

$$E[\mathbf{c}] = \|f(\mathbf{x}) - \sum_{i=1}^{N} c_i R(\mathbf{x}, \mathbf{x}_i)\|_{L_2}^2 + \lambda\|\mathbf{c}\|_{L_1} \tag{8.18}$$

yielding an approximation to f that has a similar form to Equation 8.16. Girosi (1997) shows that if, instead of the L_2 norm, we use the norm induced by R, then Basis Pursuit De-Noising is in fact equivalent to Support Vector Machine regression and identical sparse representations are obtained.

This function minimization is formulated as a quadratic programming problem (see Appendix A in Papageorgiou *et al.*, 1998) and can be solved using traditional methods. Appendix B in Papageorgiou *et al.*, 1998 presents a decomposition algorithm that allows us to quickly solve this minimization problem even when we have a large dictionary of basis functions.

Reconstruction

In the case of image reconstruction and compression when we do not assume any prior knowledge (other than that we are considering images), we can use techniques like JPEG, wavelets, and regularization using a spline or gaussian kernel. The focus of this chapter is regularization schemes for the case where we do have statistical information on the class of functions we are reconstructing. When we do have such knowledge, as in the case of the correlational structure of the class to which the image to be compressed belongs, we may be able to obtain better compression by using this information. As described in the introductory sections, we can use the set of basis functions that encode the correlational structure of the class of images we are interesed in reconstructing. For a given image that we would like to approximate, we use these *class-specific* basis functions in the SVM formulation to obtain a sparse subset with which we can encode the image.

The generalized correlation kernels are generated from a training set of 924 grey-level 32×16 images of pedestrians that have been normalized to the same scale and position. We test the correlation kernels and the SVM formulation of function approximation by analyzing the reconstruction of pedestrian images not in the training set and comparing to the widely used PCA technique. The test database of pedestrian images consists of 50 out-of-sample 32×16 grey-level images of frontal and rear views of pedestrians; as in the training set, these images have been normalized such that the pedestrian bodies are aligned in the center of the image and are scaled to the same size.

For the SVM experiments, we use the correlation kernel corresponding to $d = 1.0$ as our dictionary of basis functions, so the reconstructed signal will be a sparse linear combination of those basis functions:

$$R_{1.0}(\mathbf{x}, \mathbf{y}) = \sum_{n=1}^{M} \lambda_n \phi_n(\mathbf{x}) \phi_n(\mathbf{y}) \tag{8.19}$$

To accurately test the reconstruction performance, we need to measure the ability of the technique to reconstruct unseen data and not simply fit the data. For each image in the test set, we randomly partition the pixels into a set that has M pixels – the input set, F_{input} – and a set consisting of the remaining $(N - M)$ pixels – the test set, F_{test}.

In the case of the SVM, to find the sparse set of basis functions that minimizes the error over the input subset, F_{input}, we obtain the coefficients of reconstruction by minimizing:

$$H[f] = \frac{1}{M} \sum_{i=1}^{M} |F_{input}(\mathbf{x}_i) - f(\mathbf{x}_i)|_{\epsilon}^{2} + \frac{1}{C} \|f\|_{K}^{2} \tag{8.20}$$

where,

$$f(\mathbf{x}) = \sum_{i=1}^{M} c_i R(\mathbf{x}, \mathbf{x}_i) \tag{8.21}$$

The portion of the coefficients, c_i, that will be 0 is determined by the variable C.

For PCA-based reconstruction, we minimize L_2 error over F_{input}:

$$\min_c \sum_{i=1}^{M} \|F_{input}(\mathbf{x}_i) - \sum_{j=1}^{N} c_j \phi_j(\mathbf{x}_i)\|_{L_2}^2 \tag{8.22}$$

where c_j is given by the dot product between F_{input} and ϕ'_j is taken over the M input points:

$$c_j = \langle F_{input}, \phi'_j \rangle \tag{8.23}$$

Out-of-sample performance in each case is determined by reconstructing the full image and measuring the error over the pixels in f_{test}. We measure performance as the error achieved with respect to the number of basis functions used in the above formulations (equivalently, reconstruction error versus the sparsity of the representation). In the case of the SVM regression, the number of basis functions is varied by changing the ϵ parameter. To compare with PCA-based reconstruction, for a given ϵ, we use, as the number of principal components (ie. basis functions) for the reconstruction, the number of support vectors found in the SVM formulation. In our experiments, the size of the input set is varied as $\frac{1}{4}N$, $\frac{1}{2}N$, and $\frac{3}{4}N$; error is measured in L_2.

As a benchmark meant to ensure that the performance of the system using SVM with the correlation kernels is not due exclusively to the SVM machinery, we also show the results using SVM with gaussian kernels, yielding approximations of the form:

$$f(\mathbf{x}) = \sum_{i=1}^{M} c_i e^{\left(\frac{x - x_i}{\sigma}\right)^2} \tag{8.24}$$

where the value of σ is determined empirically over a small set of images and that same σ is used throughout. This setting of sigma for all the tests may be limiting the performance of the SVM with a gaussian kernel; on the other hand, we are also *a priori* fixing the locality parameter, *d*, in our choice of correlation kernel.

The results of these reconstructions, averaged over the 50 out-of-sample images, are shown in Figures 8.2a-c for each case of using $\frac{1}{4}$, $\frac{1}{2}$, and $\frac{3}{4}$ of the pixels as input, respectively. The SVM reconstructions using different numbers of basis functions were generated by varying ϵ. From these performance results, we can see that, even though the PCA formulation minimizes L_2 error and SVM regression is minimizing error in the RKHS induced by the epsilon insensitive norm, SVM performs better than PCA even when measuring error in L_2 over out-of-sample test data. Furthermore, SVM with the correlation kernels performs better than SVM with gaussian kernels, showing that the correlation kernels encode important prior information on the pedestrian

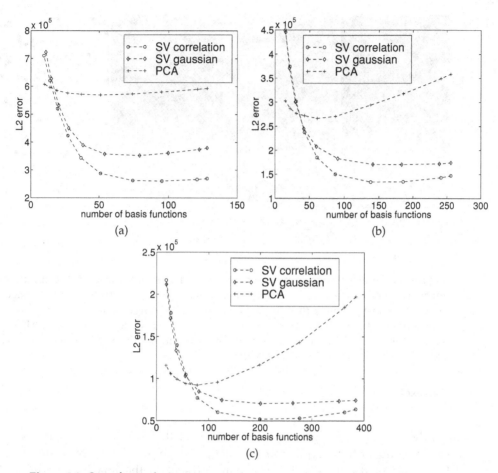

Figure 8.2: Out-of-sample L_2 reconstruction error comparison between SVM with correlation kernel $R_{1.0}$, SVM with gaussian kernel ($\sigma = 3.0$), and PCA, where the input is a random sampling of the original image. Each of these figures represents a different sized sampling, (a) $\frac{1}{4}$ of the image as input, (b) $\frac{1}{2}$ of the image as input, and (c) $\frac{3}{4}$ of the image as input.

class. The difference in performance is most pronounced for the reconstructions that use the smallest input set.

Figure 8.3 presents an extreme case where the input data is a random set of only $\frac{1}{16}$th (6.25%) of the image pixels; here, a higher resolution image (64×32) is used. The SVM reconstruction with correlation kernels recovers more of the structure of the pedestrian than PCA, due to the smoothness preserving properties of the SVM approach to function approximation (Vapnik, 1995).

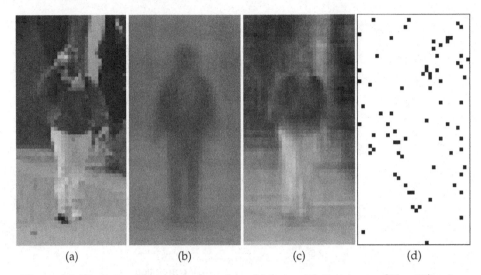

$$(a) \qquad (b) \qquad (c) \qquad (d)$$

Figure 8.3: Reconstruction comparison for a higher resolution image (64 × 32) using identical random sets of $\frac{1}{16}$ th of the original pixels as input; (a) the original image, (b) PCA reconstruction with 74 basis functions, (c) SVM reconstruction with 74 basis functions ($\epsilon = 10$ for the SVM), (d) locations of the support vectors are denoted as black values. With a small subset of the original image as input, the SVM reconstruction is clearly superior to the PCA reconstruction.

Superresolution

To further highlight the generalization power of the SVM reconstruction, we can do an experiment to determine *superresolution* capability, that is, reconstructions at a finer level of detail than was originally present in the image. Superresolution entails approximating a small image with some representation and then sampling that representation at a finer scale to recover the higher resolution image. This could be useful if, for instance, we have an image of a person's face that is too small for us to be able to recognize who it is; after superresolving the image, the details that emerge could allow us to recognize the person.

This is not possible with our generalized correlation kernels since they are discrete kernels generated from high resolution images (64 × 32) and we cannot subsample them. Therefore, to superresolve a given 32 × 16 image, we can consider it as a 64 × 32 image sampled every two pixels in both dimensions and then use the correlation kernel basis functions defined in the high resolution space (64 × 32) to recover the full high resolution image.

As input to the superresolution technique, we take a low resolution 32 × 16 image of a pedestrian and reconstruct it at high resolution (64 × 32). Figure 8.4 shows (a) an example of a 32 × 16 image of a pedestrian that has been directly scaled to 64 × 32 and (b) the true 64 × 32 pedestrian image. These are compared with (c) the

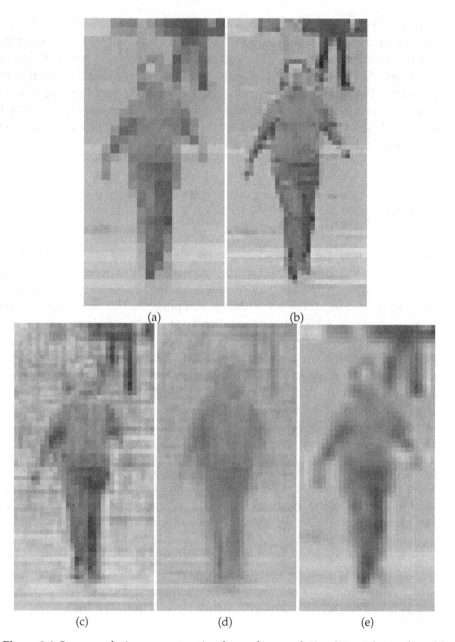

(a)　　　　　　　　(b)

(c)　　　　　　(d)　　　　　　(e)

Figure 8.4: Superresolution reconstruction from a low resolution (32×16) sampling; (a) the input 32×16 image, scaled up to 64×32 by direct scaling, (b) the actual 64×32 image, (c) SVM superresolution reconstruction using 272 basis functions from $R_{1.0}$ ($\epsilon = 10$), (d) PCA superresolution reconstruction using 272 basis functions, and (e) cubic spline interpolation.

superresolved image, reconstructed at 64×32 using the SVM with correlation kernels $R_{1.0}$, compared against both (d) a PCA reconstruction, and (e) a standard cubic spline interpolation reconstruction (Schumaker, 1981). The errors in the SVM reconstruction are 1,530,507, 22,093, and 7,302 (L_2, L_1, and L_ϵ) and for the spline reconstruction are 1,694,091, 23,631, and 7,241 (L_2, L_1, and L_ϵ). We note that here we measure error over the entire output image. Though these are still preliminary results, they indicate that the SVM with correlation kernels may yield a truer superresolved reconstruction than other techniques.

Compression

We can also investigate image *compression* using the set of correlation-based basis functions, in the same manner as the reconstruction experiments presented in the previous section. For the task of compression, the goal is to approximate the entire given signal f using as few basis functions as possible. The experiments are run as before; we compare the SVM regularization approach to compression with our benchmark, PCA-based compression. For the SVM approach, we use the correlation kernel with $d = 1.0$ and compare with using SVM with gaussian kernels. Performance is measured as the error achieved for a given number of basis functions. The number of basis functions that are used in the case of SVM regression are varied by changing the ϵ parameter. As in the reconstruction experiments, the number of eigenvectors we use to compare against PCA-based compression is the number of support vectors for given level of ϵ.

Figure 8.5 plots the reconstruction error against the number of basis functions for three different error norms: L_2, L_1, and L_ϵ. Comparing the SVM and PCA approaches to compression is less conclusive than the reconstruction experiments; the results here depend on the measure of error. PCA performs better when measured in L_2 and L_1 while SVM wins when measured in L_ϵ. The L_2 and L_ϵ results are not surprising; when error is measured in the norm that a technique is minimizing, we would expect that technique to perform better than the others. On the other hand, it is not clear which norm results in a reconstructed image that *appears* more similar to the original image; a later section contains a discussion of the different norms.

Comparing SVM and BPDN

Girosi (1997, 1998) showed that Basis Pursuit De-Noising is equivalent to Support Vector Machines when the L_2 norm in the BPDN formulation is replaced by the norm induced by the regularization kernel. Here, we empirically test the effect of the different error norms in the two approaches by comparing SVM and BPDN recon-

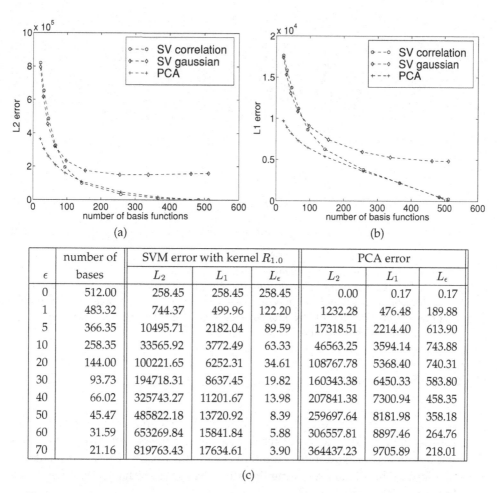

ϵ	number of bases	SVM error with kernel $R_{1.0}$			PCA error		
		L_2	L_1	L_ϵ	L_2	L_1	L_ϵ
0	512.00	258.45	258.45	258.45	0.00	0.17	0.17
1	483.32	744.37	499.96	122.20	1232.28	476.48	189.88
5	366.35	10495.71	2182.04	89.59	17318.51	2214.40	613.90
10	258.35	33565.92	3772.49	63.33	46563.25	3594.14	743.88
20	144.00	100221.65	6252.31	34.61	108767.78	5368.40	740.31
30	93.73	194718.31	8637.45	19.82	160343.38	6450.33	583.80
40	66.02	325743.27	11201.67	13.98	207841.38	7300.94	458.35
50	45.47	485822.18	13720.92	8.39	259697.64	8181.98	358.18
60	31.59	653269.84	15841.84	5.88	306557.81	8897.46	264.76
70	21.16	819763.43	17634.61	3.90	364437.23	9705.89	218.01

(c)

Figure 8.5: Comparison of compression error between SVM with correlation kernel $R_{1.0}$, SVM with gaussian kernel, and PCA; (a) L_2 error, (b) L_1 error, and (c) L_ϵ error. The L_ϵ results are presented in tabular format. The L_2 and L_1 results indicate that performance is comparable between SVM with the correlation kernel and PCA for large numbers of basis functions, but the SVM generates better sparse approximations (using less than 100 basis functions).

struction error when compressing our test set of 50 pedestrian images. Both of these techniques are evaluated using the correlation kernel $R_{1.0}$. Figure 8.6 graphs the results and indicates that the performance of the two techniques is not identical. For representations using large numbers of basis functions, the performance is comparable, but BPDN obtains more accurate *sparse* approximations, when measured in L_2, to the original image (where the number of basis functions is less than 100). Again, the reason behind this is that we are measuring error in the norm that BPDN is explicitly minimizing.

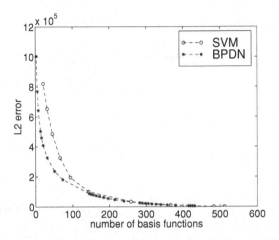

Figure 8.6: A comparison of SVM and BPDN measuring reconstruction error obtained when representing pedestrian images as a sparse set of correlation-based basis functions ($R_{1.0}$); L_2 reconstruction error is plotted against the number of basis functions found by each technique. The performance of these techniques is comparable for large numbers of basis functions, but BPDN obtains better sparse approximations, measured in L_2, to the original images (number of basis functions < 100).

Multiscale Representations

Multiscale representations allow us to represent a signal using successive levels of approximation; lower levels of resolution capture the coarse structure of the signal and finer levels resolution of resolution encode the details. These representations are standard in the signal processing literature (Mallat and Zhang, 1989; Simoncelli and Freeman, 1995; Mallat and Zhang, 1993).

In our image reconstruction experiments, we have focused on approximating a signal using a single kernel with $d = 1.0$, corresponding to coarse scale features. In certain applications, we may be able to derive class-specific basis functions for several scales; this is the case for our generalized correlation kernels where, to vary the locality of the basis functions, we simply change d. We can then use the sparsification paradigm on this larger overcomplete dictionary to obtain a sparse approximation of a given signal with a set of basis functions at several scales. The SVM formulation for multiple scales has not been derived yet, but Basis Pursuit De-Noising can be used with these multiscale dictionaries.

As we discussed previously, Basis Pursuit De-Noising is an approach to sparsification that minimizes a functional containing an term measuring the approximation error in L_2 using a linear combination of basis functions and a sparsity term in L_1. In

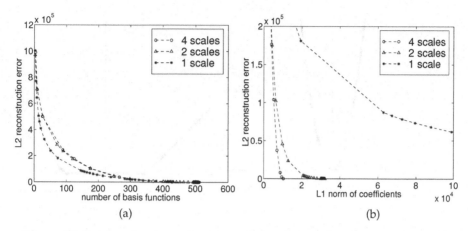

Figure 8.7: Compression error when using multiscale basis functions with BPDN; (a) L_2 error plotted against the L_0 norm of the coefficients (ie., the number of basis functions), (b) L_2 error plotted against the L_1 norm of the coefficients. These graphs imply that, in the context of sparsity, the L_1 norm is not a good approximation of L_0.

our signal and reconstruction experiments, where we have focused on using a set of basis functions ϕ_n that are at a single scale, we would minimize:

$$E[\mathbf{c}] = \|f(\mathbf{x}) - \sum_{i=1}^{N} c_i \phi_i(\mathbf{x}_i)\|_{L_2}^2 + \lambda \|\mathbf{c}\|_{L_1} \tag{8.25}$$

for some signal f.

We can formulate the BPDN functional for our case of generating a multiscale representation using correlation kernels as follows:

$$E[\mathbf{c}] = \|f(\mathbf{x}) - \sum_{i=1}^{N} \sum_{d=d_1}^{d_D} c_{i,d} R_d(\mathbf{x}, \mathbf{x}_i)\|_{L_2}^2 + \lambda \|\mathbf{c}\|_{L_1} \tag{8.26}$$

where d ranges over the elements of $\mathbf{D}$, the set of scales we are using.

The experiments compare the performance of the BPDN technique for correlation kernels using various numbers of scales: one scale ($\mathbf{D} = \{1.0\}$), two scales ($\mathbf{D} = \{0.5, 1.0\}$), and four scales ($\mathbf{D} = \{0.0, 0.5, 0.75, 1.0\}$). As before, we run the experiments on our set of 50 out-of-sample images of pedestrians. Figure 8.7a, which plots the average reconstruction error in L_2 against the number of basis functions used in the compression, seems to indicate that to achieve a certain error rate, fewer scales of basis functions are better. This is counter to our argument for using multiple scales of basis functions since we would expect that, with more scales to choose from, the minimization technique would be able to obtain a better approximation when choosing basis functions from this larger dictionary.

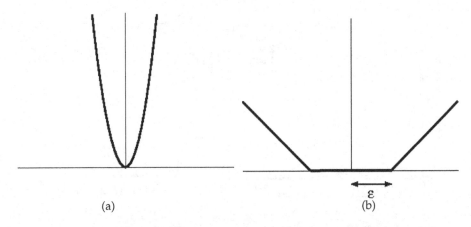

Figure 8.8: The two different error norms; (a) L_2 norm, (b) L_ϵ norm.

To explain this apparent inconsistency, Figure 8.7b plots reconstruction error against the L_1 *norm of the coefficients*, which is the measure of sparsity that BPDN minimizes. Here, the desired behavior of the one-, two-, and four-scale reconstructions is evident – for a given level of reconstruction error, starting with a multiscale dictionary affords a more sparse representation. What does this mean?

The true measure of sparsity is the L_0 norm of the coefficients, or the number of basis functions. Since this would lead to an Integer Programming problem which is computationally prohibitive for the number of basis functions we are using, the BPDN formulation approximates L_0 by L_1. These results offer empirical evidence that these norms are in fact very different and L_1 is not a good approximation of L_0.

Error Norms for Image Compression

The techniques for basis selection that we present in this chapter use fundamentally different criteria to represent signals, depending on what functional form the error term takes; PCA minimizes the traditional L_2 norm and SVM minimizes L_ϵ, an ϵ-insensitive norm (Pontil *et al.*, 1998), both plotted in Figure 8.8. While the vast majority of reports of image processing techniques ascribe to the use of the L_2 norm, it is not clear that this measure of error is the "best" for this particular domain. One important caveat: any pixel-based norm, in particular all L_p, is clearly not the "right" error metric to use since the human visual system takes into account higher order image structure; our discussion focuses on choosing the best norm when we are restricted to a "pixelwise" cost such as L_p or L_ϵ.

In the context of image reconstruction, the L_2 norm penalizes any perturbations

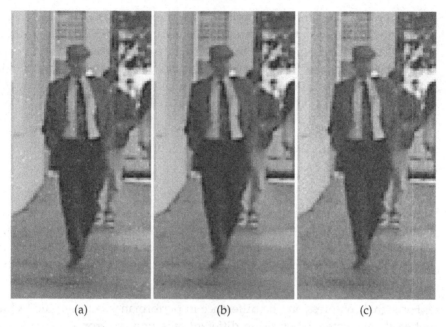

(a)   (b)   (c)

Figure 8.9: Examples of images with different types of errors; (a) low L_2 error, high L_ϵ error, relative to image (c); (b) true image; (c) high L_2 error, low L_ϵ error, relative to image (a).

from the true value, while the L_ϵ norm does not penalize values that are within ϵ of the true value, but linearly penalizes values lying outside of this region. The difference in these similarity measures is shown in Figure 8.9; Figure 8.9a has low L_2 error and high L_ϵ error, relative to 8.9c, while Figure 8.9c has high L_2 error and low L_ϵ error, relative to 8.9a; 8.9b is the true image. The deviations in Figure 8.9a seem to stand out more than those in 8.9c, but 8.9c has higher L_2 error.

How are we to reconcile this seeming inconsistency in what the traditional L_2 error tells us with what our brain tells us? It is well known that people cannot perceive differences in intensity that are very small (Schade, 1956; Campbell and Robson, 1968; Hess and Howell, 1977). In DeVore *et al.* (1992), the authors argue that the L_1 error norm is a more accurate mathematical realization of the norm embedded in the human visual system than the L_2 norm. Fundamental to their hypothesis is the structure of the Contrast Sensitivity Threshold (CST) curve that captures a person's ability to distinguish an oscillating pattern of increasing frequency at different levels of contrast. Their argument determines the value of p for which the L_p norm best fits what the geometry of the CST curve implies; they find that $p = 1$ is the best approximation of the perceptual system's norm.

We can combine their results with the fact that at low contrasts in the middle frequencies of the CST curve, it is nearly impossible to distinguish the different bands, implying the existence of some base threshold. This leads us to postulate that the L_ϵ norm may be a more perceptually accurate norm than L_1, since it encodes both the geometric constraints and threshold evident in the CST curve. In the absence of a psychophysical experiment that investigates this hypothesis, this conjecture is speculation, of course. For other more detailed perspectives on the modeling of human perception, see the chapters by Mamassian, Landy and Maloney, Schrater and Kersten, Jacobs, and Yuille and Coughlan in this book.

Conclusion

We have shown that the use of class-specific correlation-based kernels, when combined with the notion of sparsity, results in a powerful signal reconstruction technique. In a comparison to a traditional method of signal approximation, Principal Components Analysis, our approach achieves a more sparse representation for a given level of error.

For signal compression, the difference in performance between the techniques is not easily evaluated; when using different measures of error, we obtain a different "best" system. The choice of a system to use could depend on the characteristics of the different norms. The L_2 norm penalizes any difference in reconstruction. On the other hand, the L_ϵ norm does not penalize differences in the small ϵ-insensitive region around the true value, but linearly penalizes errors outside this region. One way of comparing the L_2, L_1, and L_ϵ norms could be to decide which is a more accurate description of psychophysical measures of similarity between images. Based on the arguments presented in the previous section and the references cited therein, we postulate that the L_ϵ norm may be the norm we should use in image reconstruction, superresolution, and compression.

Our approach of using a dictionary of class-specific correlation kernels to obtain sparse representation of a signal leads to an interesting question: could this sparse representation that has been generated to *approximate* a signal be used to *classify* different signals? In other words, is the representation of pedestrians via sparse sets of correlation-based basis functions different enough from the representation of other objects (or all other objects), so that it can be used as a model for that class of objects? The representations we generate are derived through an argument that minimizes error for reconstructing the image. This, however, says nothing about the ability of that same representation to be used to differentiate images of different objects. Whether or not this can be done is an open question; Appendix C in Papageorgiou *et al.*, 1998 presents a preliminary discussion of this approach.

An alternative is to use the Gaussian prior implied by the regression approach to derive features for classification in terms of its sufficient statistics (see Jaakkola & Haussler, 1998 and observations in Evgeniou *et al.*, 1999).

Acknowledgments

The authors would like to thank the following people for useful discussions and suggestions that helped improve the quality of this work: Sayan Mukherjee, Edgar Osuna, Massimiliano Pontil, and Ryan Rifkin.

The eigen-decomposition of our pedestrian class was generated using routines from *Numerical Recipes in C* (Press *et al.*, 1992). In our implementation of BPDN, as well as the associated decomposition algorithm, we used the LSSOL quadratic programming package from Stanford Business Software, Inc. (Gill *et al.*, 1986). The cubic spline superresolution reconstruction in this chapter was generated using MATLAB Version 5.2 (The MathWorks, Inc., 1998).

Research at CBCL is sponsored by a grant from the Office of Naval Research under contract No. N00014-93-1-3085, Office of Naval Research under contract No. N00014-95-1-0600, National Science Foundation under contract No. IIS-9800032, and National Science Foundation under contract No. DMS-9872936. Additional support is provided by: AT&T, Central Research Institute of Electric Power Industry, Eastman Kodak Company, DaimlerChrysler, Digital Equipment Corporation, Honda R&D Co., Ltd., NEC Fund, Nippon Telegraph & Telephone, and Siemens Corporate Research, Inc.

References

[1] B. Boser, I. Guyon, and V. Vapnik. A training algorithm for optimal margin classifier. In *Proceedings of the Fifth Annual ACM Workshop on Computational Learning Theory*, pages 144–52. ACM, 1992.

[2] C. Burges. A Tutorial on Support Vector Machines for Pattern Recognition. In Usama Fayyad, editor, *Proceedings of Data Mining and Knowledge Discovery*, pages 1–43, 1998.

[3] F.W. Campbell and J.G. Robson. Application of Fourier Analysis to the Visibility of Gratings. *Jounral of Physiology*, 197:551–566, 1968.

[4] S. Chen, D. Donoho, and M. Saunders. Atomic Decomposition by Basis Pursuit. Technical Report 479, Department of Statistics, Stanford University, May 1995.

[5] T. Evgeniou, M. Pontil, and T. Poggio. Regularization networks and support vector machines. *Advances in Computational Mathematics*, 1999. (to appear).

[6] P.E. Gill, S.J. Hammarling, W. Murray, M.A. Saunders, and M.H. Wright. User's Guide for LSSOL (Version 1.0). Technical Report SOL 86-1, Stanford University, 1986.

[7] F. Girosi. An Equivalence Between Sparse Approximation and Support Vector

Machines. A.I. Memo 1606, MIT Artificial Intelligence Laboratory, 1997.

[8]   F. Girosi. An equivalence between sparse approximation and Support Vector Machines. *Neural Computation*, 10(6):1455–1480, 1998.

[9]   R.F. Hess and E.R. Howell. The Threshold Contrast Sensitivity Function in Strabismic Amblyopia: Evidence for a Two Type Classification. *Vision Research*, 17:1049–1055, 1977.

[10] The MathWorks Inc. *Using Matlab*. 1998.

[11] T. Jaakkola and D. Haussler. Probabilistic kernel regression models. In *Proceedings of Neural Information Processing Systems*, 1998.

[12] S. Mallat and Z. Zhang. Matching Pursuit in a time-frequency dictionary. *IEEE Transactions on Signal Processing*, 41:3397–3415, 1993.

[13] S.G. Mallat. A theory for multiresolution signal decomposition: The wavelet representation. *IEEE Transactions on Pattern Analysis and Machine Intelligence*, 11(7):674–93, July 1989.

[14] Sr. O.H. Schade. Optical and Photoelectric Analog of the Eye. *Journal of the Optical Society of America*, 46(9):721–739, September 1956.

[15] M. Oren, C.P. Papageorgiou, P. Sinha, E. Osuna, and T. Poggio. Pedestrian detection using wavelet templates. In *Proceedings of Computer Vision and Pattern Recognition*, pages 193–99, 1997.

[16] E. Osuna, R. Freund, and F. Girosi. Support Vector Machines: Training and Applications. A.I. Memo 1602, MIT Artificial Intelligence Laboratory, 1997.

[17] C.P. Papageorgiou. Object and Pattern Detection in Video Sequences. Master's thesis, MIT, 1997.

[18] C.P. Papageorgiou, F. Girosi, and T. Poggio. Sparse Correlation Kernel Analysis and Reconstruction. A.I. Memo 1635, MIT Artificial Intelligence Laboratory, 1998. (CBCL Memo 162).

[19] C.P. Papageorgiou, M. Oren, and T. Poggio. A general framework for object detection. In *Proceedings of 6th International Conference on Computer Vision*, 1998.

[20] P. S. Penev and J. J. Atick. Local Feature Analysis: A general statistical theory for object representation. *Neural Systems*, 7(3):477–500, 1996.

[21] T. Poggio and F. Girosi. A Sparse Representation for Function Approximation. *Neural Computation*, 10(6):1445–1454, 1998.

[22] T. Poggio and F. Girosi. Notes on PCA, Regularization, Support Vector Machines and Sparsity. A.I. Memo 1632, MIT Artificial Intelligence Laboratory, April 1998.

[23] M. Pontil, S. Mukherjee, and F. Girosi. On the Noise Model of Support Vector Machine Regression. A.I. Memo 1651, MIT Artificial Intelligence Laboratory, October 1998.

[24] W.H. Press, S.A. Teukolsky, W.T. Vetterling, and B.P. Flannery. *Numerical Recipes*

in C. Cambridge University Press, 2 edition, 1992.

[25] L.L. Schumaker. *Spline Functions: Basic Theory.* John Wiley and Sons, New York, 1981.

[26] E.P. Simoncelli and W.T. Freeman. The steerable pyramid: A flexible architecture for multi-scale derivative computation. In *2nd Annual IEEE International Conference on Image Processing,* pages 444–447, October 1995.

[27] V. Vapnik. *The Nature of Statistical Learning Theory.* Springer Verlag, 1995.

[28] G. Wahba. *Spline Models for Observational Data.* Series in Applied Mathematics, Vol. 59, SIAM, Philadelphia, 1990.

Part II: Neural Function

9 Natural Image Statistics for Cortical Orientation Map Development

Christian Piepenbrock

Introduction

Simple cells in the primary visual cortex have localized orientation selective receptive fields that are organized in a cortical orientation map. Many models based on different mechanisms have been put forward to explain their development driven by neuronal activity [31, 30, 16, 21]. Here, we propose a global optimization criterion for the receptive field development, derive effective cortical activity dynamics and a development model from it, and present simulation results for the activity driven development process. The model aims to explain the development of (i) cortical simple cell receptive fields and (ii) orientation maps (iii) by one mechanism based on Hebbian learning (iv) driven by the viewing of natural scenes. We begin by suggesting an objective for the cortical development process, then derive models for the neuronal mechanisms involved, and finally present and discuss results of model simulations.

Practically all models that have been proposed for the development of simple cell receptive fields and the formation of cortical maps are based on the assumption that orientation selective neurons develop by some simple and universal mechanism driven by neuronal activity. The models, however, differ in the exact mechanisms they assume and in the type of activity patterns that may drive the development.

Orientation selective receptive fields are generally assumed to be a property of the geniculo-cortical projection: the simple cell receptive fields are elongated and consist of alternating On and Off responding regions. The models assume that neuronal activity is propagated from the lateral geniculate nucleus to the visual cortex and elicits an activity pattern that causes the geniculo-cortical synaptic connections to modify by Hebbian [17, 20, 21, 23] or anti-Hebbian learning rules [25].

Independently of how the cortical network exactly works, a universal mechanism for the development should modify the network to achieve optimal information processing in some sense. It has been proposed that the goal of coding should be to detect the underlying cause of the input by reducing the redundancy in the neuronal activities [1]. This is achieved to some degree in the visual system that processes natural images projected onto the retina. The images are typically highly redundant, because they contain correlations in space and time. Some of the redundancy is already reduced in the retina: the On-Off response properties of retinal ganglion cells, e.g., effectively serve as local spatial decorrelation filters. Ideally, a layer of linear On-Off ganglion cells with identical receptive field profiles could "whiten" the image power spectrum and decorrelate the activities of any pair of ganglion cells [8]. In a subsequent step, simple cells in the primary visual cortex decorrelate the input even further—they respond to typical features (oriented bars) in their input activities. These features correspond to input activity correlations of higher order, i.e., between many neurons at a time. In other words, simple cell feature detectors could result from a development model that aims to reduce the redundany between neuronal activities in a natural viewing scenario. It has been demonstrated in simulations that development models based on the independent component analysis algorithm or a sparse representation lead to orientation selective patterns that resemble simple cell receptive field profiles [23, 2]. We conclude that it is a reasonable goal for simple cell development to reduce the redundancy of neurons' responses in a natural viewing environment.

Experiments show that the development of simple cell receptive fields and the cortical orientation map depends on neuronal activity [5]. Without activity, the receptive fields remain large, unspecific, and only coarsely topographically organized. Activity leads to the emergence of orientation selective simple cells and an orientation map. The activity patterns during the first phase of the development, however, do not depend on visual stimulation and natural images [7]. Some orientation selective neurons may be found in V1 up to 10 days before the opening of the eyes in ferrets, and an orientation map is present as early as recordings can be made after eye opening [6]. The activity patterns that have been recorded before eye opening may resemble simply noise or—during some phase of the development—take the form of waves of excitation wandering across the retina [33]. These waves are autonomously generated within the retina independently of visual stimulation and it has been hypothesized that these activity patterns might serve to drive the geniculate and even cortical development. Nevertheless, the receptive fields and the orientation map are not fully developed at eye opening and remain plastic for some time [14]. A lack of stimulation causes cortical responses to fade, and rearing animals in environments with unnatural visual environments leads to cortical reorganization [7]. We conclude that visual experience is essential for a correct wiring of simple cells in V1.

The model assumptions about the type of activity patterns that drive the development process differ widely. In any case, a successful model should be able to predict the development of orientation selectivity for the types of spontaneous activity patterns present before eye opening as well as for natural viewing conditions. Whilst the activity patterns change, the mechanism that shapes simple cell receptive fields is unlikely to be very different in both phases of the development [9]. One type of models, the correlation based models, have been simulated for pre-natal white noise retinal activity [20] or for waves of neuronal activity as they appear on the retina prior to eye opening [24]. These models would predict the development of orientation selectivity under natural viewing conditions, if the model condition is fulfilled that geniculate activities are anti-correlated [24]. Another type of models, the self-organizing map, has been shown to yield an orientation selectivity map, if it is trained with short oriented edges [21]. Models based on sparse coding driven by natural images result in oriented receptive fields [23].

From the above, it becomes clear that one needs to make a few more critical assumptions to derive a simple cell development model that makes neurons' responses less redundant. The most important one is the model neurons' response function. Models have been proposed that use linear activity dynamics [20], neurons with saturating cortical activities [29], nonlinear sparse coding neurons [23], or winner-take-all network dynamics [21]. For linear neurons, a development model that leads to independent activities, in general, extracts the "principal component" from the ensemble of presented input images. The many degenerate principal components for sets of natural images filtered by ganglion cells are global patterns of alternating On and Off patches. Each of these patterns covers the whole visual field. In correlation based learning models that limit each receptive field to only a small section of the visual field [16, 20, 19] this leads to oriented simple cell receptive fields of any orientation. Models that explicitly iterate the fast recurrent cortical activity dynamics (e.g. until the activity rates reach a steady state or saturate) usually model some kind of nonlinear input-ouput relations. One variant—the sparse coding framework—leads to oriented receptive fields only, if the input patterns contain oriented edges [23]. The extreme case of a sparse coding model is the winner-take-all network: for each input pattern, only one simple cell (and its neighbors) respond. In any case, independently of whether the intracortical dynamics are explicitly simulated or just approximated by a simple expression, with respect to Hebbian development, the key property of the model is the nonlinearity in the mapping between the geniculate input and the cortical output.

Simple cells were originally defined as those feature detection cells that respond linearly to their geniculate input [13]. It has turned out, however, that the orientation tuning is sharper than can be expected from the geniculate input alone. This may be explained by a network effect of interacting cortical neurons [10]: cells that respond well to a stimulus locally excite each other and suppress the response of other neurons. Such a nonlinear network effect may be interpreted as a competition between the neurons to represent an input stimulus and has been modeled, e.g., by divisive inhibition [3].

The formation of the simple cells' arrangement in a cortical map is in most models a direct consequence of local interactions in V1. The interactions enforce the map continuity across the cortical surface by making neighboring neurons respond to similar stimuli and therefore develop similar receptive fields. Experimentally, it is known that short range connections within V1 are effectively excitatory, while long range connections up to a few millimeters are inhibitory [18]. Many models of cortical map development reduce the receptive fields to a few feature dimensions and do not model simple cell receptive field profiles at all [22, 15]. Most other models for the development of simple cell receptive fields do not explain the emergence of cortical maps [23, 2, 25].

On the one hand, the only models that lead to localized orientation selective receptive fields and realistic orientation selectivity maps are Kohonen type networks [21, 27]. They are, however, based on unrealistic winner-take-all dynamics and cannot be derived from a global objective function. On the other hand, models that explain the emergence of orientation selective receptive fields in a sparse coding framework driven by natural images have not been extended to model cortical map development [23]. To overcome these limitations, we introduce a new model in the next section that is based on soft cortical competition.

The Model

In this section, we derive a learning rule for the activity driven development of the cortical simple cell receptive fields. Our model is based on the assumptions that (i) cortical simple cell orientation selectivity is largely a property of the geniculo-cortical projection, (ii) the cortical activities are strongest at those neurons that receive the strongest afferent input, (iii) the simple cells respond nonlinearly to their input and the nonlinearity is a competitive network effect. The model's Hebbian development rule may be viewed as changing the synaptic weights to maximize the entropy of the neurons' activities subject to the constraints of limited total synaptic resources and competitive network dynamics.

The primary visual pathways

Light stimuli are picked up by the photoreceptor cells in the eyes (see Figure 9.1). Ganglion cells in the retina transform the local excitation patterns into trains of action potentials and project to the lateral geniculate nucleus (LGN). Signals from there first reach the cortex in V1. We model a patch of the parafoveal retina (with k photoreceptor cells) small enough to neglect the decrease of ganglion cell density with exccentricity. We assume that an excitation pattern in the eyes is well characterized by a log light intensity "pixel image" $\vec{u}$ (k-dimensional) with one vector component for each modeled cell. The image processing whithin the retina and the LGN may

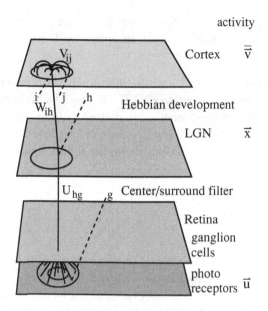

Figure 9.1: Model for the primary visual pathways.

be modeled by a linear local contrast filter U, and we represent the geniculo-cortical signals by their firing rates. In the model, we make no explicit distinction between On and Off responding cells and, instead, use values that represent the difference between the activity rates of an On and a neighboring Off cell and thus may become negative. The activity in each of l modeled geniculo-cortical fibers is consequently represented by one component of the l-dimensional vector $\vec{x} = U\vec{u}$.

During free viewing, the eyes see natural images. They fixate one point and after a few hundred milliseconds, quickly saccade to the next. The saccadic eye movements are short compared to the fixation periods. We model this natural viewing scenario by a succession of small grey valued images $\vec{u}^\mu$ randomly drawn from a set of photographs of natural images including rocks, trees, grass, etc. each representing one fixation period $\mu = 1, \ldots, t$.

Cortical processing

Our simple cell model and the development rule are derived from an abstract optimization criterion based on the following assumptions:

A geniculate activity pattern $\vec{x}$ (each component of the vector represents the activity rate in one model fiber) is projected to a layer of simple cells by a geniculo-cortical synaptic weight matrix W. Orientation selectivity emerges as a result of Hebbian learning of these effective synaptic connection strengths. In principle, this matrix allows for a full connectivity between any model geniculate and cortical cell, although experimentally the geniculo-cortical receptive fields have shown to be always localized.

The cortical simple cells recurrently interact by short range connections effectively modeled by an interaction matrix V. The m model simple cells respond nonlinearly with activities $\vec{v}^{\mu}$ (an m-dimensional vector) to their afferent input $VW\vec{x}^{\mu}$. Those cells that receive the strongest input should respond the most. Therefore, we propose that during the simple cell development, the following objective function should be minimized:

$$E\left(W, \{\vec{v}^{\mu}\}\right) = -\frac{1}{t} \sum_{\mu} (\vec{v}^{\mu})^T V W \vec{x}^{\mu} \tag{9.1}$$

The simple cells are orientation feature detectors and should compete to represent a given image. We assume that we can express all simple cells' spikes (that never *exactly* coincide in time) as a list of events in a stochastic network of interacting neurons spiking at independent times. Each cell's firing rate is the probability of firing the next spike in the cortical network times the average cortical activitiy. The firing probabilities in such a network may be modeled by the Boltzmann distribution with the normalization constant Z (partition function) and an associated mean "energy" E determined by a parameter β (the system's inverse pseudo temperature):

$$P\left(W, \{\vec{v}^{\mu}\}\right) = \frac{1}{Z} \exp\left(-\beta E(W, \{\vec{v}^{\mu}\})\right) \tag{9.2}$$

Cortical development

To obtain an expression for the model likelihood of a set of synaptic weights W, we marginalize over all possible activity states of the network (for each image μ, there are m possible activity states $\vec{v}^{\mu}$—each neuron could spike). The synaptic weights W that provide the optimal representation for a given stimulus environment should maximize

$$P(W) = \sum_{\{\vec{v}^{\mu}\}} P\left(W, \{\vec{v}^{\mu}\}\right) = \frac{1}{Z} \prod_{\mu} \vec{1}^T \exp\left(\beta V W \vec{x}^{\mu}\right) \overset{!}{=} \max, \tag{9.3}$$

where $\vec{1}$ is the vector of 1's and exp() is applied component-wise to its vector argument. Finally, we maximize this expression by gradient descent on the negative log-likelihood (with step size η) in a stochastic approximation for one pattern μ at a time and obtain an update rule for the synaptic weights

$$\Delta W(\vec{x}^{\mu}) = \eta \beta V^T \bar{\vec{v}}^{\mu}(\vec{x}^{\mu})^T \quad \text{with} \quad \bar{\vec{v}} = \frac{\exp(\beta V W \vec{x}^{\mu})}{\vec{1}^T \exp(\beta V W \vec{x}^{\mu})} \tag{9.4}$$

This is the rule that we propose for simple cell receptive field development and orientation map formation. Biologically, it (i) implements a Hebbian learning rule and (ii) cortical competition in (iii) an effective model for the cortical activity dynamics.

(i) Hebbian learning means that a synaptic connection W_{ij} becomes more efficient, if the presynaptic activity $\vec{x}_j^{\mu}$ is correlated with the postsynaptic one $\sum_l V_{li}\bar{v}_l^{\mu}$. Typically, synaptic weights under Hebbian learning rules may grow infinitely and need to be bounded. We assume that the total synaptic weight for each neuron i is limited and renormalize $\sum_j (W_{ij})^2$ after each development step to the value 1.

(ii) Cortical activity competition means that cortical simple cells are not entirely linear. Their orientation tuning is sharper than it could be expected from the geniculo-cortical input alone and it has been proposed that this is an effect of the local cortical circuitry [10, 28]. Equation 9.4 provides an *effective* model for cortical activity competition by divisive inhibition. $\bar{\vec{v}}^{\mu}$ represents the "mean field activities" of the model cells (laterally spread by the interaction weights V). The short range interactions V make neighboring neurons excite each other and the normalization term in the denominator suppresses weak signals such that only the strong signals remain in this "competition". The parameter β represents the effectiveness of this process—it models the degree of competition in the system.

(iii) The nonlinear cortical activity model $V^T \bar{\vec{v}}^{\mu}$ is a simple mathematical formulation for the effect of cortical competition. Given an input activity pattern $\vec{x}^{\mu}$, it expresses the cortical activity profile as a steady state rate code. The model has not been designed to explain exactly how and which recurrent circuits dynamically lead to such a competitive response. Nevertheless, for intermediate values of β, the model response assumes realistic values.

Technically, our approach is based on a two state (spin) model with competitive dynamics and local interactions (with interaction kernel V). The Hebbian development rule works under the constraint of limited synaptic resources and achieves minimal energy for the system by maximizing the entropy of all neurons' activities given a set of input stimuli.

Simulations

We have simulated the development of simple cell receptive fields and cortical orientation maps driven by natural image stimuli. In this section, we explain how we process the natural images, and then study the properties of the proposed developmental model.

For our simulations, we use natural images recorded with a CCD camera (see Figure 9.2a) that have an average power spectrum as shown in Figure 9.2c. The images are linearly filtered with center-surround receptive fields to resemble the image processing in the retina and the LGN. Given an input image $\vec{u}$ as a pixel grid (each $\vec{u}_i$ is one image pixel) we compute the LGN activities $\vec{x} = U\vec{x}$ using a linear convolution kernel U (a circulant matrix) with center/surround receptive fields. The receptive field is shown in Figure 9.2d and its power spectrum (Figure 9.2c) as a function of spatial frequency w (in 1/pixels) is given by $F(w) = w\exp(-(w/\phi)^4)$ where $\phi = 0.2$ is the cutoff frequency. The center/surround filters flatten the power spectrum of the images as shown in Figure 9.2g. They almost whiten the spectrum up to the cutoff frequency—an ideal white spectrum would be a horizontal line and contain no two-pixel correlations at all. All together, we use 15 different 512x512 pixel images as the basis for our simulations, filter them as described and shown in Figure 9.2b and normalize them to unit variance.

In all simulations, the model LGN consists of l =18x18 neurons and for each pattern presentation we randomly draw an 18x18 filtered pixel image patch from one of the 15 images. For computational efficiency we discard low image contrast patches with a variance of less than 0.6 that would effectively not lead to much learning anyway.

Geniculo-cortical development

The most prominent observation is that the outcome of the simulated development process critically depends on the value of β—the degree of cortical competition. For very weak competition, unstructured large receptive fields form, in the case of weak competition, the fields localize and form a topographic map, and only at strong competition, orientation selective simple cells and a cortical orientation map emerge (Figure 9.3). In all simulations, the geniculo-cortical synaptic weights are initially set to a topographic map with Gaussian receptive fields of radius 5 pixels with 30% random noise. Every pattern presentation leads to a development step as described in the "Cortical development" section. The topographic initialization is not necessary for the model but significantly speeds up convergence. We use an annealing scheme in the simulations starting with a low β and increasing it exponentially every 300000 iterations. Convergence is reached after about 1 million iterations and all simulations

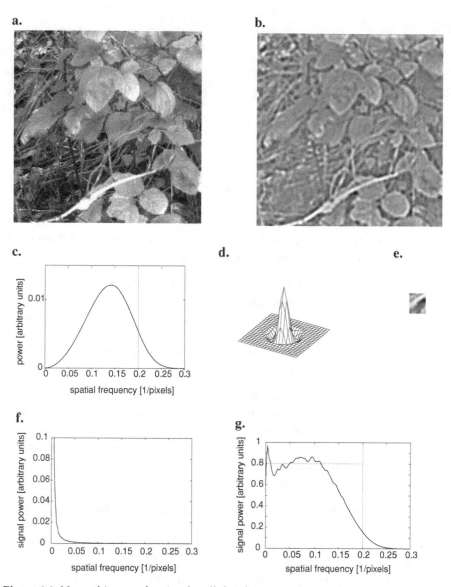

Figure 9.2: Natural images for simple cell development: **a)** Example of a natural image as used in the simulations (200x200 pixels out of whole 512x512 image). Shown are approximately log light intensities as grey values. **b)** The same image as output from retinal ganglion cells with center-surround receptive fields. **c)** Power spectrum of the model retinal ganglion cell center-surround receptive field profile. **d)** Model retinal ganglion cell center-surround receptive field profile. **e)** One example of an 18x18 pixel image patch used as cortical input in the model simulations. **f)** Average power spectrum of all the natural images used in the simulations as shown in b). **g)** Average power spectrum of all the filtered images as shown c). The ganglion cells almost whiten the spectrum (ideal horizontal line) up to the cutoff frequency 0.2.

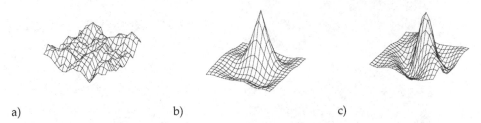

a)   b)   c)

Figure 9.3: Receptive fields from different topographic map simulations. Left: very weak competition ($\beta = 0.00001$); middle: weak competition ($\beta = 0.001$); right: strong competition ($\beta = 1$)

were run for at least 1.5 million pattern presentations. Some much longer simulations yielded no further changes in the receptive fields and cortical maps.

Extremely weak competition ($\beta = 0.00001$) leads to cortical receptive fields that cover the whole visual field and become identical for all neurons. They are completely unstructured (Figure 9.3a) or—depending on the images used—patchy with a typical spatial frequency corresponding to the peak of the power spectrum (Figure 9.2g). In any case, the fields become as large as possible and do not form a topographic map.

For weak competition ($\beta = 0.001$), the receptive fields localize and form center-surround filters (Figure 9.3b) with no orientation selectivity (or very weak selectivity with an identical orientation preference angle in all neurons). A few of the receptive field profiles from a simulation of 22×22 neurons are shown in Figure 9.4a top. Neighboring receptive fields heavily overlap and together form a smooth topographic map of the visual field (Figure 9.5a).

Strong competition ($\beta = 1$) is the regime in which orientation selective simple cells emerge (Figure 9.3c). The receptive fields are localized and have on (positive weights) and off (negative weights) subfields and may be well approximated by Gabor functions. Neighboring simple cells develop receptive fields with a similar preferred orientation (Figure 9.4a bottom) and together all simple cells form a cortical orientation map as shown in Figure 9.6. The model map has all the key properties known from real visual cortical maps: the angle of preferred orientation changes smoothly, except at pinwheel points; on the average there is an equal number of 180 degrees right-turning and 180 degrees left turning pinwheels (for the particular simulated example shown it is 9 vs. 11, but this is not a systematic bias). A systematic and statistical analysis of the map properties is difficult, however, due to the limited size of the map (28x28 neurons), the long simulation times, and the strong artifacts along the border of the map: the preferred orientation of receptive fields at map borders always aligns with the border. In addition to the orientation map, the simple cell receptive fields are localized and form a topographic map as well (Figure 9.5b). This map shows a global

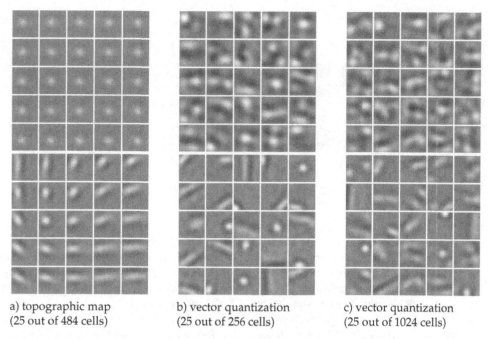

a) topographic map
(25 out of 484 cells)

b) vector quantization
(25 out of 256 cells)

c) vector quantization
(25 out of 1024 cells)

Figure 9.4: Receptive fields from different simulations. At low competition the representation is coarse (top row, $\beta = 0.001$ in a; $\beta = 0.01$ in b, c). It refines for stronger competition (bottom row, $\beta = 1$ in a; $\beta = 0.1$ in b, c) or, in the case of vector quantization (b, c), also for larger cell numbers. The results for vector quantization show completely unordered sets of receptive fields.

order, but strong local distortions. The average receptive field diameter is approximately 8 pixels (the mean standard deviation for the Gaussian fits is 4.33 in Fig. 9.5a and 4.01 in Fig. 9.5b). This allows for little more than 2 hypercolumns on a visual field of width 18 pixels as used in the simulations. The topographic distortions in Fig. 9.5b occur exactly on this scale and therefore do not constitute a topographic disorder— the simulations only suggest that topographic order may not strictly be present on a sub-hypercolumn scale.

Cortical representation of stimulus features

All modeled cortical neurons together represent the statistical properties of the input stimuli. The stronger the competition, the more stimulus properties are represented in the receptive field profiles. For very weak competition (compare Figure 9.3a), all receptive fields look identical, are not orientation selective, and have the maximal receptive field size allowed by the network. The only stimulus property represented in the receptive field profiles is the spatial frequency that dominates the power spectrum (if that is not exactly white—compare Figure 9.2g). If some weak competition

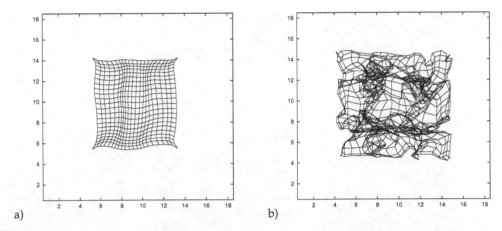

Figure 9.5: Cortical topographic maps. **a)** Simulation with weak competition. **b)** Simulation with strong competition. To obtain these maps, Gaussians are fitted to the absolute values of the weight patterns (see Figure 9.4) of each receptive field and connected by a grid. Simulations with very weak competition do not yield topographics maps. Receptive fields from different simulations of 22x22 cortical neurons.

is present (Figure 9.7 right), all receptive fields are similar: they are practically not orientation specific, have one typical spatial frequency, and a radius of about 4 pixels. Nevertheless, in addition to the spatial frequency, the fact that natural stimuli are usually localized, is represented in the model cells. At strong competition, the receptive fields are a lot more diverse: the simple cells become full input feature detectors that are orientation selective and span a range of field sizes and spatial frequencies (Figure 9.7 left) as well as orientations (Figure 9.8) much like in the real cortex. Even stronger competition cannot not qualitatively alter the receptive fields any more. Beyond $\beta = 1$, the second term of Equation 9.4 behaves much like a winner-take-all rule that lets only one neuron (and its neighbors) respond to a given stimulus.

While the development model works to optimize the cortical representation (Equation 9.1), weak competition could be viewed as "blurring" the cortex' view of the stimulus features. Strong competition, on the other hand, leads to orientation selective cells and a realistic outcome. Simulations with diffent numbers of cortical neurons show that all neurons together always fill the space of feature orientation / spatial frequency at an equal density (Figure 9.8).

The space of natural image features

It has turned out that our proposed development model yields realistic receptive field profiles and cortical maps only in the case of strong cortical competition. To gain a better understanding of the underlying reasons and the features that natural images

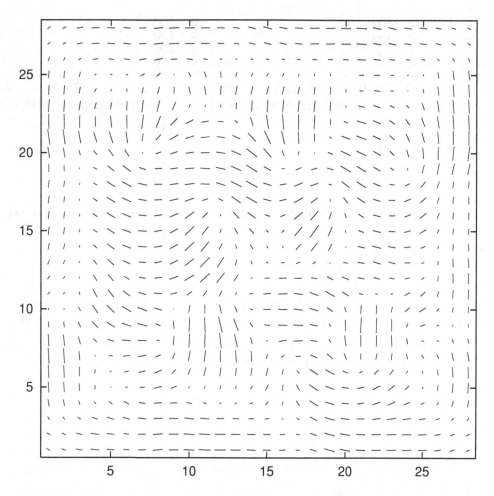

Figure 9.6: Cortical orientation map. The orientation specificity is indicated by the length of the lines. As an artifact of the model the orientation selectivity near the borders aligns with them.

typically consist of, we compare our model to some other models and data analysis techniques.

The self organizing map (SOM) is the only algorithm that has been applied to model receptive field development, as well as cortical orientation map and topographic map formation in one model [21, 27]. Our model becomes actually quite similar to the self organizing map model used in [21] for very large values of β: in the limit of $\beta \to \infty$, the term $\vec{v}$ in Equation 9.4 turns into a winner-take-all function for $VW\vec{x}^\mu$ as used in all competitive learning models. Self organizing maps aim to encode all input stimuli by representative vectors (neurons' receptive fields) that preserve the neighborhood in the input space of stimuli. The SOM algorithm, how-

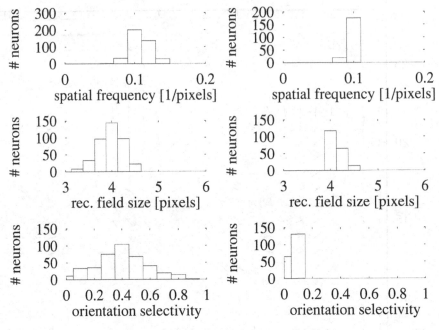

Figure 9.7: Simulations of cortical maps with 22 × 22 cells. Left: strong competition ($\beta = 1$); right: weak competition ($\beta = 0.001$)

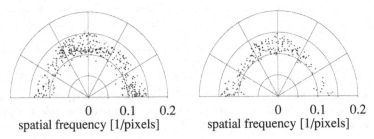

Figure 9.8: Simulations of cortical orientation maps with $\beta = 1$. Plotted is the preferred orientation vs. the preferred spatial frequency for each receptive field. Left: 28 × 28 cells; right: 22 × 22 cells.

ever, does not optimize any given global objective function such as Equation 9.1, and the winner-take-all rule is not a very realistic model for the effective cortical output dynamics.

If we discard the local cortical connectivity from our model (replace V by the identity matrix), it fails to develop cortical maps, but for large β turns into to a vector quantization algorithm [11].[1] The goal of vector quantization is to encode all given input patterns by a set of representative vectors (neurons' receptive fields), each representing an approximately equally large number of input patterns. The input space is extremely high dimensional (one dimension for each input pixel) and the receptive fields are "average patterns" for the set of input stimuli they represent. Figure 9.9 (left) shows the result of such a vector quantization simulation. Receptive fields with a diverse receptive field size, degree of orientation selectivity, spatial frequency and orientation preference emerge (compare with topographic map simulation in Figure 9.7 left). Furthermore, from the figure, it becomes evident that the ensemble of input images contains more vertical edges than edges of other directions. Examining the receptive fields directly (Figure 9.4c bottom) reveals that round receptive fields emerge as well as elongated edge detectors of different spatial frequencies and some more complex patterns. How detailed the representation is, depends also on the number of output neurons: less neurons represent the input stimuli with less detail as shown in Figure 9.4b bottom where edge detectors are present, but neurons recognizing more complex patterns are missing. In our model framework, we may also weaken the cortical competition from a winner-take-all rule ($\beta \geq 0.1$) to a softer regime ($\beta = 0.01$) which yields fuzzy, large receptive fields of lower spatial frequencies showing less detailed structure (Figure 9.4bc top and Figure 9.9 right).

The results for vector quantization are qualitatively similar to two other development models for simple cell receptive fields driven by natural images. The first, based on sparse coding [23], uses fast neuronal dynamics to model the competition among the cortical neurons and slower dynamics for the development of synaptic weights [23]. As a result, orientation selective filters emerge from natural image stimuli that resemble simple cell receptive field profiles. We follow a similar approach, but do not explicitly model the fast neuronal dynamics and instead, express only the steady state (term $\vec{v}^{\mu}$ in Equation 9.4). This allows to view the cortical output $\vec{v}^{\mu}$ simply as a nonlinear function of its geniculate input $W \vec{x}^{\mu}$ and speeds up simulations a lot. The second approach, independent component analysis (ICA), models the cortical activities by a nonlinear (but not competitive) output function [2]. Following the objective to make the cortical outputs as independent of each other as possible, a sparse cortical activation function proves to be necessary and yields a set of receptive field profiles that resemble our results from Figure 9.9 b. The simulation outcome critically depends on the right choice for the nonlinear function just as in our simulations (varying β). However, the approach is limited to square matrices W.

---

1. with normalized weights vectors W and input images with unit variance [12] and is thus equivalent to vector quantization confined to the unit hypersphere.

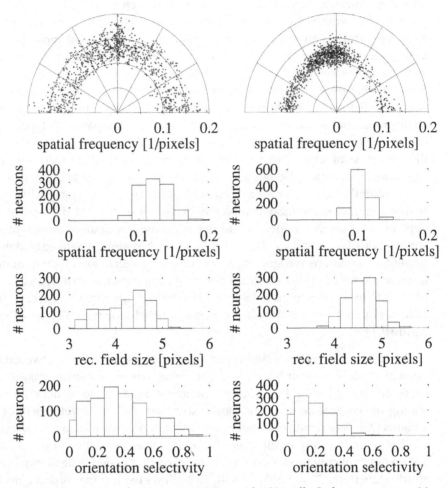

Figure 9.9: Simulations of vector quantization with 1024 cells. Left: strong competition ($\beta = 0.1$); right: weak competition ($\beta = 0.01$)

Discussion

The model proposed in this chapter explains the development of localized orientation selective receptive fields and the cortical orientation map. Localized orientation selective fields develop due to the "sparse cortical activation function" modeled by a soft competition mechanism and matched by the fact that natural images have a sparse structure and contain edges. In our simplified "vector quantization" simulations of the model, the ensemble of receptive fields forms a discrete approximation of the input pattern probability distribution and consists of round or long oriented receptive fields. In contrast, in our cortical map simulations, neighboring receptive fields are forced to represent similar features and the network "compromizes" between a faithful approximation of the input pattern probability distibution and a very smooth cortical map by forming local oriented edge filters that have less diverse and detailed features than the corresponding vector quantization receptive fields (compare Figure 9.4a with b and c).

The strongest limitation of the current model is the size of the cortical maps. Currently, due to computational limitations, they are too small to analyze the simulated maps in a statistically meaningful way, e.g., with respect to the spatial frequency, the pinwheel density, position, and orientation. Vertical and horizontal edges are overrepresented in our training images and this is reflected in the results of the vector quantization simulations. However, this result could not be established in a statistically meaningful way for our model maps due to their small receptive field size. In animal experiments, a dependence of simple cells on stimuli has been found in cat [26] and horizontal and vertical simple cells are overrepresented in normal ferrets [4].

In the introduction, we argued from an information processing point of view that images are de-correlated step by step in the primary visual pathways: the retinal on/off ganglion cells would filter out second order (two-pixel) correlations and whiten the image while the geniculo-cortical projection extracts image features and produces a sparse representation. It should be noted that the ganglion cells do not have to exactly whiten the image spectrum. The development model still works, if the cortical input does not have a whitened spectrum. The convergence of the development model is slower, but a qualitative difference in the outcome occurs only in the case of extremely low competition: completely flat receptive fields emerge instead of patchy ones. The correlation based learning models predict simple cell receptive field formation in this parameter regime and rely on constraints for the receptive field size and an input power spectrum that is neither "raw" nor exactly white, but has a pronounced peak at the typical spatial frequency of On and Off subfields. These models develop edge detecting receptive fields by receptive field size constraints, but do not extract the edge information from the input images.

We suggest a competitive mechanism for cortical dynamics and predict a sparse representation for the simple cells. From a functional point of view, a sparse code is a good strategy to represent visual stimuli, because the structure of natural images is sparse. Our model of divisive inhibition assumes global inhibition and local excitation between the neurons. It is known, however, that the long range inhibition is orientation specific and reaches only a few hypercolumns [18]. In terms of possible competitive dynamics, this could mean that competition is present in the cortex, but only as a local mechanism: neurons within one hypercolumn compete to represent a stimulus, because there is likely to be only one orientation present in one location of the visual field and spatially separated hypercolumns should be more independent. Our model could be improved by a second learning rule for the intra-cortical weights in a straight forward manner to test these hypotheses, but much larger simulations would be necessary.

The model output of the cortical neurons ($\vec{v}$ in Equation 9.4) expresses the effective neurons' steady state firing rates in a dynamic network for a given input pattern. The input signals are given as positive (On center ganglion cell response) or negative values (Off center response at the same location) and in the cortical network we do not explicitly model the inhibitory neurons. It is, of course, possible to model the cortical dynamics in more biological detail and existing models yield qualitatively similar results [20, 32]. In our model, however, each of the simple components is designed to serve a different key property: (*i*) the fraction in Equation 9.4 represents divisive inhibition as a model for self-excitation of each neuron together with long range inhibition between cortical neurons and serves as the key nonlinearity and the model's basis for competition among the cells; (*ii*) the variable competition strength β allows to steer the network from practically linear to an extremely "sparse" winner-take-all output; (*iii*) the excitation between cortical neurons (matrix V) is the basis for cortical map formation. In summary, the output term is a nonlinear competitive function of the inputs—biologically much more realistic than a winner-take-all rule—and consists of three simple mechanisms that allow an interpretation of the development outcome in terms of a global objective function.

The intra-cortical excitatory connections V of the model enforce a realistic map formation, but do not improve the model's representation of the input. This impression is a consequence of the continuous valued activity rates used for the simple cells. In the real cortex, however, the activity rates can only be estimated from the spike counts and to make the system fault tolerant and to improve the signal estimation by averaging, it is advantageous to force neighboring neurons to encode similar stimuli. Thus, the excitatory local connections (and thus cortical maps) may serve to make the representation of stimuli in the cortex fast, noise robust, and redundant—a critical condition for a network of real spiking neurons always pressed to decide which image features is currently present in the visual field. The model predicts that inhibition within the cortex serves as the basis for competition (and output gain control), whilst local excitation makes the network noise robust by enforcing map formation.

Our model and discussion have neglected any signals besides the input images that may be received by the primary visual cortex. Visual attention may play a role and be another significant source of nonlinearity that could influence the fine tuning of the receptive fields during the later stages of the development process.

We have shown that the development of localized simple cell receptive fields and cortical topographic and orientation maps may be explained in one consistent model framework derived from a global objective function based on cortical competition. In the model, competition is the key mechanism necessary for the simple cell development and finally leads to a sparse representation and the first level of image feature extraction in the brain. The activity driven development sets in after the geniculate fibers initially contact the primary visual cortex in a coarsely topographic map and we initialize the model weights in the same way. We observe that our simulations converge much faster if we use an annealing scheme that starts with weak competition slowly strengthening over time. This might also happen in the cortex: activity patterns first reach it long before eye opening when the local circuitry may not yet be able to support strong competition. At this time, a coarse map might emerge much like in Figure 9.4a (top). At the time the visual cortex receives structured waves of activity (still before the first visual stimulation), it may begin to develop the first orientation selective simple cells. This would give the cortex a head start in visual development and allow it to have the basic connectivity set up at the moment of eye opening. The key to a good representation (and ultimately an understanding) of the environment, however, seems to be the refinement of the connectivity driven by natural stimuli after birth. The mechanisms proposed in this chapter sets up a framework that could explain all the phases and, in particular, the final adaptation to the real world.

Acknowledgements

This work was supported by the Boehringer Ingelheim Fonds. The author would like to thank Martin Stetter, Thore Graepel, Klaus Obermayer, and Peter Adorjan for helpful discussions.

References

[1] H. B. Barlow. The coding of sensory messages. In *Current Problems in Animal Behavior*. Cambridge University Press, Cambridge, 1961.

[2] A. J. Bell and T. J. Sejnowski. The independent components of natural scenes are edge filters. *Vision Research*, 37:3327–38, 1997.

[3] M. Carandini, D. J. Heeger, and J. A. Movshon. Linearity and normalization in simple cells of the macaque primary visual cortex. *J. Neuroscience*, 17:8621–44, 1997.

[4] B. Chapman and T. Bonhoeffer. Overrepresentation of horizontal and vertical orientation preferences in developing ferret area 17. *Proc. Natl. Acad. Sci. USA*, 95:2609–14, 1998.

[5] B. Chapman, I. Goedecke, and T. Bonhoeffer. Development of orientation preference in the mammalian visual cortex. *J Neurobiology*, 41:18–24, 1999.

[6] B. Chapman, M. P. Stryker, and t. Bonhoeffer. Development of orientation preference maps in ferret primary visual cortex. *J. Neuroscience*, 16:6443–53,

1996.

[7]   M. C. Crair, D. C. Gillespie, and M. P. Stryker. The role of visual experience in the development of columns in cat visual cortex. *Science*, 279:566–70, 1998.

[8]   Y. Dan, J. J. Atick, and R. C. Reid. Efficient coding of natural scenes in the lateral geniculate nucleus: experimental test of a computational theory. *J. Neuroscience*, 16:3351–62, 1996.

[9]   Y. Fregnac and D. E. Shulz. Activity-dependent regulation of receptive field properties of cat area 17 by supervised hebbian learning. *J. Neurobiology*, 41:69–82, 1999.

[10]   J. L. Gardner, A. Anzai, I. Ohzawa, and R. D. Freeman. Linear and nonlinear contributions to orientation tuning of simple cells in the cat's striate cortex. *Vis. Neurosci.*, 16:1115–21, 1999.

[11]   T. Graepel, M. Burger, and K. Obermayer. Phase transitions in stochastic self-organizing maps. *Phys. Rev. E*, 56(4):3876–3890, 1997.

[12]   J. Hertz, A. Krogh, and R. G. Palmer. *Introduction to the Theory of Neural Computation*. Addison-Wesley, 1991.

[13]   D. H. Hubel and T. N. Wiesel. Receptive fields, binocular interaction and functional architecture in the cat's visual cortex. *Journal of Physiology London*, 160:106–154, 1962.

[14]   D. S. Kim and T. Bonhoeffer. Reverse occlusion leads to a precise restoration of orientation preference maps in visual cortex. *Nature*, 370:370–2, 1994.

[15]   T. Kohonen. Physiological interpretation of the self-organizing map algorithm. *Neur. Netw.*, 6:895–905, 1993.

[16]   R. Linsker. From basic network principles to neural architecture: Emergence of orientation columns. *Proc. Natl. Acad. Sci. USA*, 83:8779–8783, 1986.

[17]   R. Linsker. From basic network principles to neural architecture: emergence of spatial opponent cells. *Proc. Natl. Acad. Sci. USA*, 83:7508–7512, 1986.

[18]   J. S. Lund, Q. Wu, and J. B. Levitt. Visual cortical cell types and connections: Anatomical foundations for computational models. In M. A. Arbib, editor, *Handbook of Brain Theory*. MIT Press, Cambridge, 1995.

[19]   D. J. C. MacKay and K. D. Miller. Analysis of Linsker's application of Hebbian rules to linear networks. *Network*, 1:257–297, 1990.

[20]   K.D. Miller. A model for the development of simple cell receptive fields and the ordered arrangements of orientation columns through activity-dependent competition between ON- and OFF-center inputs. *J. Neurosci.*, 14:409–441, 1994.

[21]   K. Obermayer, H. Ritter, and K. Schulten. Large-scale simulations of self-organizing neural networks on parallel computers: Application to biological modelling. *Par. Comp.*, 14:381–404, 1990.

[22]   K. Obermayer, H. Ritter, and K. Schulten. A principle for the formation of the spatial structure of cortical feature maps. *Proc. Natl. Acad. Sci. USA*, 87:8345–

8349, 1990.

[23] B. A. Olshausen and D. J. Field. Emergence of simple-cell receptive field properties by learning a sparse code for natural images. *Nature*, 381:607–9, 1996.

[24] C. Piepenbrock, H. Ritter, and K. Obermayer. Linear correlation-based learning models require a two-stage process for the development of orientation and ocular dominance. *Neural Processing Letters*, 3:31–37, 1996.

[25] R. P. Rao and D. H. Ballard. Dynamic model of visual recognition predicts neural response properties in the visual cortex. *Neural Computation*, 9:721–63, 1997.

[26] F. Sengpiel, P. Stawinski, and T. Bonhoeffer. Influence of experience on orientation maps in cat visual cortex. *Nat. Neurosci*, 2:727–32, 1999.

[27] J. Sirosh and R. Miikkulainen. Topographic receptive fields and patterned lateral interaction in a self-organizing model of the primary visual cortex. *Neural Computation*, 9:577–94, 1997.

[28] D. Somers, S. Nelson, and M. Sur. An emergent model of orientation selectivity in cat visual cortical simple cells. *J. Neurosci.*, 1995.

[29] M. Stetter, A. Muller, and E. W. Lang. Neural network model for the coordinated formation of orientation preference and orientation selectivity maps. *Phys. Rev. E*, 50:4167–4181, 1994.

[30] N.V. Swindale. A model for the formation of orientation columns. *Proc. R. Soc. Lond. B*, 215:211–230, 1982.

[31] C. von der Malsburg. Self-organization of orientation sensitive cells in the striate cortex. *Kybernetik*, 14:85–100, 1973.

[32] S. A. J. Winder. A model for biological winner-take-all neural competition employing inhibitory modulation of nmda-mediated excitatory gain. In *Advances in Neural Information Processing Systems NIPS 11*, 1999.

[33] R. O. L. Wong, M. Meister, and C. J. Shatz. Transient period of correlated bursting activity during development of the mammalian retina. *Neuron*, 11:923–938, 1993.

10 Natural Image Statistics and Divisive Normalization

Martin J. Wainwright, Odelia Schwartz, and
Eero P. Simoncelli

Introduction

Understanding the functional role of neurons and neural systems is a primary goal
of systems neuroscience. A longstanding hypothesis states that sensory systems are
matched to the statistical properties of the signals to which they are exposed [e.g.
[4, 6]]. In particular, Barlow has proposed that the role of early sensory systems is
to remove redundancy in the sensory input, by generating a set of neural responses
that are statistically independent. Variants of this hypothesis have been formulated
by a number of other authors [e.g. [2, 52]] (see [47] for a review). The basic version
assumes a fixed environmental model, but Barlow and Foldiak later augmented
the theory by suggesting that adaptation in neural systems might be thought of
as an adjustment to remove redundancies in the responses to recently presented
stimuli [8, 7].

There are two basic methodologies for testing such hypotheses. The most direct
approach is to examine the statistical properties of neural responses under natural
stimulation conditions [e.g. [25, 41, 17, 5, 40]] or the statistical dependency of pairs
(or groups) of neural responses. Due to their technical difficulty, such multi-cellular
experiments are only recently becoming possible, and the earliest reports appear
consistent with the hypothesis [e.g. [54]]. An alternative approach is to "derive" a
model for early sensory processing [e.g. [36, 43, 20, 2, 37, 9, 49, 53]]. In such an
approach, one examines the statistical properties of environmental signals and shows
that a transformation derived according to some statistical optimization criterion
provides a good description of the response properties of a set of sensory neurons.
We follow this latter approach in this chapter.

A number of researchers [e.g. [36, 43, 3]] have used the covariance properties of natural images to derive linear basis functions that are similar to receptive fields found physiologically in primary visual cortex (i.e., localized in spatial position, orientation and scale). But these early attempts required additional constraints, such as spatial locality and/or symmetry.

Covariance properties are adequate to characterize Gaussian probability models. But when the higher-order statistical properties of natural images are examined, they are found to be strikingly non-Gaussian [19, 61, 18]. More recent work has shown that these non-Gaussian characteristics may be captured using fairly simple parametric models [e.g. [29, 48, 16, 58]]. Several authors have used higher-order statistical measures to derive linear basis functions that are similar to cortical receptive fields [e.g. [37, 9, 53]].

We have empirically examined the responses of such linear basis functions to natural images, and found that these responses exhibit striking statistical dependencies, even when the basis functions are chosen to optimize independence [e.g. [48, 11]]. Such dependencies cannot be removed through further linear processing. Rather, a nonlinear form of cortical processing is required, in which the linear response of each basis function is rectified (and typically squared) and then divided by a weighted sum of the rectified responses of neighboring neurons. Similar "divisive normalization" models have been used by a number of authors to account for nonlinear behaviors in neurons [39, 10, 21, 22, 13]. Our approach shows that natural image statistics, in conjunction with Barlow's hypothesis, lead to divisive normalization as the appropriate nonlinearity for removing dependency. That is, the type of nonlinearity found in cortical processing is well-matched to the non-Gaussian statistics of natural images.

In earlier work, we have shown that our model, with all parameters determined from the statistics of a set of natural images, can account qualitatively for recent physiological observations of suppression of V1 responses by stimuli presented outside the classical receptive field [51]. Here, we show that the model can account for responses to non-optimal stimuli. In addition, we show that adjusting the model parameters according to the statistics of *recent* visual input can account for physiologically observed adaptation effects [57].

Statistical Properties of Natural Images

As mentioned above, a number of authors have derived linear basis sets by optimizing higher-order statistical measures. For our purposes here, we find it convenient to work with a fixed linear basis that is an approximation to these optimal bases. In particular, we use a "steerable pyramid" [50], whose basis functions are translations, rotations, and dilations of a common filter kernel. This kernel has a spatial frequency

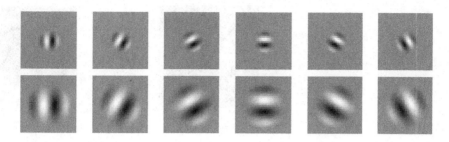

Figure 10.1. Example basis functions at two different scales, taken from a 6-orientation steerable pyramid.

bandwidth of roughly one octave, and an orientation tuning bandwidth of roughly 30 degrees. Example basis functions are shown in figure 10.1.

The marginal statistics of the coefficients obtained by projecting natural images onto such basis functions are known to be highly non-Gaussian and kurtotic [19, 29]. In addition, the joint statistics of these coefficients exhibit striking non-linear dependencies [59, 48]. We have modeled these dependencies, and used the models in a variety of image processing applications, such as compression [11] and denoising [49].

Figure 10.2 shows the joint statistics of neural responses from a typical pair of adjacent basis functions. Statistics were gathered by collecting response pairs at all spatial positions within a single natural image. A joint histogram is constructed by counting the number of response pairs that fall into each bin in the two-dimensional grid. The resulting array is displayed as a grayscale image, in which the pixel intensity is proportional to the bin counts, except that each column is independently re-scaled, thus forming a *conditional* histogram. The conditional histogram in the upper left panel of Figure 10.2 shows that this pair of neural responses is well decorrelated, since the expected value of the ordinate is approximately zero, independent of the abscissa. However, the "bowtie" shape of the histogram reveals that these coefficients are not statistically independent. Rather, the variance of the ordinate scales with the absolute value of the abscissa. We emphasize that this form of dependency cannot be captured using a traditional jointly Gaussian model, and cannot be eliminated with linear processing!

This type of statistical dependency appears in pairs of coefficients at nearby spatial positions, orientations, and scales. Figure 10.3 shows conditionalized joint histograms for a number of different basis function pairs. The strength of the dependency varies depending on the specific pair chosen. Loosely speaking, we find that the dependency is strongest for basis functions that are close in spatial position, orientation, and scale (spatial frequency), and decreases for pairs that differ markedly in one or more of these attributes.

We have observed this form of dependency in a wide variety of natural images,

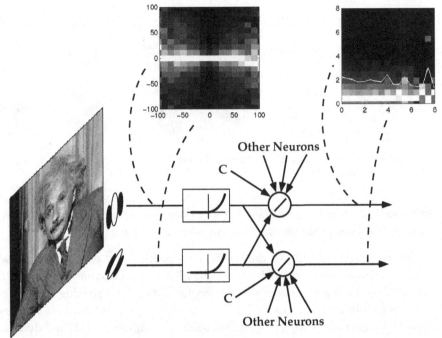

Figure 10.2. Illustration of image statistics as seen through two neighboring linear receptive fields. Left image: Joint conditional histogram of two coefficients. Pixel intensity corresponds to frequency of occurrence of a given pair of values, except that each column has been independently rescaled to fill the full intensity range. Right image: Joint histogram of divisively normalized coefficients (see text).

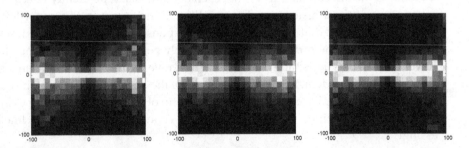

Figure 10.3. Conditional joint histograms for several different pairs of basis functions. Left: spatially adjacent pair (same orientation and scale); Middle: orthogonal orientations (same position and scale); Right: differing in scale by a factor of two.

even when we use a basis set that is optimized to produce maximally independent responses [e.g. [9]]. For a given pair of coefficients, the strength of dependency does vary slightly from image to image. Nevertheless, we emphasize that this is a property of the images themselves, and is *not* due purely to our choice of linear basis functions.

For example, no such dependency is observed when the input image consists of white noise (each pixel independent).

It should not be a surprise that one cannot decompose an image into independent components using a linear basis, since images are not formed from linear superpositions of independent patterns. Even if one assumes that the objects that constitute a scene are drawn independently, the most common combination rule for image formation is *occlusion*, which is nonlinear. The intuitive explanation for the magnitude dependency is that typical localized image structures (e.g. edges, corners) tend to have substantial power across several scales and orientations at the same spatial location. Such a structure will be represented in the wavelet domain via a superposition of the corresponding basis functions. The signs and relative magnitudes of the coefficients associated with these basis functions will depend on the precise location, orientation and scale of the structure. But all of the magnitudes will scale with the contrast of the structure. Thus, measurement of a large coefficient at one scale means that large values in nearby coefficients are more likely.

Redundancy Reduction through Divisive Normalization

In previous work [48, 51, 58], we have shown that these statistical dependencies may be reduced using a normalization operation, in which each linear coefficient, L_j, is squared (or halfwave rectified and squared) and then divided by a weighted sum of the squares of its neighbors $\{L_k\}$ and an additive constant:

$$R_j \equiv \frac{L_j^2}{\sigma_j^2 + \sum_k w_{jk} L_k^2} \tag{10.1}$$

The neighbors, $\{L_k\}$, correspond to linear responses of basis functions at nearby positions, orientations and spatial scales. The right-hand panel in figure 10.2 shows the conditional histogram of these normalized responses. Note that the probability mass is of approximately constant cross section (apart from statistical sampling errors), and the conditional variance (solid line) is approximately constant. Our current work aims to establish a more formal class of image model for which this divisive operation is optimal [58, 55].

The parameters $\{w_{jk}, \sigma_j^2\}$ used in computing the normalization signal are directly determined by statistical measurements of natural images. Intuitively, larger weights w_{jk} are associated with neighboring neurons whose responses are more predictive of the squared response of the given neuron. The constant σ_j corresponds to the residual variance that cannot be predicted from neighboring coefficients.

In order to compute explicit values for the weights and constant, we minimize the quantity

$$M(w_{jk}, \sigma_j^2) = \mathbb{E}\left\{ [\log R_j]^2 \right\},$$

(10.2)

where $\mathbb{E}$ denotes expected value, which is computed in practice by averaging over all spatial positions of a set of natural images. This procedure corresponds to maximum-likelihood (ML) estimation of the parameters, assuming a lognormal distribution for the conditional density:

$$p(L_j \mid \{L_k\}; \sigma_j, w_{j,k}) = \frac{1}{|L_j|\sqrt{2\pi\gamma^2}} \exp\left\{ -\frac{1}{2\gamma^2}\left[\log L_j^2 - \log[\sigma_j^2 + \sum_k w_{jk} L_k^2] \right]^2 \right\}$$

(10.3)

The conditional mean and standard deviation of this lognormal distribution are both proportional to $\{\sigma_j^2 + \sum_k w_{jk} L_k^2\}^{\frac{1}{2}}$. This choice of probability density is therefore consistent with the empirical observation that the standard deviation of L_j roughly scales with the absolute value of the neighbor L_k.

Related choices of error function [48, 51] yield qualitatively similar results. For our the simulations of the following sections, statistical measurements were taken over an image ensemble of four natural images. In all cases, a group of eleven neighbors was used: five orientation neighbors, four spatial neighbors, and two neighbors in scale (coarse and fine).

Physiological Modeling: Divisive Suppression

In previous work [51], we have shown that a statistically-derived weighted normalization model can account for various suppressive effects that occur when stimuli are presented outside of the classical receptive field of neurons in primary visual cortex. Parameters of the normalization model (weights and additive constant) are computed by optimizing equation (10.2) over a set of four example images. In particular, a drifting grating presented in an annular region surrounding the receptive field reduces responses to stimuli presented within the receptive field. This reduction appears to be primarily divisive (i.e., a change in gain), and is usually strongest when the parameters (eg., orientation, spatial frequency) of the annular stimulus are matched to those of the preferred excitatory stimulus of the neuron.

Here, we demonstrate examples of non-linear behavior inside the classical receptive field. In each example, we compare model simulations to electrophysiological

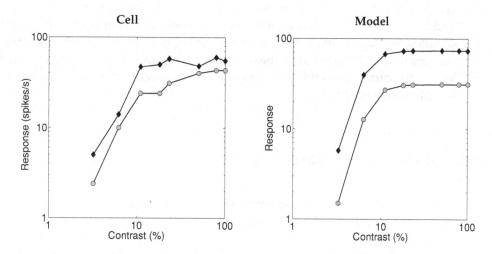

Figure 10.4. Responses to drifting sinusoidal stimuli at optimal (solid) and non-optimal (hollow) orientations. Left: Cell, taken from [13]. Right: Model.

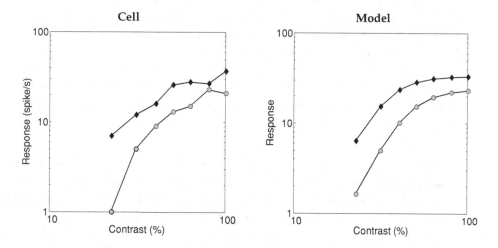

Figure 10.5. Responses to drifting sinusoidal stimuli at optimal (solid) and non-optimal (hollow) spatial frequencies. Left: Cell, taken from [13]. Right: Model.

recordings a from a typical V1 simple cell in an anesthetized Macaque monkey [13]. Figure 10.4 shows responses to a sinusoidal grating at the optimal orientation, along with responses to a grating at an orientation 30 degrees away from optimal. Figure 10.5 shows responses to to a sinusoidal grating at the optimal spatial frequency, along with responses to a grating at frequency 0.78 times the optimal. For the model neuron, we have scaled the non-optimal frequency by the ratio of bandwidths between neurons in our model (1 octave) and V1 cells (roughly 1.5 octaves). Note that in both model and cell, the contrast response curves for the non-optimal stimulus are shifted downward from those for the optimal stimulus. Compared with an optimal stimulus, the non-optimal stimulus induces stronger responses in other neurons, increasing the relative strength of the normalization signal. This changes the saturation level of the curve. In addition, the amount of shift in cell and model response curves is qualitatively matched.

Physiological Modeling: Adaptation

In the previous sections, we assumed a model with normalization parameters optimized for a generic ensemble of images. Biologically, such an optimal solution would arise through some combination of evolutionary (i.e. genetic) and developmental processes. But given that visual input is constantly changing, it is natural to ask whether the system attempts to adapt itself to the statistics of visual input over shorter time scales. Visual adaptation over relatively short periods is a well-known phenomenon. For example, very rapid adaptation occurs in the retina, where the photoreceptor response continually adjusts to the mean illumination [e.g. [26]]. Adaptation effects are also well-documented in the cortex [e.g. [34, 1]], but neither their functional purpose nor their mechanism are fully understood. A number of researchers have proposed mechanisms by which cortical adaptation could take place [e.g. [22, 60, 15]]. Barlow and Foldiak [8, 7] proposed that linear receptive field properties are adjusted in order to decorrelate responses to recently presented visual stimuli. In related work, we have recently found that optimal changes to linear responses based on signal and noise power spectra predict various psychophysical results following adaptation [56].

In this section, we examine the hypothesis that normalization parameters are adjusted based on the statistics of recent visual input. In contrast to previous approaches to cortical adaptation [e.g. [8, 7, 15, 56]], we assume that the linear receptive fields are held fixed, but that the normalization parameters are updated. We begin by showing that two canonical types of cortical adaptation can be distinguished on the basis of image statistics. We then test our adaptation hypothesis by computing a set of "adapted" normalization parameters based on a modified visual environment, and comparing the "adapted" neural responses to physiological recordings.

Types of adaptation

By considering specific types of changes to the visual environment, we find that image statistics serve to distinguish between two canonical types of adaptation, which we refer to as *contrast* and *pattern* adaptation. Each type of adaptation arises from a specific change in image statistics. In response to the statistical change, normalization parameters are altered in predictable ways, which then leads to a change in the contrast response function.

For simplicity, consider a single pair of neurons: a linear receptive field and a "neighbor" tuned for a nearby scale. First imagine that we have some "default" visual world, which we call environment A. Typically, environment A corresponds to samples of natural images. The joint conditional statistics of the pair of basis functions in this world are shown in the top left panel of Figure 10.6, where we see the familiar type of "bowtie" dependency between the two responses. Now suppose that we form a new visual world, which we call environment B, by uniformly re-scaling the contrast of environment A by a factor β. The statistical consequence of this change is a simple re-scaling of the linear responses. This change is illustrated in the bottom left panel of Figure 10.6, where the axes of the conditional histograms corresponding environment B have been scaled up by a factor of $\beta = 2$. Note that apart from this re-scaling, there is no change in the shape of the conditional histogram. From the cost function in equation (10.2), it can be seen that rescaling the linear responses by a factor β will change the optimal constant σ but not affect the weights $w_{j,k}$. In particular, the optimal constant for environment B will now be $\sigma_B = \beta \, \sigma_A$, which compensates for the factor of β in front of all the linear responses L_k. This change in the normalization constant leads to a very specific change in the contrast response function, as shown in the graph on the left side of Figure 10.6. The constant σ affects the contrast at which saturation sets in, but not the maximal response level. Therefore, the increase in σ produces a rightward shift of the contrast response. In other work, rightward shifts of these curves have been modeled by an increase in the normalization constant [e.g. [22]]. Our work establishes that such a change is in fact the optimal adjustment under a uniform re-scaling of contrast. In summary, re-scaling the contrast changes the normalization constant, which shifts the contrast response function to the right; this sequence of events will be called *contrast adaptation*.

A quite different type of change in image statistics involves changing the dependency between a model neuron and its neighbor, as shown in the right side of Figure 10.6. Such increased dependency could arise in a variety of ways. For illustration here, we constructed environment B by combining environment A with samples from a contrast-varying sinusoidal grating at a spatial frequency lying between the optimal frequencies of the two model neurons. In such an environment, the responses of the two neurons exhibit increased dependency, as reflected by the joint conditional histograms plotted in Figure 10.6. The increased dependency is shown by the greater thickness of the "bowtie" in the lower histogram (for environment B), as compared to the upper histogram (environment A). As a result, in order to eliminate the greater dependency between the neuron and its neighbor, more divisive normalization is required. Thus, the model predicts an increase in the normalization weight w, which represents the divisive influence of the neighbor on the neuron. The effect of increas-

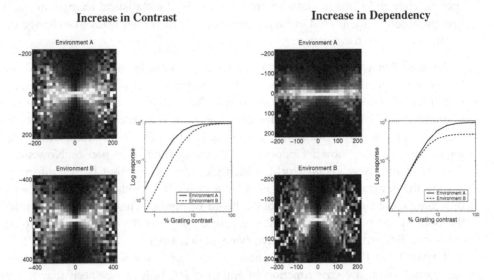

Figure 10.6. Canonical environmental changes, and the resulting adaptation effect. Left: Increase of contrast. Conditional histograms of linear receptive field responses at adjacent spatial scales (same orientation and spatial position) for two image ensembles (environments). Ensemble B is identical to Ensemble A, but with twice the contrast. The change in environmental contrast produces a change in the normalization constant σ, causing a horizontal shift in the contrast response function. Right: Increase of dependency. Ensemble B contains different spatial patterns than environment A, such that the dependency between the responses of the two linear receptive fields is increased. This is evident in the wider "bowtie" shape of the histograms. Right: the increase in dependency leads to an increase in the normalization weight w for this neighbor, causing a decrease in the saturation level of the contrast response.

ing the weight is to decrease the saturation level of the response curve, as shown in the graph on the right side of Figure 10.6. In summary, increased dependency between a neuron and its neighbor increases the corresponding normalization weight, which in turn lowers the saturation level of the curve. This sequence of events will be called *pattern adaptation*.

Simulation

Contrast and pattern adaptation, as defined here, correspond to pure forms of adaptation in response to specific changes in the visual environment. As we will see in our comparisons to physiological data, standard adaptation protocols typically lead to a mixture of contrast and pattern adaptation. To simulate a physiological adaptation experiment, we begin by computing a set of *generic* normalization parameters using equation (10.2), where the expectation is taken over a fixed ensemble of four natural images. The generic parameters are used to compute responses of neurons under normal (i.e., "unadapted") conditions, and form a baseline for comparison to the "adapted" responses.

The protocol typically used in neurophysiological experiments consists of presenting an adapting stimulus for an initial adaptation period that ranges from seconds to minutes. Brief probe stimuli are then interleaved with periods of top-up adaptation. We simulated such an adaptation protocol by creating an adapting image ensemble, consisting of the natural image ensemble augmented by the adapting stimulus. The adapting stimulus is chosen in accordance with the experimental protocol: sinusoidal grating images were used for the results reported here. The specific attributes of this grating (e.g., contrast, orientation, spatial frequency) were determined by the experiment under consideration. Note that the adapting ensemble is *not* formed by adding (pixel by pixel) the grating image to each member of the set of natural images. Rather, we collect sample responses from natural images, and mix them with sample responses from the sinusoidal grating image. This collection of responses is then used to compute an *adapted* set of normalization parameters via equation (10.2). These adapted parameters are used to simulate neural responses following adaptation.

Effect on contrast response: Different adapting contrasts

It is well-documented that prolonged stimulation of neurons in striate cortex changes their contrast-response function. When the response is measured over a limited range of contrasts, the primary effect of adapting to a high contrast grating can be described as a rightward shift on log-log axes [35]. However, measurements over a wider range of contrasts reveal that adaptation to high contrast gratings not only shifts the function to the right, but also changes its saturation level [1, 44].

Shown on the left side of Figure 10.7 are experimental measurements [1] of contrast response functions following adaptation to optimal frequency sinusoids at three different contrasts. The right side of Figure 10.7 plots the corresponding model predictions. The drop-off of the model responses are not as steep as those of the cell, because we used a fixed exponent of two, whereas typical fits to cell data yield exponents closer to three. The response curves of both the cell and model data undergo a rightward shift (contrast adaptation), as well as a change in the saturation level (pattern adaptation). In the context of our normalization model, such a mixture of effects is to be expected, because adapting to a high contrast sinusoid not only changes the contrast level experienced by the cell, but also biases the pattern statistics of recent visual input.

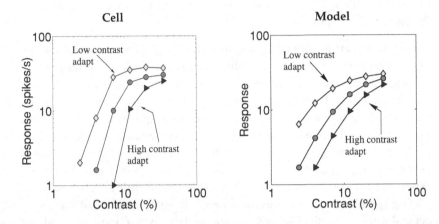

Figure 10.7. Left: Experimental data from Albrecht et al. [1], showing measured contrast response functions following adaptation to three different contrasts. Adapting stimuli were sinusoidal gratings at the optimal frequency. Right: Corresponding model predictions of changes in the response using an adapting ensemble with optimal frequency sinusoid at three different contrasts.

Effect on contrast response: Different test frequencies

An interesting feature of adaptation is that its strength depends on the relationship between the adapting and test stimulus. Albrecht et. al. studied the contingent nature of adaptation by exposing a cell to a grating of optimal spatial frequency, and then testing it with either the optimal or a non-optimal frequency [1]. Plotted in Figure 10.8 are contrast response curves, tested with either the optimal spatial frequency (left panel), or with a non-optimal spatial frequency (right panel). The corresponding model predictions under the same conditions are also shown in Figure 10.8. In each panel, the upper curve corresponds to the unadapted responses, whereas the lower curve shows the responses following adaptation to a sinusoid at the optimal spatial frequency.

As before, adaptation shifts the curves to the right, and changes the saturation level. However, note that the size of the shift is smaller when the test spatial frequency differs from the adapting frequency. The model also makes analogous predictions about changes in the responses following adaptation to different orientations, for which (to the best of our knowledge) published data is currently unavailable. That is, a close match between the test and adapting stimuli (whether in terms of orientation or frequency) leads to stronger effects of adaptation. This specificity illustrates that adaptation depends on a contingency between test and adapting stimuli.

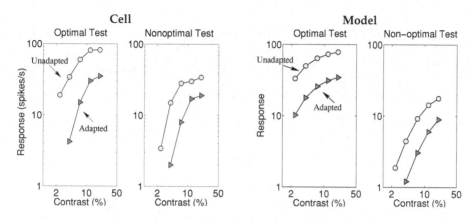

Figure 10.8. Left: Experimental data from Albrecht et al. [1]. Adaptation shifts the curves right, and changes the saturation level. The effect weakens as the test and adapting frequencies are separated (right panel). Right: Model predictions of changes in the response following adaptation to the optimal orientation and frequency. Each curve corresponds to a different spatial frequency under unadapted (top curves) and adapted (bottom curves) conditions.

Effect on tuning curves

A more dramatic illustration of the contingent nature of adaptation is provided by its effect on tuning curves. A number of researchers have reported that adaptation can alter the shape of tuning curves [e.g. [31, 1, 44, 45]]. That is, adapting to a non-optimal stimulus (either in orientation or frequency) suppresses one flank of the tuning curve, with little or no effect on the other flank. The overall effect is to skew the shape of the tuning curve. Model predictions of orientation tuning curves under such an adapting protocol are shown in Figure 10.9. The diamonds show the unadapted tuning curve; here the mild asymmetry in the tuning curve is due to mild asymmetries in the natural image statistics of our ensemble. The grey triangles show the tuning curve after adapting to the optimal stimulus at $0°$. Here the main effect of adaptation is an overall suppression of the tuning curve, corresponding to contrast adaptation. Superimposed on this main effect is the effect of pattern adaptation, which causes increased suppression at and around the optimal orientation. Adapting to the non-optimal $+14°$ stimulus causes an even more dramatic effect. Here, although the overall suppression of the tuning curve is weak, adaptation causes strong suppression in the right flank of the curve coupled with little effect on the opposite flank. The resultant skewing of the tuning curve is a nice illustration of the contingent nature of adaptation.

These types of differential effects on tuning curves were first reported by Movshon and Lennie [31]; later, Saul and Cynader [44, 45] explicitly plotted frequency tuning curves that were skewed following adaptation. More recently, Müller et al. [32]

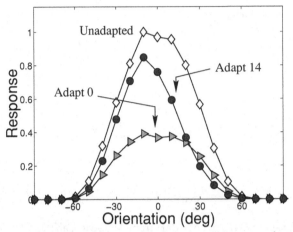

Figure 10.9. Orientation tuning curves under three conditions: unadapted, adapted to the optimal 0° stimulus, and adapted to the non-optimal +14° stimulus. The effects reflect a mixture of contrast and pattern adaptation, and illustrate the contingent nature of adaptation.

have reported such effects in some cells, but at time scales significantly shorter than those used in the previous studies. Further experimental investigation is needed to determine if these effects are due to the same adaptation mechanisms. Finally, Carandini et. al. [14] have shown that adaptation to a plaid containing both the optimally oriented grating and a perpendicular grating could increase the amount of cross-orientation suppression in V1 neurons. Such a result is completely consistent with our model, in which the increased statistical dependency in the responses of orthogonally oriented neurons would lead to an increase in the suppressive weights between them.

Discussion

Work reported in this chapter was motivated by the early proposal of Barlow [6]: namely, that a desirable goal in early sensory processing is to obtain neural responses that are independent. As emphasized by Barlow, independent neural responses lead to a more efficient representation of sensory input, and facilitate ecologically relevant tasks such as novelty detection. We began by demonstrating that the responses of linear receptive fields, when exposed to natural images, exhibit strikingly non-Gaussian dependencies. Interestingly, the type of nonlinearity suitable for removing these dependencies, per Barlow's hypothesis, also reproduces the type of nonlinear behavior observed in cortical neurons. On this basis, we developed a divisive normalization model for cortical neurons, whose parameters are entirely determined by the statistical properties of visual images. We find it remarkable that this model can account qualitatively for the suppressive effects of non-optimal stimuli, as well as for basic adaptation effects. Moreover, by considering how normalization parameters should change in response to specific changes in image statistics, we were able to distinguish between two canonical types of adaptation.

Nonetheless, there are many issues that need to be resolved. On the theoretical side, we are working to understand the class of models for which divisive normalization provides an optimal "nonlinear whitening" operation [58, 55]. Moreover, there are also fundamental problems in attempting to state the independence hypothesis more formally. In particular, quantitative testing of the hypothesis requires specification of an image ensemble from which the statistics are taken. We have chosen a small set of generic scenes, but it could be the case that neurons are specialized for particular subclasses of images. Also lacking is a clear statement of which groups of neurons are meant to produce an ensemble of statistically independent responses. Even within cortical area V1, response properties vary considerably from layer to layer, and even within layers. A sensible assumption might be that each stage of processing in the system takes the responses of the previous stage and attempts to eliminate as much statistical redundancy as possible, within the limits of its computational capabilities. This "successive whitening" version of the theory naturally leads one to ask: How far can this bottom-up theory go to explain higher levels of sensory processing? Surely, at some level, the tasks that the organism performs must have some influence on the design of the system.

There are a number of open questions concerning both temporal aspects of the model, as well as the mechanistic implementation of normalization. The current model addresses only steady-state behavior, and the normalization signal is computed and applied instantaneously. Clearly, a more realistic implementation must perform the normalization of a population of neurons using recursive lateral or feedback connections, thereby introducing temporal dynamics. Recent experiments on V1 neurons reveal temporal dynamics that seem consistent with such delayed normalization signals [e.g. [42, 32]]. Such recurrent connections might directly provide shunting inhibition [e.g. [23, 12]], but the divisive form of the steady-state model does not necessarily require this. We have recently begun to explore models that incorporate delayed feedback mechanisms, but produce steady-state responses consistent with the weighted normalization model described in this paper [30].

Regarding adaptation, our current work does not address the time course or mechanism of such processes. It is possible that several forms of adaptation occur simultaneously on different time scales. Moreover, we have not yet specified a local update (or "learning") rule to instantiate the optimization specified in equation (10.2).

Our model is fundamentally suppressive. But a number of authors have reported facilitatory influences from beyond the classical receptive field [e.g. [28, 33, 24]]. Facilitation can arise in our model in several ways. First, facilitation of low-contrast optimal stimuli can occur when the secondary (non-optimal) stimulus slightly excites the linear kernel of a model neuron (e.g. when the facilitating stimulus overlaps the classical receptive field). This could explain a number of published results, in which interactions have been shown to be facilitatory at low contrast and suppressive at high contrast [e.g. [27, 38]]. Second, a recurrent implementation of our model might lead to dis-inhibition effects (those neurons that usually suppress responses in the recorded neuron are themselves being suppressed by the facilitating stimulus, leading to an increase in response). As our implementation is currently not recurrent, we have not examined this possibility in detail.

We believe the statistically derived decomposition we have described here may be applicable to other sensory modalities. In particular, we have recently found interesting parallels in the statistics of natural sounds, and the response properties of auditory nerve fibers [46]. Finally, it is our hope that elaboration of the independence hypothesis might benefit future experimental studies. In particular, we are working to design specialized stochastic stimuli for characterizing normalization models, as well as their behavior under various adaptation conditions.

References

[1] D G Albrecht, S B Farrar, and D B Hamilton. Spatial contrast adaptation characteristics of neurones recorded in the cat's visual cortex. *J. Physiology*, 347:713–739, 1984.

[2] J J Atick. Could information theory provide an ecological theory of sensory processing? *Network: Computation in Neural Systems*, 3:213–251, 1992.

[3] J J Atick and A N Redlich. Convergent algorithm for sensory receptive field development. *Neural Computation*, 5:45–60, 1993.

[4] F Attneave. Some informational aspects of visual perception. *Psych. Rev.*, 61:183–193, 1954.

[5] R Baddeley, L F Abbott, M C Booth, F Sengpiel, T Freeman, E A Wakeman, and E T Rolls. Respones of neurons in primary and inferior temporal visual cortices to natural scenes. *Proc. Roy. Soc. (Lond.)*, B264:1775–1783, 1998.

[6] H B Barlow. Possible principles underlying the transformation of sensory messages. In W A Rosenblith, editor, *Sensory Communication*, page 217. MIT Press, Cambridge, MA, 1961.

[7] Horace B Barlow. A theory about the functional role and synaptic mechanism of visual aftereffects. In C Blakemore, editor, *Vision: Coding and Efficiency*. Cambridge University Press, 1990.

[8] Horace B Barlow and P Foldiak. Adaptation and decorrelation in the cortex. In R Durbin, C Miall, and G Mitchinson, editors, *The Computing Neuron*, chapter 4, pages 54–72. Addison-Wellesley, New York, 1989.

[9] A J Bell and T J Sejnowski. The 'independent components' of natural scenes are edge filters. *Vision Research*, 37(23):3327–3338, 1997.

[10] A B Bonds. Role of inhibition in the specification of orientation of cells in the cat striate cortex. *Visual Neuroscience*, 2:41–55, 1989.

[11] R W Buccigrossi and E P Simoncelli. Image compression via joint statistical characterization in the wavelet domain. *IEEE Trans Image Proc*, 8(12):1688–1701, December 1999.

[12] M Carandini and D J Heeger. Summation and division by neurons in primate visual cortex. *Science*, 264:1333–1336, 1994.

[13] M Carandini, D J Heeger, and J A Movshon. Linearity and normalization in simple cells of the macaque primary visual cortex. *Journal of Neuroscience*, 17:8621–8644, 1997.

[14] M Carandini, J A Movshon, and D Ferster. Pattern adaptation and cross-orientation interactions in the primary visual cortex. *Neuropharmacology*, 37:501–511, 1998.

[15] F S Chance, S B Nelson, and L F Abbott. Synaptic depression and the temporal response characteristics of V1 cells. *Journal of Neuroscience*, 18:4785–4799, 1998.

[16] M S Crouse, R D Nowak, and R G Baraniuk. Wavelet-based statistical signal processing using hidden Markov models. *IEEE Trans. Signal Proc.*, 46:886–902, April 1998.

[17] Y Dan, J J Atick, and R C Reid. Efficient coding of natural scenes in the lateral geniculate nucleus: Experimental test of a computational theory. *J. Neuroscience*, 16:3351–3362, 1996.

[18] John G. Daugman. Entropy reduction and decorrelation in visual coding by oriented neural receptive fields. *IEEE Trans. Biomedical Engineering*, 36(1):107–114, 1989.

[19] D J Field. Relations between the statistics of natural images and the response properties of cortical cells. *J. Opt. Soc. Am. A*, 4(12):2379–2394, 1987.

[20] P Foldiak. Forming sparse representations by local anti-hebbian learning. *Biol. Cybernetics*, 64:165–170, 1990.

[21] W S Geisler and D G Albrecht. Cortical neurons: Isolation of contrast gain control. *Vision Research*, 8:1409–1410, 1992.

[22] D J Heeger. Normalization of cell responses in cat striate cortex. *Visual Neuroscience*, 9:181–198, 1992.

[23] D J Heeger. Modeling simple cell direction selectivity with normalized, half-squared, linear operators. *Journal of Neurophysiology*, 70(5):1885–1898, 1993.

[24] M K Kapadia, M Ito, C D Gilbert, and G Westheimer. Improvement in visual sensitivity. *Neuron*, 15(4), Oct 1995.

[25] S B Laughlin. A simple coding procedure enhances a neuron's information capacity. *Z. Naturforsch.*, 36c:910–912, 1981.

[26] S.B. Laughlin. The role of sensory adaptation in the retina. *Journal of Experimental Biology*, 146:39–62, 1989.

[27] J B Levitt and J S Lund. Contrast dependence of contextual effects in primate visual cortex. *Nature*, 387:73–76, 1997.

[28] L Maffei and A Fiorentini. The unresponsive regions of visual cortical receptive fields. *Vision Research*, 16:1131–1139, 1976.

[29] S G Mallat. A theory for multiresolution signal decomposition: The wavelet representation. *IEEE Pat. Anal. Mach. Intell.*, 11:674–693, July 1989.

[30] S Mikaelian and E Simoncelli. Modeling temporal response characteristics of V1 neurons with a dynamic normalization model. In *Proc. Computational Neuroscience*, Brugge, Belgium, 2000. To appear.

[31] J A Movshon and P Lennie. Pattern-selective adaptation in visual cortical neurones. *Nature*, 278:850–852, 1979.

[32] J R Müller, A B Metha, J Krauskopf, and P Lennie. Rapid adaptation in visual cortex to the structure of images. *Science*, 285:1405–1408, Aug 1999.

[33] J I Nelson and B J Frost. Intracortical facilitation among co-oriented, coaxially aligned simple cells in cat striate cortex. *Exp. Brain Res.*, 61:54–61, 1985.

[34] I Ohzawa, G Sclar, and R D Freeman. Contrast gain control in the cat visual cortex. *Nature*, 298:266–268, 1982.

[35] I Ohzawa, G Sclar, and R D Freeman. Contrast gain control in the cat's visual system. *J. Neurophysiology*, 54:651–667, 1985.

[36] E Oja. A simplified neuron model as a principal component analyzer. *Journal of Mathematical Biology*, 15:267–273, 1982.

[37] B A Olshausen and D J Field. Emergence of simple-cell receptive field properties by learning a sparse code for natural images. *Nature*, 381:607–609, 1996.

[38] U Polat, K Mizobew, M W Pettet, T Kasamatsu, and A J Norcia. Collinear stimuli regulate visual responses depending on cell's contrast threshold. *Nature*, 391:580–584, February 1998.

[39] W Reichhardt and T Poggio. Figure-ground discrimination by relative movement in the visual system of the fly. *Biol. Cybern.*, 35:81–100, 1979.

[40] P Reinagel and R C Reid. Temporal coding of visual information in the thalamus. *J Neuroscience*, 2000. In Press.

[41] F Rieke, D A Bodnar, and W Bialek. Naturalistic stimuli increase the rate and efficiency of information transmission by primary auditory afferents. *Proc. R. Soc. Lond. B*, 262:259–265, 1995.

[42] D L Ringach, M J Hawken, and R Shapley. The dynamics of orientation tuning in macaque primary visual cortex. *Nature*, 387:281–284, May 1997.

[43] T D Sanger. Optimal unsupervised learning in a single-layer network. *Neural Networks*, 2:459–473, 1989.

[44] A B Saul and M S Cynader. Adaptation in single units in the visual cortex: The tuning of aftereffects in the spatial domain. *Visual Neuroscience*, 2:593–607, 1989.

[45] A B Saul and M S Cynader. Adaptation in single units in the visual cortex: The tuning of aftereffects in the temporal domain. *Visual Neuroscience*, 2:609–620, 1989.

[46] O Schwartz and E Simoncelli. Natural sound statistics and divisive normalization in the auditory system. In *Adv. Neural Information Processing Systems*, volume 13, Cambridge, MA, 2001. MIT Press. Presented at Neural Information Processing Systems, Dec 2000.

[47] E Simoncelli and B Olshausen. Statistical properties of natural images. *Annual Review of Neuroscience*, 24, May 2001. To Appear.

[48] E P Simoncelli. Statistical models for images: Compression, restoration and synthesis. In *31st Asilomar Conf on Signals, Systems and Computers*, pages 673–678, Pacific Grove, CA, November 1997. IEEE Computer Society. Available from http://www.cns.nyu.edu/~eero/publications.html.

[49] E P Simoncelli. Bayesian denoising of visual images in the wavelet domain. In P Müller and B Vidakovic, editors, *Bayesian Inference in Wavelet Based Models*, chapter 18, pages 291–308. Springer-Verlag, New York, Spring 1999. Lecture Notes in Statistics, vol. 141.

[50] E P Simoncelli, W T Freeman, E H Adelson, and D J Heeger. Shiftable multi-scale transforms. *IEEE Trans Information Theory*, 38(2):587–607, March 1992. Special Issue on Wavelets.

[51] E P Simoncelli and O Schwartz. Image statistics and cortical normalization models. In M. S. Kearns, S. A. Solla, and D. A. Cohn, editors, *Adv. Neural Information Processing Systems*, volume 11, pages 153–159, Cambridge, MA, 1999. MIT Press. Presented at Neural Information Processing Systems, 1-3 Dec 1998.

[52] J H van Hateren. A theory of maximizing sensory information. *Biol. Cybern.*, 68:23–29, 1992.

[53] J H van Hateren and A van der Schaaf. Independent component filters of natural images compared with simple cells in primary visual cortex. *Proc. R. Soc. Lond. B*, pages 359–366, 1998.

[54] W E Vinje and J L Gallant. Sparse coding and decorrelation in primary visual cortex during natural vision. *Science*, 287, Feb 2000.

[55] M Wainwright, E Simoncelli, and A Willsky. Random cascades on wavelet trees and their use in modeling and analyzing natural imagery. *Applied and Computational Harmonic Analysis*, 2001. Special issue on wavelet applications. To appear.

[56] M J Wainwright. Visual adaptation as optimal information transmission. *Vision Research*, 39:3960–3974, 1999.

[57] M J Wainwright and E P Simoncelli. Explaining adaptation in V1 neurons with a statistically optimized normalization model. In *Investigative Opthalmology and Visual Science Supplement (ARVO)*, volume 40, pages S–573, May 1999.

[58] M J Wainwright and E P Simoncelli. Scale mixtures of Gaussians and the statistics of natural images. In S. A. Solla, T. K. Leen, and K.-R. Müller, editors, *Adv. Neural Information Processing Systems*, volume 12, pages 855–861, Cambridge, MA, May 2000. MIT Press. Presented at Neural Information Processing Systems, Dec 1999.

[59] B Wegmann and C Zetzsche. Statistical dependence between orientation filter outputs used in an human vision based image code. In *Proc SPIE Visual Comm. and Image Processing*, volume 1360, pages 909–922, Lausanne, Switzerland, 1990.

[60] H R Wilson and R Humanski. Spatial frequency adaptation and contrast gain control. *Vis. Res.*, 33(8):1133–1149, 1993.

[61] C Zetzsche and W Schönecker. Orientation selective filters lead to entropy reduction in the processing of natural images. *Perception*, 16:229, 1987.

11 A Probabilistic Network Model of Population Responses

Richard S. Zemel and Jonathan Pillow

Introduction

An important debate in computational neuroscience centers on the origin of selectivities in populations of cortical cells. A focus of this debate has been an extensive set of empirical data on orientation selectivity in primary visual cortex. A central question concerns how the observed sharp tuning of striate cells arises from broadly-tuned LGN input that is purely excitatory and grows monotonically with contrast. One class of network models posits that the sharp tuning is primarily due to the effects of recurrent connections within the striate population. These *recurrent* models (e.g., Ben-Yishai, Bar-Or, & Sompolinsky, 1995; Somers, Nelson, & Douglas, 1995) can account for a wide range of the empirical data (reviewed in Sompolinsky and Shapley, 1997). Other models, such as *feedforward* models (Troyer, Krukowski, & Miller, 1998) and *gain-control* models (Carandini, Heeger, & Movshon, 1997), emphasize a variety of other mechanisms.

We suggest that some insight into these models can be gained by comparing their answers to the following question: What information is presumed to be contained in the population response? A model that presumes that the population provides a noisy encoding of a single value will focus on methods of removing the noise that would suggest an incorrect value. A model that assumes that the input signal is confounded by irrelevant dimensions, such as contrast variation when the encoded dimension is orientation, will focus on filtering out those other dimensions.

In this paper, we propose a different answer to this question. Our hypothesis is that the population response is designed to preserve full information about relevant dimensions in the stimulus. This information could be a single unambiguous value, an ambiguous value (where the ambiguity in orientation could be due to low contrast, fuzzy edges, curved edges, etc.), or more than one value.

We have shown previously that population responses can represent this additional information, by interpreting the population response as a probability distribution over the underlying stimulus dimension (Zemel, Dayan, & Pouget, 1998). This work did not say anything about how this information could arise in the population, but instead simply assumed that it was there. In this chapter, we show how to generate population responses that contain this additional information, in a neural network model using a combination of feedforward and recurrent connections. A novel computational aspect of this approach is that we use the preservation of this information as an objective in training the weights in the model.

The proposal that a model population can faithfully encode more than one value is not without controversy. Carandini and Ringach (1997) studied a simple recurrent model of a hypercolumn of striate cells. Their model successfully and succinctly captures a range of experimental results, including sharp orientation tuning and contrast-invariant tuning width. However, their model makes several peculiar predictions when the input contains more than a single orientation. If the input contains two orientations differing by less than 45°, the model responds as to a single orientation at the mean of the two values; if the two orientations differ by more than 45°, the model responds as if they were nearly orthogonal. The model also cannot signal the presence of three orientations, and generates a spurious orthogonal response to noisy single-orientation inputs. These authors analyzed their model and showed that these effects, termed *attraction* and *repulsion* between orientations, are unavoidable in a broad class of recurrent models of orientation selectivity.

The aim of the model presented here is to explore if a broader range of activity patterns can be maintained within a population, to convey additional relevant stimulus information. We first describe the probabilistic formulation of the information that underlies the population response, then provide details of the model. We then compare the results of our model and several others to a variety of stimuli, and analyze the key differences.

Our Approach

The heart of our model is a probabilistic formulation of population responses. We have previously used this formulation to interpret the responses of a population of units in the model. Here, we apply this same formulation to adjust the weights in the model to produce the desired responses.

Probabilistic formulation

We recently developed a *distribution population coding* (DPC) model (Zemel et al., 1998) that generalizes the standard population coding model to the situation in which a probability distribution underlies the population activity. Decoding in DPC, like the standard statistical decoding methods, is based on a probabilistic model of observed responses, which allows the formulation of a decoding method that is optimal in a statistical sense. The key contribution of our model concerns the fact that most models of population codes assume that the population response encodes a single value, and therefore discard information about multiple values and/or ambiguity. By recovering a full distribution, our model preserves this information.

The DPC model begins from the same starting point as the standard model: the neurophysiological finding that in many cases responses of cells within a cortical area can be predicted based on their *tuning curves*. Cell i's tuning curve, $f_i(\mathbf{x})$, describes its expected firing rate, typically defined as a spike count, as a function of the relevant dimension(s) $\mathbf{x}$. These tuning curves are estimated by observing the cell's response on many trials using a set of stimuli that vary along $\mathbf{x}$. A *population code* is defined to be a population of cells whose tuning curves span the space of $\mathbf{x}$ values; this population can thus be considered as a basis for encoding the dimensions $\mathbf{x}$ underlying a set of stimuli. Here, we will focus on the case where $\mathbf{x}$ is a single dimension θ, such as the orientation of a grating.

The standard model of population responses (e.g., Seung & Sompolinsky, 1993) assumes that firing rates vary, even for a fixed input. The recorded activity r_i of each unit i is characterized as a stochastic function of its tuning curve $f_i(\theta)$, where the noise n_i is typically zero-mean Gaussian or Poisson, and the responses of the different units are conditionally independent given θ. This leads to the simple *encoding* model, describing how θ is coded in $\mathbf{r}$:

$$r_i = f_i(\theta) + n_i \tag{11.1}$$

Bayesian *decoding* inverts the encoding model to find the posterior distribution $\mathcal{P}(\theta|\mathbf{r})$, which describes how likely each direction is given the observed responses (Földiák, 1994; Salinas & Abbott, 1994; Sanger, 1996). For example, under an independent Poisson noise assumption,

$$\mathcal{P}[\theta|\mathbf{r}] \sim \log \left\{ \mathcal{P}[\theta] \prod_i \mathcal{P}[r_i|\theta] \right\} \sim \sum_i r_i \log f_i(\theta) \tag{11.2}$$

This method thus provides a multiplicative kernel density estimate, tending to produce a sharp distribution for a single value of θ. A single estimate $\hat{\theta}$ can then be extracted from $\mathcal{P}[\theta|\mathbf{r}]$ using some criterion (e.g., the orientation with the highest probability, or the value that maximizes the data likelihood), and interpreted as the most likely single value in the stimulus. Figure 11.1A illustrates the framework used for standard decoding.

We are interested in cases where the activities **r** code a whole distribution $\mathcal{P}[\theta]$ over the underlying variable, as opposed to a single value θ. A simple associated *encoding* model extends the standard model, positing that the expected response of the cell is the average of its response to the set of values described by $\mathcal{P}[\theta]$:

$$\langle r_i \rangle = \int_\theta \mathcal{P}[\theta] f_i(\theta) d\theta \tag{11.3}$$

Evidence for this encoding model comes from studies of cells in area MT using stimuli containing multiple motions within the cell's receptive field. The general neurophysiological finding is that an MT cell's response to these stimuli can be characterized as a scaled sum of its responses to the individual components (van Wezel, Lankheet, Verstrate, Maree, & van de Grind, 1996; Recanzone, Wurtz, & Schwarz, 1997; Treue, Hol, & Rauber, 1999).

Decoding in this model is more complicated than in the standard model. Bayesian *decoding* takes the observed activities and produces a probability distribution over probability distributions over θ, i.e., $\mathcal{P}[\mathcal{P}[\theta]|\mathbf{r}]$. Figure 11.1B illustrates the framework used for decoding in DPC. In Zemel et al. (1998), we proposed decoding using an approximate form of maximum likelihood in distributions over θ, finding the $\hat{\mathcal{P}}^{\mathbf{r}}(\theta)$ that maximizes

$$L\left[\mathcal{P}(\theta)|\mathbf{r}\right] \sim \sum_i r_i \log\left[f_i(\theta) * \mathcal{P}(\theta)\right] - \alpha g\left[\mathcal{P}(\theta)\right] \tag{11.4}$$

where $\mathcal{P}[\theta]$ is the , prior probability distribution over θ, and the smoothness term $g[]$ acts as a regularizer.

This decoding method is not meant to model neural processing, as it involves complicated and non-neural operations. Simpler decoding methods, such as linear decoding from a set of basis functions, may be used. However, the primary focus in this paper is to understand what information in principle may be conveyed by a population code under the interpretation that populations are encoding distributions. This leads to the interpretation that the extracted distribution $\hat{\mathcal{P}}^{\mathbf{r}}(\mathbf{x})$ describes the information about $\mathcal{P}[\theta]$ available in the population response **r**. A sensible objective for the population then is that its response to a stimulus characterized by $\mathcal{P}[\theta]$ should faithfully encode this true distribution, i.e., $\hat{\mathcal{P}}^{\mathbf{r}}(\mathbf{x})$ should provide a good approximation to $\mathcal{P}[\theta]$. Indeed, a range of simulations with this model have shown that if activities are generated according to the encoding model (Equation 11.3), then the decoded distribution $\hat{\mathcal{P}}^{\mathbf{r}}(\mathbf{x})$ does preserve most of the information in the original $\mathcal{P}[\theta]$ (Zemel et al., 1998; Zemel & Dayan, 1999).

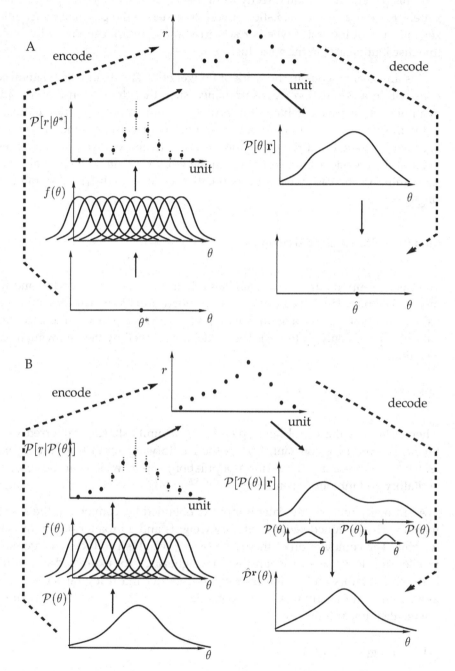

Figure 11.1. (A) The standard Bayesian population coding framework assumes that a single value is encoded in a set of noisy neural activities. (B) The distribution population coding framework shows how a distribution over θ can be encoded and then decoded from noisy population activities. From Zemel and Dayan (1999).

In this paper, rather than directly using the encoding model to specify a response pattern **r**, we use a more realistic network to generate the population activities. The key question of interest if whether activities in a network can faithfully encode the true distribution $\mathcal{P}[\theta]$ in the stimulus.

This aim is analogous to the work of Pouget et al. (1998), in which lateral connections within a population were formulated such that the response of a population to a noisy input was a stable hill of activity, where its peak position corresponded to the most likely direction estimate based on the decoding model (Equation 11.2). That work showed that the population could actively remove noise in its response to faithfully encode a single estimate. In the work presented here, we aim to do the same thing in the case where the population encodes a distribution rather than a single value.

Model architecture and dynamics

The basic set-up in our model resembles others, such as the Carandini and Ringach model. The population is a group of rate-coded units identical except in preferred value, where the response of units with preferred value ϕ to a stimulus containing a value θ depends only on $(\theta - \phi)$. The model is governed by the following mean-field equation:

$$\tau\frac{dV}{dt} + V = V^{FF} + V^{LAT} \tag{11.5}$$

where $V(\theta, t)$ is the membrane potential of all units sharing preferred value θ at time t, τ is the time constant, V^{FF} is the feedforward input from the layer below, and V^{LAT} represents lateral (intra-population) input, which can be resolved into excitatory and inhibitory components: $V^{LAT} = V^{LAT\_E} - V^{LAT\_I}$.

As in many models, the lateral input is obtained by convolving the responses **r** with a narrowly tuned set of excitatory weights and a broader profile of inhibitory weights. The combination of these two sets of weights produces a center-surround profile. Thus $V^{LAT} = w*\mathbf{r}$, where the net weights w can be expressed as the difference between excitatory and inhibitory weights. Finally, unit firing rates **r** are computed as a function of the unit membrane potential, $\mathbf{r} = g(V)$. We use an approximation to the rectified linear function:

$$g(V) = a\log(1 + \exp(b(V + c))), \tag{11.6}$$

where $a, b,$ and c are constants (Zhang, 1996). Rectification is a nonlinear operation necessary to prevent negative firing rates; this function $g(V)$ has the added desirable property that it is easy to invert analytically. We can therefore express the lateral input as

$$V^{LAT} = w * g(V) \tag{11.7}$$

The primary differences in our model from the standard ones arise from the probabilistic formulation described above. We apply this probabilistic formulation in two ways. First, we use it to optimize the lateral weights in the model, so that the population activity patterns provide a faithful encoding of the true information about θ contained in the stimulus. Second, we use the probabilistic model to read out, or interpret the information conveyed about the underlying variable θ by the population response. This is accomplished via the distribution decoding method described by Equation 11.4. These points are discussed in more detail below.

Weight optimization

In order for the network response to encode information about θ, we need to be able to specify target response patterns as a function of the evidence for orientation θ in the input. We use the distribution encoding model described by Equation 11.3 to determine the targets. We defined $\mathcal{P}[\theta]$ as the information about θ in the input. If this is known for a given input, then an activity pattern

$$\mathbf{r} = \{r_i\} = \left\{ \int_\theta \mathcal{P}[\theta] f_i(\theta) d\theta \right\} \tag{11.8}$$

is the appropriate target, where f_i is the unit tuning function. Each cell's tuning function (describing its expected response to a singular stimulus, containing only one value of the relevant variable) is a circular normal distribution about its preferred value:

$$f_i(\theta) = A + B \exp(K \cos(2 * (\theta - \theta_i))), \tag{11.9}$$

where θ_i is the i'th unit's preferred orientation, A is baseline (stimulus-independent) firing rate, and B and K determine the amplitude and sharpness of tuning, respectively. We used the values $A = 1$, $B = .013$, and $K = 8$ during weight optimization, giving the cell a maximal firing rate of 40 spikes per second and a relatively sharp tuning profile.

Two important aspects of this approach bear comment here. First, in our model, these tuning functions are used only to generate the target responses; for decoding purposes we use a function based on the model's actual response to a single-orientation stimulus $\mathcal{P}[\theta] = \delta(\theta)$. These two activity patterns may not be the same, as the true stable states of the network may not exactly match the shape of tuning functions used to train it. In this case, decoding must be based on the information available in the observed population responses. Second, any decoding model based on inverting the encoding model should obtain a $\hat{\mathcal{P}r}(\mathbf{x})$ that approximates the true $\mathcal{P}[\theta]$. Optimization in our model is thus only a function of the encoding method, and does not depend on the particular decoding method.

The recurrent weights, both excitatory and inhibitory, are optimized based on a set of examples. Each example consists of: (a) the feedforward input for a stimulus containing 1, 2, or 3 values, and (b) target output values for the model units, obtained from Equation 11.8 based on the units' tuning curves (Equation 11.9) and the values in the stimulus. In our simulations, $\mathcal{P}[\theta]$ is a scaled sum of sharp normal distributions centered on the set of values present in the stimulus. The training set contained 100 examples each of single, double, and triple orientation stimuli, with the orientations selected randomly.

The weights are modified such that the targets are the stable activity profiles of the differential state update equation (Equation 11.5). This can be implemented in the Fourier domain as

$$\hat{w} = \left\langle \frac{(\hat{\mathbf{V}}(j) - \hat{\mathbf{V}}^{FF})\hat{\mathbf{r}}(j)}{\|\lambda + \hat{\mathbf{r}}(j)\|^2} \right\rangle_{j=1}^{m} \tag{11.10}$$

where $\mathbf{V}(j)$ is the target membrane voltage (computed as $\mathbf{V} = g^{-1}(\mathbf{r})$), λ is a regularization parameter, and $\langle \ldots \rangle$ denotes the mean over the set of examples.

Read-out

A second important facet of our model involves a different way of interpreting the activities of the population. In order to determine what information about orientation is present in the unit responses, we apply the statistical decoding approach in the framework outlined above. The method we use here is described by Equation 11.4. This method takes into account the units' tuning functions in finding the distribution over θ most likely to have generated the observed responses.

The decoding procedure produces a distribution over orientations, $\hat{\mathcal{P}r}(\mathbf{x})$, that is meant to describe the evidence across the range of orientations in an input stimulus. An additional step is required to match this to the true orientations present in the stimulus. We adopt a simple procedure of picking out the modes of the extracted distribution, and assuming that each mode corresponds to a separate orientation in the input.

Results

Other models

Many different models for orientation selectivity in primary visual cortex have been proposed (Ben-Yishai et al.1995; Somers et al.1995; Carandini & Ringach, 1997; Troyer et al., 1999; Adorjan et al., 2000). We have selected three of these models in order to analyze the significance of different assumptions about the population response and to compare the performance of our model with several others.

The Carandini-Ringach model is the first model for comparison. It contains an architecture and dynamics similar to our model, and its performance on orientation stimuli containing multiple values and noisy values has already been analyzed. A second model we explore here is the Ben-Yishai et al. (1995) model. This model ssumes that a single orientation underlies the input, and endeavors to generate a population response whose tuning is nearly independent of both the contrast and the strength of the orientation bias (anisotropy) in the stimulus. The third and final comparison model is the Pouget et al. (1998) model; as stated above, the primary aim of this model closely resembles ours. Both models attempt to use the recurrent weights in a population to settle on an activity pattern that is an expected pattern under the encoding model. We discuss the main features of these three models and our implementations of them below.

The populations of all models are set up to contain identical, independent units, which differ only in their preferred values θ_i, ranging from $-\pi/2$ to $\pi/2$. Each model contains a dynamic update equation, external input specified as a function of stimulus orientation, a set of recurrent weights, and an activation function for converting membrane potential V into a spike rate r. In all models, feedforward input to a unit depends only on the difference between its preferred value and the orientations in the input, and the recurrent weights are a symmetric function of the difference in preferred values between units.

(1). *Carandini-Ringach model*: This model uses the same update equation as ours (Equation 11.5), but has a semilinear activation function. The recurrent weights have a center-surround profile given by a weighted difference of Gaussians, clipped at $\pm 60°$. Input to the model is a broadly-tuned Gaussian, and is kept constant during the dynamic updates.

(2). *Ben-Yishai et al.model*: This model uses the update equation (Equation 11.5) and a semilinear activation function. The recurrent weights have a cosine profile of the form $w(\theta) = -J_0 + J_2 \cos(2\theta)$, where $-J_0$ represents a uniform level of recurrent inhibition and J_2 determines the strength of orientation-dependent feedback. Input to the model is given by another cosine function, $c(1-\epsilon+\epsilon \cos(2\theta))$, where c represents contrast, and ϵ gives the strength of the orientation bias in the input. This input is constant over time.

(3). *Pouget et al. model*: This model uses an invertible nonlinear activation function like ours (Equation 11.6). It has no constant external input—the input specifies only the initial state of the network, and has the shape of the unit tuning function. Dynamic updates are performed according to $V_t = (1 - \gamma)V_{t-1} + \gamma V_{t-1}^{LAT}$, where γ specifies the rate of change between time steps. Weights in this model are determined by an optimization procedure that seeks to make the tuning functions into stable states of the network. As in our model, tuning functions have the shape of a circular normal distribution.

For the Ben-Yishai et al. model, we performed simulations with the values $J_0 = 86$ and $J_2 = 112$. These parameters specify a regime in which the model's tuning is dominated by cortical interactions and (as desired) is relatively independent of contrast and orientation anisotropy. The results described below all use model populations containing $N = 512$ units, except for the Pouget et al. model, which contained $N = 64$ units. We have since tested this model with 512 units, and found no significant difference in the results.

Test stimuli

Comparing these models is somewhat complicated for the fact that they make different assumptions about the form of the input they receive. All of the models are capable of generating a narrowly tuned response from a stimulus with a weak single orientation signal. However, the models vary greatly in the tuning width and amplitude of the input they expect to receive. Under the Pouget et al model, expected input has the narrow profile of the unit tuning function, while the Ben-Yishai et al model expects broadly tuned cosine input (in fact, this input is unimodal even when multiple orientations are present). In order to make comparisons fair, for the simulations reported in this paper, each model is given the inputs it expects. For our model, we used input with a circular normal shape, but matched the amplitude and tuning to that of the Gaussian input used in the Carandini-Ringach model. (Parameters: $A = 0$, $B = .182$, $K = 1.7$). This input was at least twice as broad as our unit tuning functions, and is intermediate between the narrow input profile of the Pouget et al model and the broad input of the Ben-Yishai et al model.

We sought to compare the models using test stimuli that simulate basic properties of LGN responses to various complex stimuli, including stimuli containing two or three orientations, or a single, noisy orientation. Although little is known about the actual LGN input to a V1 cell for such stimuli, a reasonable first guess is to use the sum of the responses to each orientation contained in the stimulus. To this end, we generated test input for comparing models by using each model's expected input

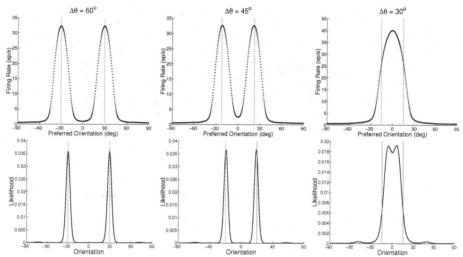

Figure 11.2. The top row of plots depicts stable response profiles of our model population to stimuli containing two values. The three columns correspond to stimuli with differing angular spread between the pair of orientations. Note that the model can stably maintain bimodal activity patterns even when the modes are far from orthogonal. The bottom row of plots depicts the information about the underlying variable decoded from those response profiles. In both rows of plots, the vertical gray lines are the values of the true orientations contained in the stimulus. The lower right plot demonstrates that information about multiple values may be preserved, even when the population response is itself unimodal.

profile convolved with the orientations present in the stimulus. For noisy input, we used each model's expected input profile corrupted with Gaussian noise.

Responses to two-value stimuli

The response of our model to stimuli containing two values, of varying angular difference, is shown in Figure 11.2. Our model forms different stable activity patterns to all three pairs, and the decoding method accurately recovers the original values present in the stimulus. In contrast, none of the other three models is able to veridically encode any of these stimuli, as demonstrated in Figure 11.3.

The qualitative performance of the different models is highlighted in Figure 11.4, which represents their responses to all possible two-orientation stimuli. Each horizontal slice represents the response to a particular stimulus, and the angular spread between the two orientations increases from 0° to 90° along the y-axis. Note that our model contains a smooth transition from uni- to bimodal response patterns. The response profile broadens and flattens as the two orientations in the stimulus become more distinct, and then separate into two hills of activity as the spread grows beyond 30°. The Carandini-Ringach model is the only other model capable of generating a

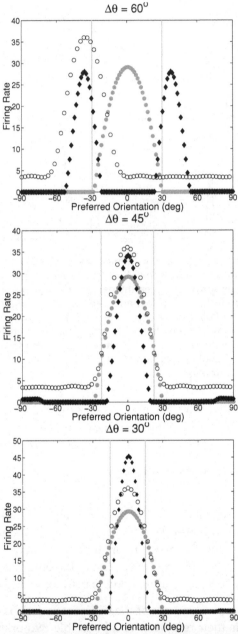

Figure 11.3. These plots show the response profiles of the comparison models when presented the same stimuli used to generate the responses shown in Figure 11.2. The open circles correspond to unit responses of the Pouget et al. (1998) model; the gray circles are for the Ben-Yishai et al. (1995) model; and black triangles are for the Carandini and Ringach (1997) model. The vertical gray lines again represent the orientations the models are attempting to encode.

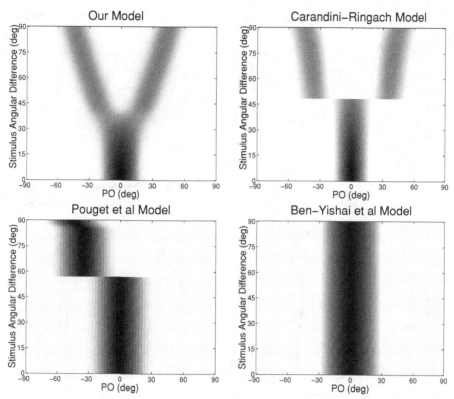

Figure 11.4. Summary of responses to all 2-value stimuli for all four models. In each plot, the model units are arranged according to their preferred orientation value (PO). Each horizontal slice shows the unit activities to a particular 2-value stimulus. The vertical axis represents the difference between the two values in the stimulus, ranging from identical to orthogonal orientations. The response at the top of the plots is therefore to a stimulus with two orientations present at ±45°. The "correct" encoding of the stimuli corresponds to a pair of lines running diagonally from 0° at the bottom of a plot to ±45° at the top. Note that the Carandini-Ringach model response is discontinuous near 45°, while our model contains a smooth transition. The Pouget et al. and Ben-Yishai et al. models both give unimodal responses to all stimuli.

stable bimodal response pattern, but note that it contains a significant discontinuity near 45°, where the response jumps from being uni- to bimodal. This shows that the model successfully encodes two orientations when they are nearly orthogonal, but has difficulty with intermediate values.

The behavior of the Ben-Yishai et al. model is determined by the cosine shape of its recurrent weights, together with the fact that recurrent input so strongly dominates its response. A cosine weight profile ensures that recurrent input is really just a measurement of the F1 component of the current population activity, leading to a response centered at the phase of the F1 component of the input. The F1 phase is zero for all stimuli shown here, so the model's response is approximately invariant.

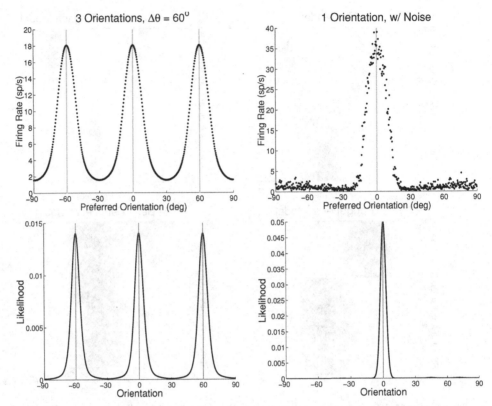

Figure 11.5. The top row of plots shows the response of our model to stimuli containing three values (left), and a single value plus noise (right). The noise added was Gaussian with mean and standard deviation 33% and 20% of the amplitude of the input. The decoding of these responses is shown below. Vertical gray lines show the location of the orientations in the stimulus.

The Pouget et al. model contains a discontinuity in its response and is also incapable of maintaining a bimodal activity profile. For separations smaller than 45° the orientations "attract" and the response is centered at the mean of the two orientations in the stimulus (0°). For larger separations, the two modes in the original input "repel" before one finally wins out, resulting in a response that is centered near either +45° or -45° (these two outcomes are equally likely, though Figure 11.4 only shows those resulting in a final response centered near -45°).

Responses to three-value and noise stimuli

Our model is also able to maintain a stable response profile for stimuli containing three values, as well as a clean unimodal response to noisy single-value stimuli (see Figure 11.5). In both cases, the decoding method reconstructs the values present in the stimulus.

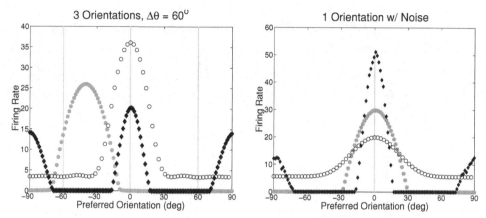

Figure 11.6. The response of comparison models to inputs containing three values (left), and a single value plus noise (right) (lines labeled as in Figure 11.3). The three orientations in the left plot are located at 0 and ±60°. The noise added in the right plot was Gaussian with mean and standard deviation (33%, 20%) relative to the magnitude of the input to each model. Note the spurious response to the orthogonal value in the Carandini-Ringach model.

None of the comparison models is able to encode three values (Figure 11.6). The Carandini-Ringach model's response is bimodal, with a peak at one of the stimulus value and at the orientation orthogonal to this value. Because the three orientations used in Figure 11.6 were evenly spaced (60° apart), noise alone determined which stimulus orientation dominated the model response. The Ben-Yishai et al. model and Pouget et al. models both give unimodal responses to all multi-orientation stimuli. For three evenly-spaced orientations, the input to the Ben-Yishai et al. model is completely isotropic (it is the weighted sum of 3 cosines), so the location of the response peak is entirely random, as seen in Figure 11.6. The Pouget et al. model response is centered at one of the three input orientations, though also determined arbitrarily. For all three models, the exact location of the response peak(s), for unevenly spaced orientations, is a complicated function of the orientations present in the stimulus, which depends in part on the response discontinuities revealed in Figure 11.4. However, responses to these stimuli never convey more than the mean, median, or mode of the stimulus values present.

The models fare better when exposed to a single orientation corrupted by input noise (Figure 11.6). The Ben-Yishai et al. and Pouget et al. models both generate a very smooth population response, resulting from the fact that both models are dominated by recurrent activity and have only weak external input. The Carandini-Ringach model response is somewhat noisier, but the most important difference is that added noise leads to a spurious response at the orthogonal orientation.

The optimized recurrent weights in our model (see Figure 11.7) have a similar shape to the center-surround weights used by most recurrent models. The wiggles in the surround of the weights gives them some power at higher frequencies. We

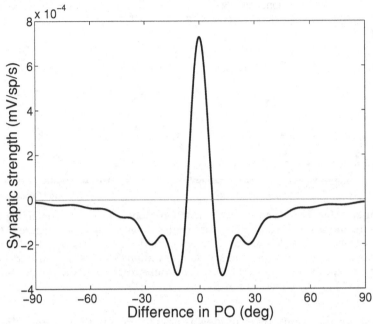

Figure 11.7. The optimized recurrent connection strengths between pairs of units in the population are plotted as a function of the difference in their preferred values (POs). Recurrent input is computed by convolving this weight profile with the current firing rates. The weights' center-surround profile sharpens the weak bias present in the feedforward input without destroying information about multiple values.

are currently analyzing these differences in greater detail. A crucial difference not apparent in this figure is that the relative strength of the recurrent versus feedforward weights is smaller in our model than the Carandini-Ringach model. This difference likely underlies our model's reduced ability to remove noise and remain strongly contrast invariant, but enhanced ability to encode multiple orientations.

Discussion

We have proposed a novel network model of population responses that can support a variety of response profiles, and veridically encodes multiple values. The significant contribution of this model lies in the proposal that the role of the population is to represent the full range of information about orientation present in the input. Previous work established that a population can represent information including uncertainty and multiple values about a variable like orienation, under the hypothesis that a distribution over the variable gives rise to the population activity. Whereas this earlier work took such population activities as given, here we show how these activities can be produced in a standard network model. In this paper, the probabilistic formulation leads both to an objective used to adapt the recurrent weights in the population, and a method for reading out the full information about orientation contained in the population activity.

We have applied this model to the issue of orientation selectivity in striate cortex. We have not yet considered even a fraction of the extensive studies on this issue, but instead our focus is on questions that have received little attention, such as responses to multi-orientation or ambiguous-orientation stimuli. Our model can replicate the cross-orientation effects observed in one of the only empirical investigations into primary visual cortex responses to multiple orientations (DeAngelis, Robson, Ohzawa, & Freeman, 1992). It also makes a number of new predictions concerning responses of these cells to stimuli containing multiple orientations: (1) a range of stable activity patterns will be produced for stimuli containing two orientations with differing angular spread; (2) inputs containing three orientations separated by 60° will produce trimodal activity patterns; and (3) noisy stimuli containing single orientations will only rarely give rise to spurious bimodal response profiles.

Each of these points differs from predictions derived from other models of orientation selectivity. The results presented in this paper show that a range of other models, such as those proposed by Carandini and Ringach (1997), Ben-Yishai et al. (1995), and Pouget et al. (1998) behave differently than our model when the input contains multiple orientation values or noisy single orientations. The brief synopsis of these results is that our model can veridically encode this information while the others cannot. The differences in behavior are somewhat surprising, since at first glance our model closely resembles th eothers. Indeed, the main elements of our models are identical to these models: the activation and tuning functions are the same as in Pouget et al. (1998), while the update equations are the same as in the other two models.

These differences in behavior may primarily be traced to two feature of the models: the relative roles of feedforward and recurrent inputs, and the recurrent weight profile. The models considered here differ greatly along these crucial dimensions. At one extreme of the first dimension lies a model such as Pouget et al. (1998), in which the input is shut off after the initial step. This allows the recurrent lateral connections to force the population activity profile to fit a specified template. At the opposite extreme lies a purely feedforward model. The other models considered here lie at different points along this dimension. The Carandini-Ringach model maintains the input at a constant level throughout the simulation duration, and gives this input a relatively strong weighting, which allows the model to encode multiple orientations when they are sufficiently separated. The Ben-Yishai et al. model also maintains a constant input, but weights it much less than the recurrent inputs, leading to an almost input-invariant response. Other models not considered here may also be partially understood by characterizing their balance of feedforward and recurrent inputs. The model proposed by Troyer et al. (1998) is primarily a feedforward model, which makes it sensitive to variations in the input, but a different formulation of recurrent connections that allows it to filter out large changes in the DC component of the inputs. Finally, a recent model by Obermayer and colleagues (Adorjan, Schwabe, Piepenbrock, & Obermayer, 2000) proposes a mixed answer to this issue. In their model, the roles change over time, as the recurrent weights dominate during the first phase of processing, but the feedforward weights dominate later.

With respect to the second crucial dimension, the recurrent weight profile, the models also differ greatly. Of particular note is the Ben-Yishai et al. model, in which the cosine tuning of the recurrent weights makes the model's response insensitive to the angular difference between orientations in multiple-orientation stimuli.

In our model, we specifically tune the recurrent weights to support multiple orientations and even ambiguity in orientations. We derive an objective function that measured the degree to which this information in the input was preserved in the population, and adjust the weights to maximize this objective. Thus the weight profile is tailored to the underlying hypothesis about the role of the population. Note that this also allows the model to optimize the balance between recurrent and feedforward inputs by adjusting the overall strength of the recurrent weights.

The main conclusions from this study then are that: (1) various orientation selectivity models can be characterized by their assumptions about what information underlies the population responses in V1, which is reflected in their balance between feedforward and recurrent inputs, and in the recurrent weight profile; (2) it is possible to devise a network model that optimizes the recurrent weights and balances these two forces to preserve information about multiple values in the input; and (3) the distribution population coding provides a natural framework for understanding the information encoded in a population response, and for formulating objectives for preserving and manipulating this information.

We conclude by discussing three final issues and current directions. First, an important and largely neglected aspect of processing in population codes that we have also ignored here is the role of time. It is known that the population response significantly changes during the time-course of a stimulus presentation. The aforementioned model by Adorjan et al. (2000) suggests one method by which the population activity may change over time, initially encoding a single value and then multiple values in a later processing phase. A promising direction for future studies is to incorporate dynamics in the encoded information into the distribution population coding framework studied here. This would considerably extend the applicability o fthe framework. For example, it would permit a natural formulation of ambiguity resolution over time in the population.

Second, an important unresolved issue in the current model concerns the readout of orientations from the decoded distribution. We adopted a simple approach of assigning a different orientation to each mode of the decoded distribution. However, other interpretations are possible: a distribution with two modes may not represent two orientations but may instead represent a single orientation that has two potential values. This ambiguity between multiplicity and uncertainty may be resolved by using a different encoding (and decoding) model in the DPC framework (Sahani & Dayan, personal communication).

A third and final point concerns the consequences of preserving the full range of orientation information, such as uncertainty and multiplicity. Our model has established that a population can potentially encode this information, but it remains to be seen how this information can be utilized in the next stage of processing, particularly without invoking any complicated non-neural decoding method. We are currently developing a model to investigate how preserving this orientation information may affect processing downstream from V1. It is known that V2 cells respond to illusory contours and figure-ground information; the underlying hypothesis of this new model is that preserving information about multiple orientations within individual V1 populations plays an important role in V2 responses.

Acknowledgements

This work was funded by ONR Young Investigator Award N00014-98-1-0509 to RZ. We thank Peter Dayan and Alexandre Pouget for many useful discussions of statistical population coding.

References

[1] Adorjan, P., Schwabe, L., Piepenbrock, C., & Obermayer, K. (2000). Recurrent cortical competition: Strengthen or weaken? In *Advances in Neural Information Processing Systems 12*, pp. 89–95. Cambridge, MA: MIT Press.

[2] Ben-Yishai, R., Bar-Or, R. L., & Sompolinsky, H. (1995). Theory of orientation tuning in visual cortex. *Proceedings of the National Academy of Sciences, USA, 92*, 3844–3848.

[3] Carandini, M. & Ringach, D. L. (1997). Predictions of a recurrent model of orientation selectivity. *Vision Research, 37:21*, 3061–3071.

[4] Carandini, M., Heeger, D. J., & Movshon, J.A. (1997) Linearity and normalization in simple cells of the macaque primary visual cortex. *Journal of Neuroscience, 17:21*, 8621–8644.

[5] DeAngelis, G. C., Robson, J. G., Ohzawa, I., & Freeman, R. D. (1992). Organization of suppression in receptive fields of neurons in cat visual cortex. *Journal of Neurophysiology, 68:1*, 144–163.

[6] Földiák, P. (1993). The 'ideal homunculus': statistical inference from neural population responses. In Eeckman, F. H. and Bower, J., editors, *Computation and Neural Systems 1992*, pp. 55–60. Norwell, MA: Kluwer Academic Publishers.

[7] Pouget, A., Zhang, K., Deneve, S., & Latham, P.E. (1998). Statistically efficient

estimation using population codes. *Neural Computation, 10,* 373–401.

[8] Recanzone, G. H., Wurtz, R. H., & Schwarz, U. (1997). Responses of MT and MST neurons to one and two moving objects in the receptive field. *Journal of Neurophysiology, 78:6,* 2904–2915.

[9] Salinas, E. and Abbott, L. F. (1996). A model of multiplicative neural responses in parietal cortex. *Proceedings of the National Academy of Sciences, USA, 93,* 11956–11961.

[10] Sanger, T. D. (1996). Probability density estimation for the interpretation of neural population codes. *Journal of Neurophysiology, 76:4,* 2790–2793.

[11] Seung, H. S. & Sompolinsky, H. (1993). Simple models for reading neuronal population codes. *Proceedings of the National Academy of Sciences, USA, 90,* 10749–10753.

[12] Somers, D. C., Nelson, S. B., & Douglas, R. J. (1995). An emergent model of orientation selectivity in cat visual cortical simple cells. *Journal of Neuroscience, 15,* 6700–6719.

[13] Sompolinsky, H. & Shapley, R. (1997). New perspectives on the mechanisms for orientation selectivity. *Current Opinion in Neurobiology, 7,* 514–522.

[14] Treue, S., Hol, K., & Rauber, H-J. (1999). Seeing multiple directions of motion—physiology and psychophysics. *Nature Neuroscience, 3:3,* 270–276.

[15] Troyer, T. W., Krukowski, A. E., & Miller, K. D. (1998). Contrast-invariant orientation tuning in cat visual cortex: Thalamocortical input tuning and correlation-based intracortical connectivity. *Journal of Neuroscience, 18:15,* 5908–5927.

[16] Van Wezel, R. J., Lankheet, M. J., Verstraten, F. A., Maree, A. F., & van de Grind, W. A. (1996). Responses of complex cells in area 17 of the cat to bi-vectorial transparent motion. *Vision Research, 36:18,* 2805–13.

[17] Zemel, R. S., Dayan, P., & Pouget, A. (1998). Probabilistic interpretation of population codes. *Neural Computation, 10,* 403–430.

[18] Zemel, R. S. & Dayan, P. (1999). Distributional population codes and multiple motion models. In *Advances in Neural Information Processing Systems 11,* pp. 174–180. Cambridge, MA: MIT Press.

[19] Zhang, K. (1996). Representation of spatial orientation by the intrinsic dynamics of the head-direction cell ensemble: A theory. *Journal of Neuroscience, 16,* 2112–2126.

12 Efficient Coding of Time-Varying Signals Using a Spiking Population Code

Michael S. Lewicki

Introduction

Representing time varying signals is a fundamental problem in processing any signal originating from the natural environment, but there is no natural way to encode such signals, and traditional methods each have their limitations. A common method of describing temporal signal is to divide it into a sequence of blocks. The data within each block is then fit or decomposed with standard basis such as a Fourier or wavelet. Blocking the data has the limitation that the components of the bases are arbitrarily aligned with respect to structure in the time series. Figure 12.1 shows a short segment of speech data and the boundaries of the blocks. Although the structure in the signal is largely periodic, each large oscillation appears in a different position within the blocks and is sometimes split across blocks. This problem is particularly acute for acoustic events with sharp onset, such as consonants in speech. It also presents difficulties for encoding the signal efficiently, because there is no compact way to describe phase-dependent structure. This can be somewhat circumvented by techniques such as windowing or averaging sliding blocks, but it would be more desirable if the representation were phase or shift invariant [15].

An example of a shift invariant representation is a filter bank, shown in figure 12.2. Each unit convolves the input signal to produce a time-varying output signal. This type of representation is implicit in many models of neural processing where the input and output signals are represented by average firing rates, and the convolutions performed by the different units correspond to the spatio-temporal receptive fields of different neurons.

The limitation of this representation is that it doesn't capture any of the temporal structure of the signal, it simply converts one time varying signal into many. If the input is a *set* of time-varying signals, the situation is somewhat different, because

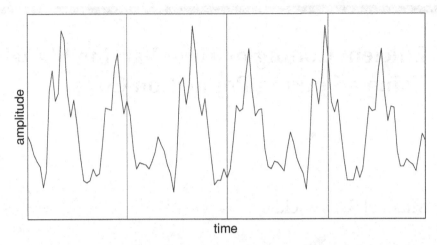

Figure 12.1: Blocking results in arbitrary phase alignment of the underlying structure.

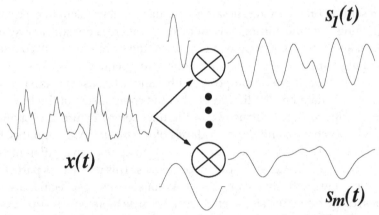

Figure 12.2. A filter bank representation of time-varying signals. The time-varying signal is convolved with different filters (represented by the $\otimes$ symbol), resulting in m different output signals. This representation is shift-invariant, but does not compactly represent structure in the original signal.

then one can attempt to find the set of transformations or filters that minimize the statistical dependencies among the outputs. This is exactly the goal of independent component analysis [9, 4] and approaches that seek factorial codes [3, 1, 17, 19]. Although some methods have been developed to make use of temporal structure for improving the statistical independence of the output signals [20, 2], here we focus on the problem of encoding the temporal structure in the signal.

The Model

Our goal is to develop a model that will efficiently represent temporal structure in a time-varying input signal. This is accomplished by modeling the signal with a small set of *kernel* functions that can be placed at arbitrary time points. Ultimately, we want to find the minimal set of functions and time points that fit the signal within a given noise level. We expect this type of model to work well for signals composed of events whose onset can occur at arbitrary temporal positions. Examples of these include musical instruments sounds with sharp attack or plosive sounds in speech.

We assume time series $x(t)$ is modeled by

$$x(t) = \sum_i s_i \phi_{m[i]}(t - \tau_i) + \epsilon(t), \qquad (12.1)$$

where τ_i indicates the temporal position of the ith kernel function, $\phi_{m[i]}$, which is scaled by s_i. The notation $m[i]$ represents an index function that specifies which of the M kernel functions is present at time τ_i. A single kernel function can occur at multiple times during the time series. Additive noise at time t is given by $\epsilon(t)$.

A more general way to express (12.1) is to assume that the kernel functions exist at all time points during the signal, and let the non-zero coefficients determine the positions of the kernel functions. In this case, the model can be expressed in convolutional form

$$x(t) = \sum_m \int s_m(\tau)\phi_m(t - \tau)d\tau + \epsilon(t) \qquad (12.2)$$

$$= \sum_m s_m(t) * \phi_m(t) + \epsilon(t), \qquad (12.3)$$

where $s_m(\tau)$ is the coefficient at time τ for kernel function ϕ_m.

It is also helpful to express the model in matrix form using a discrete sampling of the continuous time series:

$$x = As + \epsilon. \qquad (12.4)$$

The basis matrix, A, is defined by

$$A = [C(\phi_1)\, C(\phi_2)\, \cdots\, C(\phi_M)]\,, \qquad (12.5)$$

where $C(a)$ is an N-by-N circulant matrix parameterized by the vector a. This matrix is constructed by replicating the kernel functions at each sample position

$$C(a) = \begin{bmatrix} a_0 & a_{N-1} & \cdots & a_2 & a_1 \\ a_1 & a_0 & \cdots & a_3 & a_2 \\ \cdots & & \cdots & & \cdots \\ a_{N-2} & a_{N-3} & \cdots & a_0 & a_{N-1} \\ a_{N-1} & a_{N-2} & \cdots & a_1 & a_0 \end{bmatrix} \quad (12.6)$$

The kernels are zero padded to be of length N. The length of each kernel is typically much less than the length of the signal, making A very sparse. This can be viewed as a special case of a Toeplitz matrix. Note that the size of A is MN-by-N, and is thus an example of an overcomplete basis, i.e. a basis with more basis functions than dimensions in the data space [21, 8, 18, 16].

A Probabilistic Formulation

The optimal coefficient values for a signal are found by maximizing the posterior distribution

$$\hat{s} = \arg\max_s P(s|x, A) = \arg\max_s P(x|A, s)P(s) \quad (12.7)$$

where $\hat{s}$ is the most probable representation of the signal. Note that omission of the normalizing constant $P(x|A)$ does not change the location of the maximum. This formulation of the problem offers the advantage that the model can fit more general types of distributions and naturally "denoises" the signal. Note that the mapping from x to $\hat{s}$ is *nonlinear* with non-zero additive noise and an overcomplete basis [7, 16]. Optimizing (12.7) essentially selects out the subset of basis functions that best account for the data.

To define a probabilistic model, we follow existing conventions for linear generative models with additive noise [6, 16]. We assume the noise, ϵ, to have a Gaussian distribution which yields a data likelihood for a given representation of

$$\log P(x|A, s) \propto -\frac{1}{2\sigma^2}(x - As)^2. \quad (12.8)$$

The function $P(s)$ describes the a priori distribution of the coefficients. Under the assumption that $P(s)$ is sparse (highly peaked around zero), maximizing (12.7) results in very few nonzero coefficients. A compact representation of $\hat{s}$ is to describe the values of the non-zero coefficients and their temporal positions

$$P(s) = \prod_m P(u_m, \tau_m) = \prod_{m=1}^{M} \prod_{i=1}^{n_m} P(u_{m,i}) P(\tau_{m,i}),$$ (12.9)

where the prior for the non-zero coefficient values, $u_{m,i}$, is assumed to be Laplacian, and the prior for the temporal positions (or intervals), $\tau_{m,i}$, is assumed to be a gamma distribution.

Finding the Best Encoding

A difficult challenge presented by the proposed model is finding a computationally tractable algorithm for fitting it to the data. The brute-force approach of generating the basis matrix A produces an intractable number of basis functions for signals of any reasonable length, so we need to look for ways of reducing the computational cost of optimizing (12.7). We start with the gradient of the log posterior

$$\frac{\partial}{\partial s} \log P(s|A, x) \propto A^T(x - As) + z(s),$$ (12.10)

where $z(s) = (\log P(s))'$. A basic operation required is $v = A^T u$. We saw that $x = As$ can be computed efficiently using convolution (12.2). Because A^T is also block circulant

$$A^T = \begin{bmatrix} C(\phi_1') \\ \dots \\ C(\phi_M') \end{bmatrix}$$ (12.11)

where $\phi'(1:N) = \phi(N:-1:1)$. Thus, terms involving A^T can also be computed efficiently using convolution

$$v = A^T u = \begin{bmatrix} \phi_1(-t) * u(t) \\ \dots \\ \phi_M(-t) * u(t) \end{bmatrix}$$ (12.12)

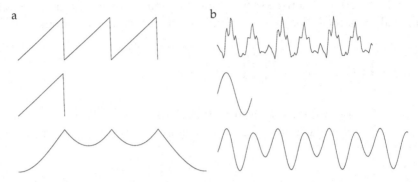

Figure 12.3. Convolution using the fast Fourier transform is an efficient way to select an initial solution for the temporal positions of the kernel functions. (**a**) The convolution of a sawtooth waveform with a sawtooth-shaped kernel function (middle). (**b**) Convolution of a speech segment with a single period sine-wave kernel function.

Obtaining an initial representation

An alternative approach to optimizing (12.7) is to make use of the fact that if the kernel functions are short enough in length, direct multiplication is faster than convolution, and that, for this highly overcomplete basis, most of the coefficients will be zero after being fit to the data. The central problem in encoding the signal then is to determine which coefficients are non-zero, ideally finding a description of the time series with the minimal number of non-zero coefficients. This is equivalent to determining the best set of temporal positions for each of the kernel functions (12.1).

A crucial step in this approach is to obtain a good initial estimate of the coefficients. One way to do this is to consider the projection of the signal onto each of the basis functions, i.e. $A^T x$. This estimate will be exact (i.e. zero residual error) in the case of zero noise and orthogonal A. For the non-orthogonal, overcomplete case the solution will be approximate, but for certain choices of the basis matrix, an exact representation can still be obtained efficiently [10, 21].

Figure 12.3 shows examples of convolving two different kernel functions with data. One disadvantage with this initial solution is that the coefficient functions, $s_m(t)$, are not sparse. For example, even though the signal in figure 12.3a is composed of only three instances of the kernel function, the convolution is mostly non-zero.

A simple procedure for obtaining a better initial estimate of the most probable coefficients is to select the time locations of the maxima (or extrema) in the convolutions. These are positions where the kernel functions capture the greatest amount of signal structure and where the optimal coefficients are likely to be non-zero. Figure 12.4 shows the result of using this procedure to obtain an initial fit to a speech segment. This can generate a large number of kernel positions, but their number can be reduced further by selecting only those that contribute significantly, i.e. where the

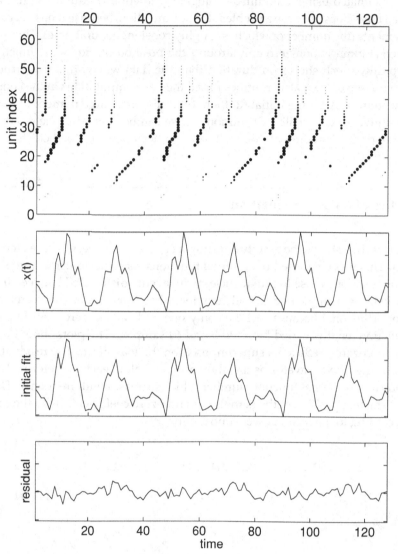

Figure 12.4. The initial fitting procedure of selecting kernel function positions at convolution peaks. The dots in the upper plot indicate positions of kernels (right axis) with size scaled by the mean power contribution. The original and initial reconstructed speech signal are plotted below, with the bottom plot showing the residual error (12 dB SNR). The residual error can be improved to 70dB SNR after optimizing the coefficient magnitudes (figure 12.5a).

average power is greater than some fraction of the noise level. From these, a basis for the entire signal is constructed by replicating the kernel functions at the appropriate time positions.

Once an initial estimate and basis are formed, the most probable coefficient values are estimated using a modified conjugate gradient procedure. The size of the generated basis does not pose a problem for optimization, because it has very few non-zero elements (the number of which is roughly constant per unit time). This arises because each column is non-zero only around the position of the kernel function, which is typically much shorter in duration than the data waveform. This structure affords the use of sparse matrix routines for all the key computations in the conjugate gradient routine. After the initial fit, there typically are a large number of basis functions that give a very small contribution. These can be pruned to yield, after refitting, a more probable representation that has significantly fewer coefficients.

Properties of the Representation

Figure 12.5 shows the results of fitting a segment of speech with a sine wave kernel set. This was composed of 64 kernel functions constructed using a single period of a sine function whose log frequencies were evenly distributed between 0 and Nyquist (4 kHz), which yielded kernel functions that were minimally correlated (they are not orthogonal because each has only one cycle and is zero elsewhere). The kernel function lengths varied between 5 and 64 samples. The plots show the positions of the non-zero coefficients superimposed on the waveform. The residual error curves from the fitted waveforms are shown offset below each waveform. The right axes indicate the kernel function number which increases with frequency. The dots show the starting position of the kernels with non-zero coefficients, with the dot size scaled according to the mean power contribution.

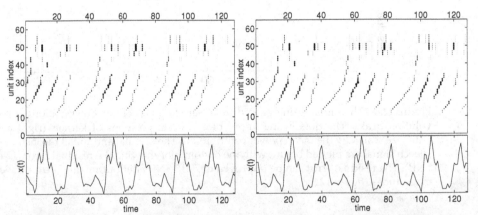

Figure 12.5. Fitting a shift-invariant model to a segment of speech, x(t). (a) Shows the fit to the original unshifted signal. The accuracy of the fit is 70 dB SNR. (b) The fit to a shifted version of the same signal.

Figure 12.5a shows that the structure in the coefficients repeats for each oscillation in the waveform. Adding a delay leaves the relative temporal structure of the non-zero coefficients mostly unchanged (figure 12.5b). The small variations between the two sets of coefficients are due to variations in the fitting of the small-magnitude coefficients. Representing the signal in figure 12.5b with a standard complete basis would result in a very different representation.

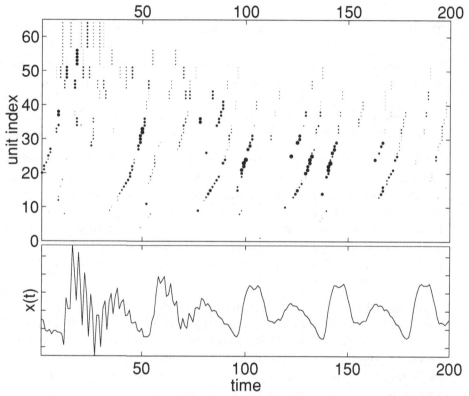

Figure 12.6. An example showing how, in the case of sinusoid kernel functions, the decomposition performs a fine-grained time-frequency analysis.

Fine-scale time frequency analysis

In contrast to Fourier or wavelet decompositions, this type of representation or decomposition can place the kernel functions at arbitrary time points. In the special case of sinusoid kernel functions, the decomposition performs a fine-scale time-frequency analysis, an example of which is illustrated in figure 12.6. The plot of the kernel function positions show how the representation picks up the high frequency structure near the beginning of the waveform. In a Fourier decomposition, the high frequency energy would only be localized to the window. A wavelet decomposition would allow better temporal localization, but would still be limited to a set of discrete temporal positions.

Neural Implementations

The initial representation is implemented using a simple convolution plus threshold. How could coefficient magnitudes be coded with fixed amplitude action potentials? We consider several models of biologically plausible models of spike coding [13]. Figure 12.7 shows several possibilities. In figure 12.7a, coefficient magnitude is encoded by the average firing rate. This is a classic model of neural coding of analogue values and can be implemented simply by making firing probability increase with increasing input. The disadvantage of this model is that temporal precision is lost.

Figure 12.7b shows a model that encodes the magnitude of the kernel functions using a distributed population code. In this model, several neurons with the same or similar convolution properties firing probabilistically in response to the input magnitude. The analog signal is transmitted using a population of spikes, but can be recovered at the post-synaptic neural simply by summation. In contrast to the average firing rate model, this model preserves temporal precision, but at the expense of addition units. This type of model offers on explanation for why overcomplete representations might be useful in neural coding.

The model in figure 12.7c encodes magnitude using the position relative to a common background oscillation that influences the firing times of neurons in the population. Neurons that receive strong input (magnitude) will fire earlier, thus encoding magnitude in terms of relative spike timing. Having a common background oscillation can serve both to establish a common reference for the population and to reduce the variability in the relative firing times.

Figure 12.7d shows a model that makes use of the same mechanisms as that in 12.7c, i.e. neurons receiving larger magnitude input will reach the spiking threshold faster, but does not use a common oscillation. Magnitude information is conveyed in the relative timing or synchrony of the spikes, and could be decoded by giving more weight to earlier action potentials. An assumption of this model is that random timing coincidences will be interpreted as noise. An advantage of this and the previous model is that no temporal precision is lost and redundancy in the unit response properties is not required, although that may still be advantageous for compensating for intrinsic noise in the population or limitations of spike timing precision.

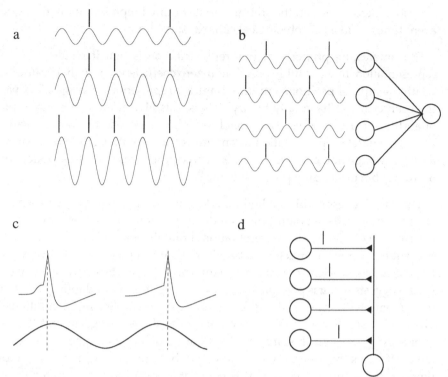

Figure 12.7. (a) Spike frequency model. Convolution magnitude is encoded by the average firing rate, with some loss of temporal precision. (b) Population spike model. Convolution magnitude is encoded by a population of neurons with similar kernels. If each unit fires probabilistically, the magnitude of the convolution is recovered in the post-synaptic sum. (c) Phase model. Convolution magnitude is encoded by the timing of the action potential relative to a common oscillation using the property that larger magnitude inputs will reach the spiking threshold faster. (d) Relative timing model. Magnitude is again coded by relative spike timing, but without a common oscillation.

Discussion

The model presented here can be viewed as an extension of the shiftable transforms of [21]. One difference is that here no constraints are placed on the kernel functions. Furthermore, this model accounts for additive noise, which yields automatic signal denoising and provides sensible criteria for selecting significant coefficients. An important unresolved issue is how well the algorithm works for increasingly non-orthogonal kernels.

Representing a time-varying signal in terms of a sparse set of kernel functions is exactly the model assumed in the approach of reverse correlation or stimulus reconstruction models [11, 12, 5], but the goals are converse, i.e. rather than going from a single spike train to an estimate of the stimulus, the model and algorithm described here transform the stimulus to its optimal representation in a *population* of event times or, in a neurobiological context, spike trains.

One interesting property of this representation is that it results in a spike-like representation. In the resulting set of non-zero coefficients, both their values and their relative temporal positions are important for representing the signal. If we restrict the coefficients to have only binary values, this algorithm shares many properties of auditory nerve models. The model described here also has the capacity to have an overcomplete representation at any given timepoint, e.g. a kernel basis with an arbitrarily large number of frequencies. These properties make this model potentially useful for binaural signal processing applications.

The effectiveness of this method for efficient coding remains to be proved. A trivial example of a shift-invariant basis is a delta-function model. For a model to encode information efficiently, the representation should be non-redundant. Each basis function should "grab" as much structure in the data as possible and achieve the same level of coding efficiency for arbitrary shifts of the data. The matrix form of the model (12.4) suggests that it is possible to achieve this optimum by adapting the kernel functions themselves using methods for adapting overcomplete representations [16, 14]. The results presented in the next chapter by Olshausen suggest that this approach is promising. Beyond this, it is evident that modeling the higher-order structure in the coefficients themselves will be necessary both to achieve an efficient representation and to capture structure that is relevant to such tasks as speech recognition or auditory stream segmentation.

Acknowledgments

We thank Tony Bell, Bruno Olshausen, and David Donoho for helpful discussions.

References

[1] Atick, J. J. (1992). Could information-theory provide an ecological theory of sensory processing. *Network-Computation in Neural Systems*, 3(2):213–251.

[2] Attias, H. (1998). Blind source separation and deconvolution: the dynamic component analysis algorithm. *Neural Computation*, (10):1373–1424.

[3] Barlow, H. B. (1989). Unsupervised learning. *Neural Computation*, 1:295–311.

[4] Bell, A. J. and Sejnowski, T. J. (1995). An information maximization approach to blind separation and blind deconvolution. *Neural Computation*, 7(6):1129–1159.

[5] Bialek, W., Rieke, F., de Ruyter van Steveninck, R. R., and Warland, D. (1991).

Reading a neural code. *Science*, 252(5014):1854–1857.

[6] Cardoso, J.-F. (1997). Infomax and maximum likelihood for blind source separation. *IEEE Signal Processing Letters*, 4:109–111.

[7] Chen, S., Donoho, D. L., and Saunders, M. A. (1996). Atomic decomposition by basis pursuit. Technical report, Dept. Stat., Stanford Univ., Stanford, CA.

[8] Coifman, R. R. and Wickerhauser, M. V. (1992). Entropy-based algorithms for best basis selection. *IEEE Transactions on Information Theory*, 38(2):713–718.

[9] Comon, P. (1994). Independent component analysis, a new concept? *Signal Processing*, 36(3):287–314.

[10] Daubechies, I. (1990). The wavelet transform, time-frequency localization, and signal analysis. *IEEE Transactions on Information Theory*, 36(5):961–1004.

[11] de Boer, E. and Kuyper, P. (1968). Triggered correlation. *IEEE Trans. Biomed. Eng.*, 15(3):169–179.

[12] de Ruyter van Steveninck, R. R. and Bialek, W. (1988). Real-time performance of a movement-sensitive neuron in the blowfly visual system: coding and information transfer in short spike sequences. *Proc. R. Soc. B,*, 234:379–414.

[13] Gerstner, W. (1999). Spiking neurons. In Maass, W. and Bishop, C. M., editors, *Pulsed Neural Networks*, pages 3–53. MIT Press.

[14] Lewicki, M. S. and Olshausen, B. A. (1999). A probabilistic framework for the adaptation and comparison of image codes. *J. Opt. Soc. of Am. A: Optics, Image Science, and Vision*, 16(7):1587–1601.

[15] Lewicki, M. S. and Sejnowski, T. J. (1999). Coding time-varying signals using sparse, shift-invariant representations. In *Advances in Neural Information Processing Systems*, volume 11, pages 730–736. MIT Press.

[16] Lewicki, M. S. and Sejnowski, T. J. (2000). Learning overcomplete representations. *Neural Computation*, 12(2):337–365.

[17] Linsker, R. (1992). Local synaptic rules suffice to maximize mutual information in a linear network. *Neural Computation*, 4:691–702.

[18] Mallat, S. G. and Zhang, Z. F. (1993). Matching pursuits with time-frequency dictionaries. *IEEE Transactions on Signal Processing*, 41(12):3397–3415.

[19] Nadal, J.-P. and Parga, N. (1994). Nonlinear neurons in the low-noise limit: A a factorial code maximizes information transfer. *Network*, 5:565–581.

[20] Pearlmutter, B. A. and Parra, L. C. (1996). A context-senstive generalization of ICA. In *International Conference on Neural Information Processing*, pages 151–157.

[21] Simoncelli, E. P., Freeman, W. T., Adelson, E. H., and Heeger, D. J. (1992). Shiftable multiscale transforms. *IEEE Trans. Info. Theory*, 38:587–607.

13 Sparse Codes and Spikes

Bruno A. Olshausen

Introduction

In order to make progress toward understanding the sensory coding strategies employed by the cortex, it will be necessary to draw upon guiding principles that provide us with reasonable ideas for what to expect and what to look for in the neural circuitry. The unifying theme behind all of the chapters in this book is that *probabilistic inference*—i.e., the process of inferring the state of the world from the activities of sensory receptors and a probabilistic model for interpreting their activity—provides a major guiding principle for understanding sensory processing in the nervous system. Here, I shall propose a model for how inference may be instantiated in the neural circuitry of the visual cortex, and I will show how it may help us to understand both the form of the receptive fields found in visual cortical neurons as well as the nature of spiking activity in these neurons.

In order for the cortex to perform inference on retinal images, it must somehow implement a generative model for explaining the signals coming from optic nerve fibers in terms of hypotheses about the state of the world (Mumford, 1994). I shall propose here that the neurons in the primary visual cortex, area V1, form the first stage in this generative modeling process by modeling the structure of images in terms of a linear superposition of basis functions (figure 13.1). One can think of these basis functions as a simple "feature vocabulary" for describing images in terms of additive functions. In order to provide a vocabulary that captures meaningful structure within time-varying images, the basis functions are adapted according to an unsupervised learning procedure that attempts to form a representation of the incoming image stream in terms of *sparse, statistically independent* events. Sparseness is desired because it provides a simple description of the structures occurring in natural image sequences in terms of a small number of vocabulary elements at any point in time (Field, 1994). Such representations are also useful for forming associations at later stages of processing (Foldiak, 1995; Baum, 1988). Statistical independence reduces the redundancy of the code, in line with Barlow's hypothesis for achieving a representation that reflects the underlying causal structure of the images (Barlow, 1961; 1989).[1]

I shall show here that when a sparse, independent code is sought for time-varying natural images, the basis functions that emerge resemble the receptive field properties of cortical simple-cells in both space and time. Moreover, the model yields a representation of time-varying images in terms of sparse, spike-like events. It is suggested that the spike trains of sensory neurons essentially serve as a *sparse code in time*, which in turn forms a more efficient and meaningful representation of image structure. Thus, a single principle may be able to account for both the receptive properties of neurons and the spiking nature of neural activity.

The first part of this chapter presents the basic generative image model for static images, and discusses how to relate the basis functions and sparse activities of the model to neural receptive fields and activities. The second part applies the model to time-varying images and shows how space-time receptive fields and spike-like representations emerge from this process. Finally, I shall discuss how the model may be tested and how it would need to be further modified in order to be regarded as a fully neurobiologically plausible model.

Sparse Coding of Static Images

Image model

In previous work (Olshausen & Field, 1997), we described a model of V1 simple-cells in terms of a linear generative model of images (figure 13.1a). According to this model, images are described in terms of a linear superposition of basis functions plus noise:

$$I(x,y) = \sum_i a_i \, \phi_i(x,y) + \nu(x,y) \,. \tag{13.1}$$

An image $I(x,y)$ is thus represented by a set of coefficient values, a_i, which are taken to be analogous to the activities of V1 neurons. Importantly, the basis set is *overcomplete*, meaning that there are more basis functions (and hence more a_i's) than effective dimensions in the images. Overcompleteness in the representation is important because it allows for the joint space of position, orientation, and spatial-frequency to

1. Although it is not possible in general to achieve complete independence with the simple linear model we propose here, we can nevertheless seek to reduce statistical dependencies as much as possible over both space (i.e., across neurons) and time.

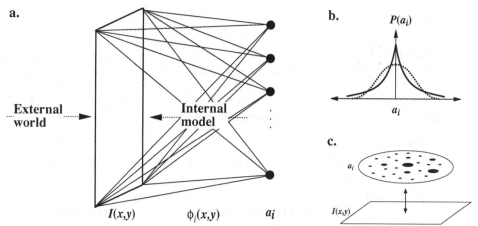

Figure 13.1. Image model. *a*, Images of the environment are modeled as a linear super-position of basis functions, ϕ_i, whose amplitudes are given by the coefficients a_i. *b*, The prior probability distribution over the coefficients is peaked at zero with heavy tails as compared to a Gaussian of the same variance (overlaid as dashed line). Such a distribution would result from a sparse activity distribution over the coefficients, as depicted in *c*.

be tiled smoothly without artifacts (Simoncelli et al., 1992). More generally though, it allows for a greater degree of flexibility in the representation, as there is no reason to believe a priori that the number of causes for images is less than or equal to the number of pixels (Lewicki & Sejnowski, 2000).

With non-zero noise, ν, the correspondence between images and coefficient values is probabilistic—i.e., some solutions are more probable than others. Moreover, when the basis set is overcomplete, there are an infinite number of solutions for the coefficients in equation 13.1 (even with zero noise), all of which describe the image with equal probability. This degeneracy in the representation is resolved by imposing a prior probability distribution over the coefficients. The particular form of the prior imposed in our model is one that favors an interpretation of images in terms of sparse, independent events:

$$P(\mathbf{a}) = \prod_i P(a_i) \tag{13.2}$$

$$P(a_i) = \frac{1}{Z_S} e^{-S(a_i)} \tag{13.3}$$

where S is a non-convex function that shapes $P(a_i)$ so as to have the requisite "sparse" form—i.e., peaked at zero with heavy tails, or positive kurtosis—as shown in figure 13.1*b*. The posterior probability of the coefficients for a given image is then

$$P(\mathbf{a}|\mathbf{I}, \theta) \propto P(\mathbf{I}|\mathbf{a}, \theta) P(\mathbf{a}|\theta) \tag{13.4}$$

$$P(\mathbf{I}|\mathbf{a}, \theta) = \frac{1}{Z_{\lambda_N}} e^{-\frac{\lambda_N}{2}|\mathbf{I} - \mathbf{\Phi}\mathbf{a}|^2} \tag{13.5}$$

$$P(\mathbf{a}|\theta) = \prod_i \frac{1}{Z_S} e^{-S(a_i)} \tag{13.6}$$

where $\mathbf{\Phi}$ is the basis function matrix with columns ϕ_i and λ_N is the inverse of the noise variance σ_ν^2. θ denotes the entire set of model parameters $\mathbf{\Phi}$, λ_N, and S.

Since the relation between images and coefficients is probabilistic, there is not a single unique solution for choosing the coefficients to represent a given image. One possibility, for example, is to choose the mean of the posterior distribution $P(\mathbf{a}|\mathbf{I}, \theta)$. This is difficult to compute, though, since it requires some form of sampling from the posterior. The solution we propose here is to choose the coefficients that maximize the posterior distribution (MAP estimate)

$$\hat{\mathbf{a}} = \arg \max_{\mathbf{a}} P(\mathbf{a}|\mathbf{I}, \theta) \tag{13.7}$$

which is accomplished via gradient ascent on the log-posterior:

$$\dot{\mathbf{a}} \propto \nabla_{\mathbf{a}} \log P(\mathbf{a}|\mathbf{I}, \theta)$$

$$= -\nabla_{\mathbf{a}} \left[\frac{\lambda_N}{2} |\mathbf{I} - \mathbf{\Phi}\mathbf{a}|^2 + \sum_i S(a_i) \right] \tag{13.8}$$

$$= \lambda_N \mathbf{\Phi}_i^T \mathbf{e} - S'(\mathbf{a}) . \tag{13.9}$$

where $\mathbf{e}$ is the residual error between the image and the model's reconstruction of the image, $\mathbf{e} = \mathbf{I} - \mathbf{\Phi}\mathbf{a}$. When S is a non-convex function appropriate for encouraging sparseness, such as $\beta \log(1 + (a_i/\sigma)^2)$, or $\beta|a_i/\sigma|^q, q \leq 1$, its derivative, S', provides a form of non-linear self-inhibition for coefficient values near zero. A recurrent neural network implementation of this differential equation (13.9) is shown in figure 13.2.

Learning

The basis functions of the model are adapted by maximizing the average log-likelihood of the images under the model, which is equivalent to minimizing the model's estimate of code length, $\mathcal{L}$:

$$\mathcal{L} = -\langle \log P(\mathbf{I}|\theta) \rangle \tag{13.10}$$

where

$$P(\mathbf{I}|\theta) = \int P(\mathbf{I}|\mathbf{a}, \theta) \, P(\mathbf{a}|\theta) \, da . \tag{13.11}$$

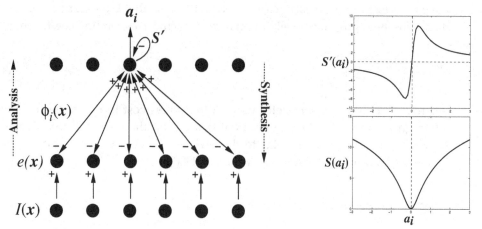

Figure 13.2. A simple network implementation of inference. The outputs a_i are driven by a sum of two terms. The first term takes a spatially weighted sum of the current residual image using the function $\phi_i(\vec{x})$ as the weights. The second term applies a non-linear self-inhibition on the outputs according to the derivative of S, that differentially pushes activity towards zero. Shown at right is the derivative of the sparse cost function $S(a_i) = \beta \log(1 + (a_i/\sigma)^2)$, $\beta = 2.5$, $\alpha = 0.3$.

$\mathcal{L}$ provides an upper bound estimate of the entropy of the images, which in turn provides a lower bound estimate of code length.

A learning rule for the basis functions may be obtained via gradient descent on $\mathcal{L}$:

$$\Delta\Phi \propto -\frac{\partial\mathcal{L}}{\partial\Phi} \tag{13.12}$$

$$= \lambda_N \left\langle \langle \mathbf{e}\,\mathbf{a}^T \rangle_{P(\mathbf{a}|\mathbf{I},\theta)} \right\rangle \,. \tag{13.13}$$

Thus, the basis functions are updated by a Hebbian learning rule, where the residual error **e** constitutes the pre-synaptic input and the coefficients **a** constitute the post-synaptic outputs. Instead of sampling from the full posterior distribution, though, we utilize an simpler approximation in which a single sample is taken at the posterior maximum, and so we have

$$\Delta\Phi \propto \langle \mathbf{e}\,\hat{\mathbf{a}}^T \rangle \,. \tag{13.14}$$

The price we pay for this approximation is that the basis functions will grow without bound, since the greater their norm, $|\phi_i|$, the smaller each a_i will become, thus decreasing the sparseness penalty in (13.8). This trivial solution is avoided by rescaling the basis functions after each learning step (13.14) so that their L2 norm, $g_i = |\phi_i|_{L2}$, maintains an appropriate level of variance on each corresponding coefficient a_i:

$$g_i^{new} = g_i^{old} \left[\frac{\langle a_i^2 \rangle}{\sigma^2} \right]^{\alpha} , \tag{13.15}$$

where σ is the scaling parameter used in the sparse cost function, S. This method, although an approximation to gradient descent on the true objective $\mathcal{L}$, has been shown to yield solutions similar to those obtained with more accurate techniques involving sampling (Olshausen & Millman, 2000).

Does V1 do sparse coding?

When the model is adapted to static, whitened[2] natural images, the basis functions that emerge resemble the Gabor-like spatial profiles of cortical simple-cell receptive fields (figure 13.3, similar results were also obtained with van Hateren & Ruderman's ICA model). That is, the functions become spatially localized, oriented, and bandpass (selective to structure at different spatial scales). Because all of these properties emerge purely from the objective of finding sparse, independent components for natural images, the results suggest that the receptive fields of V1 neurons have been designed according to a similar coding principle. The result is quite robust, and has been shown to emerge from other forms of independent components analysis (ICA). Some of these also make an explicit assumption of sparseness (Bell & Sejnowski, 1997; Lewicki & Olshausen, 1999) while others seek only independence among the coefficients, in which case sparseness emerges as part of the result (van Hateren & van der Schaaf, 1998; Olshausen & Millman, 2000).

We are comparing the basis functions to neural receptive fields[3] here because they are the feedforward weighting functions used in computing the outputs of the model, a_i (see figure 13.2). However, it is important to bear in mind that the outputs are not computed purely via this feedforward weighting function, but also via a non-linear, recurrent computation (13.9), the result of which is to *sparsify* neural activity. Thus, a neuron in our model would be expected to respond less often than one that simply

---

2. Whitening removes second-order correlations due to the $1/f^2$ power spectrum of natural images, and it approximates the type of filtering performed by the retina (see Atick & Redlich, 1992).

3. It should be noted that term 'receptive field' is not well-defined, even among physiologists. Oftentimes it is taken to mean the feedforward, linear weighting function of a neuron. But in reality, the measured receptive field of a neuron reflects the sum total of all dendritic non-linearities, output non-linearities, as well as recurrent computations due to horizontal connections and top-down feedback from other neurons.

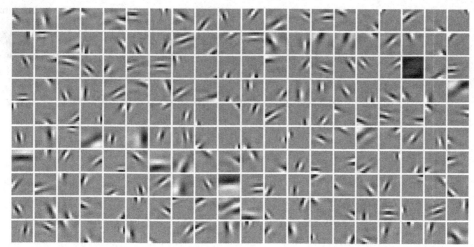

Figure 13.3. Basis functions learned from static natural images. Shown is a set of 200 basis functions which were adapted to 12 × 12 pixel image patches, according to equations (13.14) and (13.15). Initial conditions were completely random. The basis set is approximately 2×'s overcomplete, since the images occupy only about 3/4 of the dimensionality of the input space. (See Olshausen & Field, 1997, for simulation details.)

computes the inner product between a spatial weighting function and the image, as shown in figure 13.4*a*.

How could one tell if V1 neurons were actively sparsifying their activity according to the model? One possibility is to measure a neuron's receptive field via reverse correlation, using an artificial image ensemble such as white noise, and then use this measured receptive field to predict the response of the neuron to natural images via convolution. If neural activities were being sparsified as in the model, then one would expect the actual responses obtained with natural images to be non-linearly related to those predicted from convolution, as shown in figure 13.4*c*. The net effect of this non-linearity is that it tends to suppress responses where the basis function does not match well with the image, and it amplifies responses where the basis function does match well. This form of non-linearity is qualitatively consistent with the "expansive power-function" contrast response non-linearity observed in simple cells (Albrecht & Hamilton, 1982; Albrecht & Geisler, 1991). Note however that this response property emerges from the sparse prior in our model, rather than having been assumed as an explicit part of the response function. Whether or not this response characteristic is due to the kind of dynamics proposed in our model, as opposed to the application of a fixed pointwise non-linearity on the output of the neuron, would require more complicated tests to resolve.

The above method assumes that the analog valued coefficients in the model (or positively rectified versions of these quantities) correspond to spike rate. However, recent studies have demonstrated that spike rates, which are typically averaged over

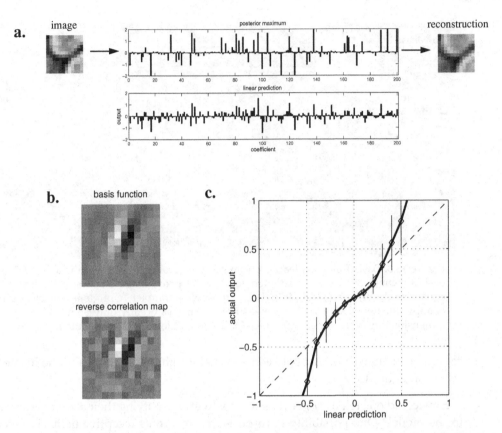

Figure 13.4. Effect of sparsification. *a*, An example 12 × 12 image and its encoding obtained by maximizing the posterior over the coefficients. The representation obtained by simply taking the inner-product of the image with the best linear predicting kernel for each basis function is not nearly as sparse by comparison. *b*, Shown is one of the learned basis functions (row 6, column 7 of figure 13.3) together with its corresponding "receptive field" as mapped out via reverse correlation with white noise (1440 trials). *c*, The response obtained by simply convolving this function with the image is non-linearly related to the actual output chosen by posterior maximization. Specifically, small values tend to get suppressed and large values amplified (the solid line passing through the diamonds depicts the mean of this relationship, while the error bars denote the standard deviation).

epochs of 100 ms or more, tend to vastly underestimate the temporal information contained in neural spike trains (Rieke et al., 1997). In addition, we are faced with the fact that the image on the retina is constantly changing due to both self-motion (eye, head and body) and the motions of objects in the world. The model as we have currently formulated it is not well-suited to deal with such dynamics, since the procedure for maximizing the posterior over the coefficients requires a recurrent computation, and it is unlikely that this will complete before the input changes appreciably. In the next section, we show how these issues may be addressed, at least in part, by reformulating the model to deal directly with time-varying images.

Sparse Coding of Time-Varying Images

Image model

We can reformulate the sparse coding model to deal with time-varying images by explicitly modeling the image stream $I(x, y, t)$ in terms of a superposition of space-time basis functions $\phi_i(x, y, \tau)$. Here we shall assume shift-invariance in the representation over time, so that the same basis function $\phi_i(x, y, \tau)$ may be used to model structure in the image sequence around any time t with amplitude $a_i(t)$. Thus, the image model may be expressed as the convolution of a set of time-varying coefficients, $a_i(t)$, with the basis functions:

$$I(x, y, t) = \sum_i \sum_{t'} a_i(t')\, \phi_i(x, y, t - t') + \nu(x, y, t) \tag{13.16}$$

$$= \sum_i a_i(t) * \phi_i(x, y, t) + \nu(x, y, t) \tag{13.17}$$

The model is illustrated schematically in figure 13.5.

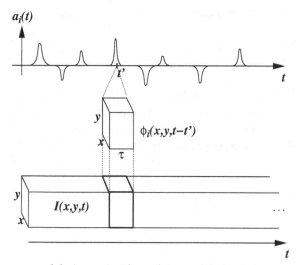

Figure 13.5. Image model. A movie $I(x, y, t)$ is modeled as a linear superposition of spatio-temporal basis functions, $\phi_i(x, y, \tau)$, each of which is localized in time but may be applied at any time within the movie sequence.

The coefficients for a given image sequence are computed as before by maximizing the posterior distribution over the coefficients

$$\hat{\mathbf{a}} = \arg \max_{\mathbf{a}} P(\mathbf{a}|\mathbf{I}, \theta) \tag{13.18}$$

which is again achieved by gradient descent, leading to the following differential equation for determining the coefficients:

$$\dot{a}_i(t) \propto \lambda_N \sum_{x,y} \phi_i(x,y,t) \star e(x,y,t) - S(a_i(t)) \tag{13.19}$$

$$e(x,y,t) = I(x,y,t) - \sum_i a_i(t) \ast \phi_i(x,y,t) . \tag{13.20}$$

where $\star$ denotes correlation. Note however that in order to be considered a causal system, $\phi(x,y,\tau)$ must be zero for $t > 0$. For now though we shall overlook the issue of causality, and in the discussion we shall consider some ways of dealing with this issue.

This model differs from the ICA (independent components analysis) model for time-varying images proposed earlier by van Hateren and Ruderman (1998) in an important respect: namely, the basis functions are applied to the image sequence in a shift-invariant manner, rather than in a blocked fashion. In van Hateren and Ruderman's ICA model, training data is obtained by extracting blocks of size 12x12 pixels and 12 samples in time from a larger movie, and a set of basis functions were sought that maximize independence among the coefficients (by seeking extrema of kurtosis) averaged over many such blocks. An image block is described via

$$I(x,y,t) = \sum_i a_i \, \phi_i(x,y,t) . \tag{13.21}$$

and the coefficients are computed by multiplying the rows of the pseudo-inverse of Φ with each block extracted from the image stream (akin to convolution). By contrast, our model assumes shift-invariance among the basis functions—i.e., a basis function may be applied to describe structure occurring at any point in time in the image sequence. In addition, since the basis set is overcomplete, the coefficients may be sparsified, giving rise to a non-linear, spike-like representation that is qualitatively different from that obtained via linear convolution (see "Results from natural movie sequences").

Learning

The objective function for adapting the basis functions is again the code length $\mathcal{L}$,

$$\mathcal{L} = - \langle \log P(\mathbf{I}|\theta) \rangle \tag{13.22}$$

$$P(\mathbf{I}|\theta) = \int P(\mathbf{I}|\mathbf{a},\theta) P(\mathbf{a}|\theta) d\mathbf{a} \tag{13.23}$$

where now the image likelihood and prior are defined as

$$P(\mathbf{I}|\mathbf{a},\theta) = \frac{1}{Z_{\lambda_N}} e^{-\frac{\lambda_N}{2}|I(x,y,t) - \sum_i a_i(t) * \phi_i(x,y,t)|^2} \tag{13.24}$$

$$P(\mathbf{a}|\theta) = \prod_{i,t} \frac{1}{Z_S} e^{-S(a_i(t))} \tag{13.25}$$

and θ refers to the model parameters ϕ_i, λ_N, and $S()$.

By using the same approximation to the true gradient of $\mathcal{L}$ discussed in the previous section, the update rule for the basis functions is then

$$\Delta \phi_i(x,y,\tau) \propto a_i(\tau) \star e(x,y,\tau) \tag{13.26}$$

Thus, the basis functions are adapted over space and time by Hebbian learning between the time-varying residual image and the time-varying coefficient activities.

Results from natural movie sequences

The model was trained on moving image sequences obtained from Hans van Hateren's natural movie database (`http://hlab.phys.rug.nl/vidlib/vid_db`). The movies were first whitened by a filter that was derived from the inverse spatio-temporal amplitude spectrum, and lowpass filtered with a cutoff at 80% of the Nyquist frequency in space and time (see also Dong & Atick, 1995, for a similar whitening procedure). Training was done in batch mode by loading a 128×128 pixel, 64 frame sequence into memory and randomly extracting a spatial subimage of the same temporal length. The coefficients were fitted to this sequence by maximizing the posterior distribution via eqs. (13.19) and (13.20). The statistics for learning were averaged over ten such subimage sequences and the basis functions were then updated according to (13.26), again subject to rescaling (13.15). After several hours of training on a 450Mhz Pentium, the solution reached equilibrium.

The results for a set of 96 basis functions, each 8x8 pixels and of length 5 in time, are shown in figure 13.6. Spatially, they share many of the same characteristics of the basis functions obtained previously with static images (figure 13.3). The main dif-

time

basis
function

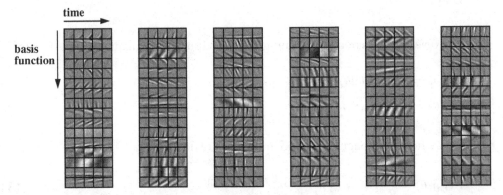

Figure 13.6. Space-time basis functions learned from time-varying natural images. Shown are a set of 96 basis functions arranged into six columns of 16 each. Each basis function is 8 × 8 pixels in space and 5 frames in time. Each row shows a different basis function, with time proceeding left to right. The translating character of the functions is best viewed as a movie, which may be viewed at `http://redwood.ucdavis.edu/bruno/bfmovie/bfmovie.html`.

ference is that they now also have a temporal characteristic, such that they tend to *translate* over time. Thus, the vast majority of the basis functions are direction selective (i.e., their coefficients will respond only to edges moving in one direction), with the high spatial-frequency functions biased toward lower velocities. These properties are typical of the space-time receptive fields of V1 simple-cells (Jones & Palmer, 1989; DeAngelis et al., 1995), and also of those obtained previously with ICA (van Hateren & Ruderman, 1998).

Because the outputs of the model are sparsified over both space and time, the model yields a qualitatively different behavior than linear convolution, as in ICA. Figure 13.7 illustrates this difference by comparing the time-varying coefficients obtained by maximizing the posterior to those obtained by straightforward convolution (similar to the linear prediction discussed in the previous section). The difference is striking in that the sparsified representation is characterized by highly localized, punctate events. Although still analog, it bears a strong resemblance to the the spiking nature of neural activity. At present though, this comparison is merely qualitative.

Discussion

We have shown in this chapter how both the spatial and temporal response properties of neurons may be understood in terms of a probabilistic model which attempts to describe images in terms of sparse, independent events. When the model is adapted to time-varying natural images, the basis functions converge upon a set of

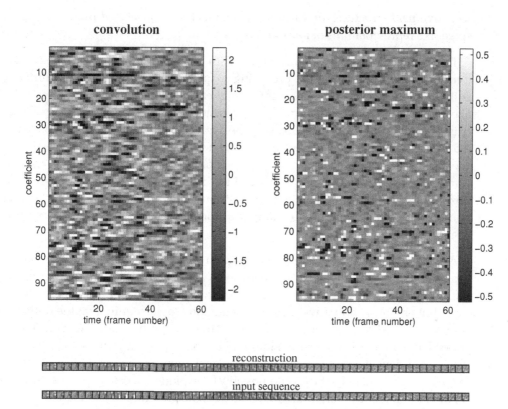

Figure 13.7. Coefficients computed by convolving the basis functions with the image sequence (*left*) vs. posterior maximization (*right*) for a 60 frame image sequence (*bottom*).

space-time functions which are spatially Gabor-like and translate with time. Moreover, the sparsified representation has a spike-like character, in that the coefficient signals are mostly zero and tend to concentrate their non-zero activity into brief, punctate events. These brief events represent longer spatiotemporal events in the image via the basis functions. The results suggest, then, that both the *receptive fields* and *spiking activity* of V1 neurons may be explained in terms of a single principle, that of sparse coding in time.

The interpretation of neural spike trains as a sparse code in time is not new. Most recently, Bialek and colleagues have shown that sensory neurons in the fly visual system, frog auditory system, and the cricket cercal system, essentially employ about one spike per "correlation time" to encode time-varying signals in their environment (Rieke et al., 1997). In fact, the image model proposed here is identical to their linear stimulus reconstruction framework used for measuring the mutual information between neural activity and sensory signals. The main contribution of this paper, beyond this previous body of work, is in showing that the particular spatiotemporal receptive field structures of V1 neurons may actually be *derived* from such sparse, spike-like representations of natural images.

This work also shares much in common with Lewicki's shift-invariant model of auditory signals, discussed in the preceding chapter in this book. The main difference is that Lewicki's model utilizes a much higher degree of overcompleteness, which allows for a more precise alignment of the basis functions with features occurring in natural sounds. Presumably, increasing the degree of overcompleteness in our model would yield even higher degrees of sparsity and basis functions that are even more specialized for the spatio-temporal features occurring in images. But learning becomes problematic in this case because of the difficulties inherent in properly maximizing or sampling from the posterior distribution over the coefficients. The development of efficient methods for sampling from the posterior is thus an important goal of future work.

Another important yet unresolved issue in implementing the model is how to deal with causality. Currently, the coefficients are computed by taking into account information both in the past and in the future in order to determine their optimal state. But obviously any physical implementation would require that the outputs be computed based only on past information. The fact that the basis functions become two-sided in time (i.e., non-zero values for both negative and positive time) indicates that a coefficient at time t_0 is making a statement about the image structure expected in the future ($t > t_0$). This fact could possibly be exploited in order to make the model predictive. That is, by committing to respond at the present time, based only on what has happened in the past, a unit will be making a prediction about what is to happen a short time in the future. An additional challenge in learning, then, is to adapt an appropriate decision function for determining when a unit should become active, so that each unit serves as a good predictor of future image structure in addition to being sparse.

Acknowledgements

This work benefited from discussions with Mike Lewicki and was was supported by NIMH grant R29-MH57921. I am also indebted to Hans van Hateren for making his natural movie database freely available.

References

[1]   Albrecht DG, Hamilton DB (1982) Striate cortex of monkey and cat: Contrast response function. *Journal of Neurophysiology, 48*: 217-237.

[2]   Atick JJ, Redlich AN (1992) What does the retina know about natural scenes?

Neural Computation, 4: 196-210.

[3] Barlow HB (1961) Possible principles underlying the transformations of sensory messages. In: *Sensory Communication,* W.A. Rosenblith, ed., MIT Press, pp. 217-234.

[4] Barlow HB (1989) Unsupervised learning, *Neural Computation, 1*: 295-311.

[5] Baum EB, Moody J, Wilczek F (1988) Internal representations for associative memory, *Biological Cybernetics, 59*: 217-228.

[6] Bell AJ, Sejnowski TJ (1997) The independent components of natural images are edge filters, *Vision Research, 37*: 3327-3338.

[7] DeAngelis GC, Ohzawa I, Freeman RD (1995) Receptive-field dynamics in the central visual pathways. *Trends in Neurosciences, 18(10),* 451-458.

[8] Dong DW, Atick JJ (1995) Temporal decorrelation: a theory of lagged and nonlagged responses in the lateral geniculate nucleus, *Network: Computation in Neural Systems, 6*: 159-178.

[9] Field DJ (1994) What is the goal of sensory coding? *Neural Computation, 6*: 559-601.

[10] Foldiak P (1995) Sparse coding in the primate cortex, In: *The Handbook of Brain Theory and Neural Networks,* Arbib MA, ed, MIT Press, pp. 895-989.

[11] Lewicki MS, Olshausen BA (1999) Probabilistic framework for the adaptation and comparison of image codes, *J. Opt. Soc. of Am., A, 16(7)*: 1587-1601.

[12] Lewicki MS, Sejnowski TJ (2000) Learning overcomplete representations. *Neural Computation, 12*:337-365.

[13] McLean J, Palmer LA (1989) Contribution of linear spatiotemporal receptive field structure to velocity selectivity of simple cells in area 17 of cat. *Vision Research, 29(6)*:675-9.

[14] Mumford D (1994) Neuronal architectures for pattern-theoretic problems, In: *Large Scale Neuronal Theories of the Brain,* Koch C, Davis, JL, eds., MIT Press, pp. 125-152.

[15] Olshausen BA, Field DJ (1997). Sparse coding with an overcomplete basis set: A strategy employed by V1? *Vision Research, 37,* 3311-3325.

[16] Olshausen BA, Millman KJ (2000). Learning sparse codes with a mixture-of-Gaussians prior. In: *Advances in Neural Information Processing Systems, 12,* S.A. Solla, T.K. Leen, K.R. Muller, eds. MIT Press, pp. 841-847.

[17] Rieke F, Warland D, de Ruyter van Stevenick R, Bialek W (1997) *Spikes: Exploring the Neural Code.* MIT Press.

[18] Simoncelli EP, Freeman WT, Adelson EH, Heeger DJ (1992) Shiftable multiscale transforms, *IEEE Transactions on Information Theory, 38(2)*: 587-607.

[19] Tadmor Y, Tolhurst DJ (1989) The effect of threshold on the relationship between the receptive field profile and the spatial-frequency tuning curve in sim-

ple cells of the cat's striate cortex, *Visual Neuroscience, 3*: 445-454.

[20] van Hateren JH, van der Schaaff A (1998) Independent component filters of natural images compared with simple cells in primary visual cortex, *Proc. Royal Soc. Lond. B, 265*: 359-366.

[21] van Hateren JH, Ruderman DL (1998) Independent component analysis of natural image sequences yields spatio-temporal filters similar to simple cells in primary visual cortex. Proc.R.Soc.Lond. B, 265:2315-2320.

14 Distributed Synchrony: A Probabilistic Model of Neural Signaling

Dana H. Ballard, Zuohua Zhang, and Rajesh P. N. Rao

Introduction

In the classical model of a neuron, the number of spikes produced is a function of the input rate [16]. This coding is well established in the peripheral nervous system and brain stem. It is also widely accepted as a model for cortical neurons. The rate code model is implicitly used by experimentalists in characterizing the neural output by the post-stimulus histogram. In addition, it has been widely used in computational learning models that use model neurons as primitive units. The rate code model fits experimental data well, but it has a crucial computational problem of slowness. Cortical firing rates are typically low, from 10 to 100 Hertz, so that decoding the spike rate at recipient neurons would take on the order of 10-100 milliseconds. Given that the neural signal has to go through many layers of neurons, the model is impractical for describing rapid behavioral responses. This is because at each soma, there would be delays in decoding the input, and we know that complete motor responses to visual input can occur within 200-400 milliseconds. Thus there is tremendous incentive for a model that could circumvent the speed problem by using single spikes in computation. It would allow contact with experimental data on a more fundamental level. The model could in principle stand in for the animal in that any measurement made on the animal system could be duplicated using the model.

Although rate code models have been popular for a long time, there has been a recent increase in experiments showing the importance of spike timing. These experiments provide motivation for our theoretical studies. *In vitro* experiments have shown that neurons fire with millisecond reliability when stimulated with realistic simulated input [11]. In the retina, the efficacy of synchronous codes has been noted as a way of retinal encoding of visual signals [10]. Retinal ganglion cells have overlapping receptive fields, so there exists the possibility of communicating information via synchronous subsets of firing patterns. Meister reviews the evidence for this idea and analyzes the efficacy of the synchronous data as an encoding scheme [10]. Synchronous codes trade off communication rate with increased signal fidelity. The retinal data provides an example of the type of encoding scheme that we propose here as a general signaling mechanism for the cortex.

Reid, Alonso, and Usrey have observed precise timing in cortico-thalamic connections [13, 2, 19]. The synchronization of activity for visual inputs has also been reported by Singer's group [5] and by Livingstone [9]. This activity seems to be part of a network as it is observed in the local field potential. In addition, Bair et al. have observed reliable spike train sequences in area MT for repeated motion stimuli [3]. Gallant et al. have also observed repeated spike train activity for repeated stimuli [8]. Additional evidence that volleys of synchronized spikes might be generated comes from experiments by Sillito et al. [17]. In anesthetized cats, neuron outputs in the LGN were correlated in the presence of the cortex, but uncorrelated (even though their firing rates were undisturbed), when the cortex was removed. In a *tour de force* experiment, Castelo-Branco et al. [5] observed correlations between the retina LGN and cortical areas 17 and 18 in the anesthetized cat. Their data show that the LGN exhibits correlations in the 60-120 Hz range and that the cortex exhibits correlations in two ranges: the 60-120 Hz range seen in the LGN and also a 30-60 Hz range.

Additional evidence for coincident firing comes from the Abeles group [12]. They show convincingly that precise spike timing can be observed at the level of a millisecond in many motor cortex cells. Furthermore, this timing is related to behavioral state, occurring in a specific interval during a complicated task. Schall [18], in more conventional post-stimulus histograms, has also shown that single neural recordings exhibit different task dependencies at different times.

Communicating with Spike Volleys

The cortex needs to communicate quickly and reliably over long distances. The central idea behind coincident firing is that neurons are more efficaciously fired if their arriving spikes are precisely timed [1]. Furthermore, this signal can be made reliable in that each individual neuron can be fired with great certainty. Thus, a neuron A can be made to fire a neuron B if there is a chain of intervening neurons where each receives synchronous input as shown in Figure 14.1. Abeles termed these *synfire chains* [1]. The synfire chain provides fast communication as the neurons in the chain are fired with a single arriving volley of spikes. As the spike velocities are on the order of 5-8cm/sec, communication along axons (ignoring delays at the somas) is fast, taking on the order of a few milliseconds. To propagate such a signal reliably, there must be several neurons at each synchronous stage. This is to ensure that the

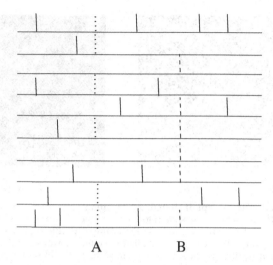

Figure 14.1. The basic idea of multiprocessing. The spike train from a single neuron is very difficult to interpret as it is the disjunction of many different processes. However, if the neurons at a stage in the path are known, then the meaning of the path can be recovered by intersecting all the individual spike trains. Here, two processes denoted by dotted (A) and dashed (B) spikes can be interpreted by intersecting the spikes on their respective paths. For the dotted path shown, interference would come when a rival path or set of paths connected to the neurons used by those on a path, or alternatively through random connections. For very wide paths of 100 neurons, interference is extremely unlikely.

firing chain is not broken. Aertsen et al. have recently shown that groups of neurons of about 100 are able to propagate a volley and maintain its precise timing [6]

Surprisingly, the message carried by a spike can be interpreted even though the collection of spikes represents the disjunction of many different signals [4]. The interpretation is actually easy but requires that one have access to all the neurons at a stage on a path. If that is possible, then the interpretation of the path is just the conjunction of all its spike trains. This is shown in Figure 14.2. A one-millisecond window of multi-cell data can be thought of as a binary "image" of spikes **S** and the particular set of axons comprising a path as another binary "image" **P**. The signal is being sent if every non zero element of **S** has a corresponding non-zero element in **P**. Despite its simplicity, this representation scheme is very difficult to interpret at the single cell level for at least three reasons:

1. The traffic through a single neuron represents all the active paths within a given time window.

2. This traffic is non-stationary in that different temporal samples may yield very different traffic patterns.

3. In a behaving animal, the computations may have a short lifetime. In a vision task for a primate, the computations need be done within a single 300 millisecond fixation.

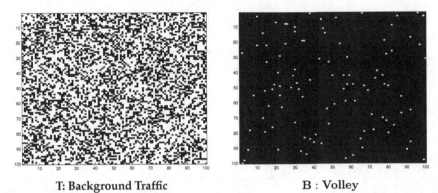

T: Background Traffic   **B : Volley**

Figure 14.2. A. The concept of shared coding along paths. A binary "image" of spikes along a set of 100 × 100 neural axons is shown for 50 independent processes, each using 100 overlapping sets of neurons. White denotes a spike.**B. Decoding a specific signal.** The signal along a specific path in a volley can still be recognized if all of the relevant axons simultaneously carry a spike, as shown in this image for a particular path (each white dot denotes an axon carrying a spike).

Cortical connections are both feed forward and feedback [7]. It is thus crucial for paths to be able to handle feedback. This is a challenging problem for communication with volleys because the feedback will necessarily be delayed by several means, and cannot arrive coincident with the spike that caused it. The solution we adopt is to delay the next input by an equal amount. Thus, the feedback spike arrives at the same time as the subsequent spike for the relevant path. The feedback is also encoded as part of the relevant path. What this means is that you can effectively think of the entire path including its feedback branches as a separate *sample data system*. In standard sample data systems, time is discrete and the system variables are analog quantities. Here is a special case where the variables are also discrete, being individual spikes. Thus in a negative feedback circuit, a volley may set up a feedback chain that cancels a subsequent volley. Since the propagation time is small, most of the delays must be realized by neurons' somas. Figure 14.3 shows this case. The important point here is that now we are adding the supposition that the volleys, where they use feedback for modification, are repeatedly sent in synchronous packets, that is, sets of volleys, each separated by a delay Δ. The length of the sets is governed by the needs of the current computation.

By incorporating delays, large-scale neural circuits could potentially be built that manipulate analog quantities according to algorithmic rules. In other words, this strategy provides a general communication protocol upon which behaviorally useful operations can be coded. Furthermore, neural circuits can exploit the security of overlapping paths to run several different computations in parallel. Each such computation needs to be sampled at an interval Δ, but they can share the same networks. Thus, in principle, vast numbers of paths can exist independently in the brain, even when they have feedback loops, without interfering with each other. The key assumptions here are the following three:

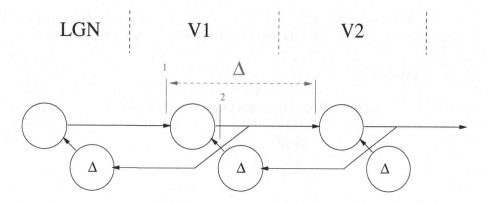

Feedforward spike 1 and feedback spike 2 are timed to arrive simultaneously

Figure 14.3. Handling Feedback. Owing to processing times, there will be delays at neuron's somas. Thus in a feedback circuit, such as the LGN-V1-V2 circuit, the feedback will arrive delayed with respect to the input. The solution is to delay the subsequent input volley by an equal amount. The feedback delay Δ is chosen by design to make the sampled data system work and should not be confused with smaller delays needed to adjust synchrony.

1. The delay Δ used in the feedback circuit is long with respect to individual traffic. (In the interim specified by Δ, many other signals can be sent that represent other variables).

2. The volleys generated by the incoming data, for example, from the thalamus, are repeated, i.e. they are in the form $\{b_t, b_{t+\Delta}, b_{t+2\Delta}, ...\}$.

3. The neurons are approximately memoryless. The calculations that decide whether or not to send a spike are not influenced by previous spikes outside of a very short time window of a few milliseconds.

The ability of the thalamo-cortical system to send synchronous volleys repeatedly might have seemed far-fetched until just recently. Weliky has demonstrated such ability in eight-channel electrode recordings from ferrets [20]. These recordings, made to study development, reveal synchronization in the LGN that is mediated by cortex on a time scale of about 10 seconds. This time scale could potentially be made faster following development.

Probabilistic Predictive Coding

Consider the problem of learning specific models of image data. We suppose that the task is to have a predictive model that can reconstruct incoming data. This has already been developed in the context of a rate model [14, 15]. In a synchronous firing model, given a set of volleys $\{b_1, b_2, ...b_T\}$, the goal of the model is to produce *answering feedback volleys* $\{\hat{b}_{1+\Delta}, \hat{b}_{2+\Delta}, ..., \hat{b}_{T+\Delta}\}$ such that $b_1 = \hat{b}_{1+\Delta}$ and so on. We do this by using an internal model consisting of units r with the goal that

$$b_t = U p(r)_t$$

Here, U is a matrix of synapses connecting the units r_t to the units that produce the $\{b_t\}$. The value of $p(r_t)$ is between 0 and 1. In this formula, r can be thought of as a neuron's membrane potential which determines a probability of firing. The model uses a sigmoid function to interpret r, i.e. $p(r) = \sigma(r)$, where

$$\sigma(r) = \frac{1}{1 + e^{-r}}$$

Following [14], one can use the Minimum Description Length principle to trade off reconstruction error cost with the cost of the reconstruction units. This leads to minimizing an error of the form

$$E = ||b_t - U\sigma(r_t)||^2 + \alpha ||r_t||^2 + \beta ||U||^2$$

In the above expression, the first term is the squared reconstruction error and the next two represent the cost of the machinery doing the reconstruction. The term $||r_t||^2$ measures the cost of producing spikes and the term $||U||^2$ measures the cost of the synaptic memory. The appropriate synaptic weights may be found by training on an image data set. These b_t are then used repeatedly in training. The MDL-based learning algorithm computes a stable set of responses r_t by using a form of gradient descent on E.

To train the synapses, sets of binary images were used in a repeated sequence. The synapses were shared between all the images so that they have to work for each volley from each image in the set. Note that the input is assumed to be appropriately interlaced, i.e. for the k-th image, the input volleys appear in a repeated sequence of what we term packets. Thus for image k,

$$..., b_1^k, b_2^k, b_3^k, ..., b_8^k, b_1^k, b_2^k, b_3^k, ..., b_8^k, b_1^k, ...$$

This is done for a time that simulates the time that the k-th image would be on the retina.

Simulation Results

To illustrate these principles using natural image patches, a network of 8×8 ON-center and 8×8 OFF-center input units and 80 coding units was trained on approximately 1000 natural image patches. The sampling strategy from [15] was used. Patches from natural images were filtered using the difference-of-Gaussians filter described therein. Next that result was converted to volleys by thresholding the resultant image. Image samples greater than zero were each assigned to an ON-center LGN model cell and image samples less than zero were each assigned to an OFF-center cell. This input was used to train the network by using the algorithm described above.

Simulation results show clearly that after training, the network can generate feedback volleys that cancel the incoming binary images (Figure 14.4). In this figure the feed forward input from the LGN is compared with the feedback signal from model cortical cells. The fact that they are comparable shows that the cancellation strategy is effective.

Figure 14.5 shows the most interesting feature of the simulation by plotting the response of the 80 coding neurons to four repeated edge image patterns. The onset of the patterns is shown by the transient firing increase on the trace. Although the communication is entirely synchronous, the patterns appear random as the routing of spikes goes through different neurons at each time step.

Although the communication is synchronous, the network can still produce data similar in form to that observed in experimental recordings. To show this, we sum the spikes over the 80 units to produce a time histogram. Single cell experiments would produce a similar histogram but with the difference that the experimentally-derived histogram is obtained by averaging over 80 trials. Here, the average is taken over 80 cells in a single trial.

The multi-unit time histogram, shown in Figure 14.6, has several interesting features. One is the onset of the four patterns shown by the phasic increases in average firing rate. Another is that the firing patterns for the repeated patterns, e.g. the first and the fifth or the second and the sixth, show some overall similarity suggesting that the cells are differentially tuned to the different patterns. A third feature is the average firing rate per pattern which stabilizes to about ten neurons (per time step). This feature is important from the modeling standpoint as it shows the sparse coding nature of the network. The input pattern contains $8 \times 8 = 64$ samples which are coded by an average of 10 cells at any instant, although all 80 cells participate in the coding.

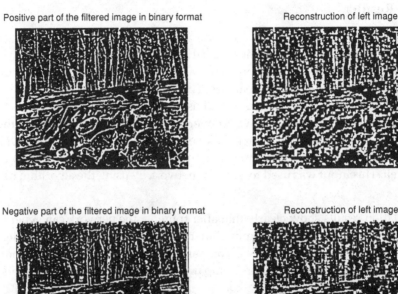

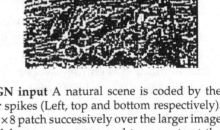

Figure 14.4. Reconstructing the model LGN input A natural scene is coded by the model LGN into ON-center and OFF-center spikes (Left, top and bottom respectively). The reconstruction is done by stepping the 8×8 patch successively over the larger image without overlap. At each location, the model responses were used to reconstruct the input. The right hand side images show the reconstruction, obtained by thresholding the feedback signal.

Conclusion

For a long time, the rate coding model has dominated the interpretation of experiments on single cortical cells. This model describes the fundamentally digital nature of the communication between cells as a form of analog signal. Interpreting the output as a single rate in this way ties up the neuron's axon and cannot account for the observed random spike patterns seen in cortical cells. The model proposed here suggests that neurons represent analog quantities, but that they communicate information about these quantities in a digital manner. The relevant calculations are done every time period in a fixed sampling interval. Empirical evidence suggests that this interval is on the order of 20 milliseconds.

In a purely synchronous model, one would expect to see periodic signals, so the lack of such direct evidence at the single cell level has been interpreted as reason

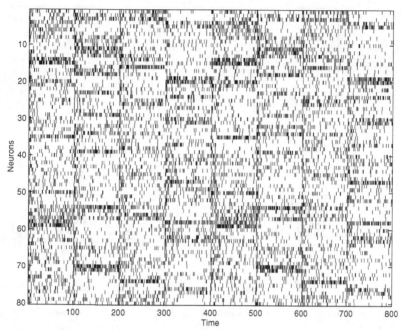

Figure 14.5. Distributed Synchrony. Four input patterns are repeated twice in sequence (in increments of 100 ms, starting at 0ms). The response of 80 model cortical cells is shown.

to reject the synchronous hypothesis. However, our model overcomes this objection as communication is shared by cells with similar receptive fields. At any sampling instant, many cells are capable of sending the desired spike and those that do are chosen probabilistically. The result is that although the overall communication is synchronous, the spikes through any particular cell appear random.

Our synchronous predictive model requires that cortico-thalamic feedback create repeated volleys in the feedforward pathway. The evidence for this comes from developmental experiments on ferrets [20]. These experiments show that cortico-thalamic connections produce synchronous firing and that severing these connections eliminates the synchrony between left and right eye signals. In addition, it has been suggested that in cortical area V1, the time to experience feedback can be as long as 100-200 milliseconds [21]. This is much longer than the theoretical time needed to propagate the signal through the neurons themselves. The suggestion, as hypothesized by our model, is that the delays are planned and play an important role in cortical signaling and computation.

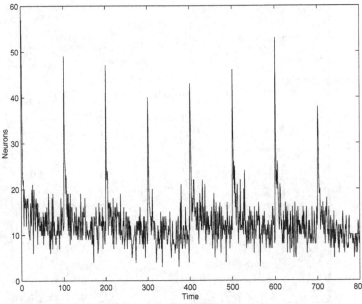

Figure 14.6. Multi-unit time histogram. This graph shows the summation of the spikes from Figure 14.5.

References

[1] M. Abeles. *Corticonics*. Cambridge University Press, 1991.

[2] J.-M. Alonso, W. M. Usrey, and R. C. Reid. Precisely correlated firing in cells of the lateral geniculate nucleus. *Nature*, 383:815–819, 1996.

[3] W. Bair, C. Koch, W. T. Newsome, and K. H. Britten Reliable temporal modulation in cortical spike trains in the awake monkey. *Proceedings of Dynamics of Neural Processing*, International Symposium (CNRS), June, 1994, Washington D.C. Lestienne R, (ed.) pp. 84-88, 1994.

[4] E. Bienenstock. A model of neocortex. *Network*, 6:179, 1995.

[5] M. Castelo-Branco, S. Neuenschwander, and W. Singer. Synchronization of visual responses between the cortex, lateral geniculate nucleaus, and retina in the anesthetized cat. *The Journal of Neuroscience*, 18:6395–6410, 1998.

[6] M. Diesmann, M.-O. Gewaltig, and A. Aertsen. Stable propagation of synchronous spiking in cortical neural networks. *Nature*, 402:529, 1999.

[7] D. J. Felleman and D. C. Van Essen. Distributed hierarchical processing in the primate cerebral cortex. *Cerebral Cortex*, 1:1–47, 1991.

[8] J. L. Gallant, C. E. Conner, and D. C. Van Essen. Neural activity in areas V1, V2, and V4 during free viewing of natural scenes compared to controlled viewing. *Neuroreport*, 9:2153, 1998.

[9] M. Livingstone. Oscillatory firing and interneuronal correlations in squirrel monkey striate cortex. *Journal of Neurophysiology*, 75:2467–2485, 1996.

[10] M. Meister. Multineuronal codes in retinal signaling. *Proceedings of the National Academy of Sciences*, 93:609–614, 1996.

[11] Z. F Mainen and T. J. Sejnowski. Reliability of spike timing in neocortical neurons. *Science*, 268:1503, 1995.

[12] Y. Prut, E. Vaadia, H. Bergman, I. Haalman, H. Slovin, and M. Abeles. Spatiotemporal structure of cortical activity: Properties and behavioral relevance. *Journal of Neurophysiology*, 79:2857–2874, 1998.

[13] R. C. Reid and J.-M. Alonso. Specificity of monosynaptic connections from thalamus to visual cortex. *Nature*, 378:281–284, 1995.

[14] R. P. N. Rao and D. H. Ballard. Dynamic model of visual processing predicts neural response properties of visual cortex. *Neural Computation*, 9:721–763, 1996.

[15] R. P. N. Rao and D. H. Ballard. Predictive coding in the visual cortex: a functional interpretation of some extra-classical receptive field effects. *Nature Neuroscience*, 2:79–87, 1998.

[16] F. Rieke, D. Warland, R. de Ruyter van Steveninck, and W. Bialek. *Spikes*. MIT Press, 1997.

[17] A. M. Sillito, H. E. Jones, G. L. Gerstein, and D. C. West. Feature-linked synchronization of thalamic relay cell firing induced by feedback from visual cortex. *Nature*, 369:479–482, 1994.

[18] K. G. Thompson, N. P. Bichot, and J. D. Schall. Dissociation of visual discrimination from saccade programming in macaque frontal eye field. *Journal of neurophysiology*, 77:1046, 1997.

[19] W. M. Usrey, J. B. Reppas, and R. C. Reid. Paired-spike interactions and synaptic efficacy of retinal inputs to the thalamus. *Nature*, 395:384–387, 1998.

[20] M. Weliky and L. C. Katz. Correlational structure of spontaneous neuronal activity in the developing lateral geniculate nucleus in vivo. *Science*, 265:599, 1999.

[21] K. Zipser, V. A. F. Lamme, and P. N. Schiller. Contextual modulation in primary visual cortex. *Journal of Neuroscience*, 16:7376, 1997.

15 Learning to Use Spike Timing in a Restricted Boltzmann Machine

Geoffrey E. Hinton and Andrew D. Brown

Population Codes and Energy Landscapes

A perceived object is represented in the brain by the activities of many neurons, but there is no general consensus on how the activities of individual neurons combine to represent the multiple properties of an object. We start by focussing on the case of a single object that has multiple instantiation parameters such as position, velocity, size and orientation. We assume that each neuron has an ideal stimulus in the space of instantiation parameters and that its activation rate or probability of activation falls off monotonically in all directions as the actual stimulus departs from this ideal. The semantic problem is to define exactly what instantiation parameters are being represented when the activities of many such neurons are specified.

Hinton, Rumelhart, and McClelland (1986) consider binary neurons with receptive fields that are convex in instantiation space. They assume that when an object is present it activates all of the neurons in whose receptive fields its instantiation parameters lie. Consequently, if it is known that only one object is present, the parameter values of the object must lie within the feasible region formed by the *intersection* of the receptive fields of the active neurons. This will be called a *conjunctive* distributed representation. Assuming that each receptive field occupies only a small fraction of the whole space, an interesting property of this type of "coarse coding" is that the bigger the receptive fields, the more accurate the representation. However, large receptive fields lead to a loss of resolution when several objects are present simultaneously.

When the sensory input is noisy, it is impossible to infer the exact parameters of objects so it makes sense for a perceptual system to represent the probability distribution across parameters rather than just a single best estimate or a feasible region. The full probability distribution is essential for correctly combining information from different times or different sources. One obvious way to represent this distribution (Anderson and van Essen, 1994) is to allow each neuron to represent a fairly compact probability distribution over the space of instantiation parameters and to treat the activity levels of neurons as (unnormalized) mixing proportions. The semantics of this *disjunctive* distributed representation is precise, but the percepts it allows are not because it is impossible to represent distributions that are sharper than the individual receptive fields and, in high-dimensional spaces, the individual fields must be broad in order to cover the space. Disjunctive representations are used in Self-Organizing Maps (Kohonen, 1995) and the Generative Topographic Maps (Bishop, Svensen and Williams, 1998) which is why they are restricted to very low-dimensional latent spaces.

Zemel, Dayan, and Pouget (1998) generalize coarse coding to neurons which have smooth unimodal tuning functions in the instantiation parameter space (see the chapter by Zemel and Pillow in this book). The tuning function determines the neuron's probability of emitting a spike by setting the rate parameter of a Poisson distribution. Given the number of spikes emitted by each neuron in a population in some time interval, it is possible to estimate a probability distribution over the entire space of possible instantiation parameters. Zhang *et. al.* (1998) show that an approach of this kind provides a good fit to data on hippocampal place cells.

The disjunctive model can be viewed as an attempt to approximate arbitrary probability distributions by adding together probability distributions contributed by each active neuron. Coarse coding suggests a multiplicative approach in which the addition is done in the domain of energies (negative log probabilities). Each active neuron contributes an energy landscape over the whole space of instantiation parameters. The activity level of the neuron multiplies its energy landscape and the landscapes for all neurons in the population are added (Figure 15.1). If, for example, each neuron has a full covariance Gaussian tuning function, its energy landscape is a parabolic bowl whose curvature matrix is the inverse of the covariance matrix. The activity level of the neuron scales the inverse covariance matrix. If there are k instantiation parameters then only $k+k(k+1)/2$ real numbers are required to span the space of means and inverse covariance matrices. So the real-valued activities of $O(k^2)$ neurons are sufficient to represent arbitrary full covariance Gaussian distributions over the space of instantiation parameters.

Treating neural activities as multiplicative coefficients on additive contributions to energy landscapes has a number of advantages. Unlike disjunctive codes, vague distributions are represented by low activities so significant biochemical energy is only required when distributions are quite sharp. A central operation in Bayesian inference is to combine a prior term with a likelihood term or to combine two

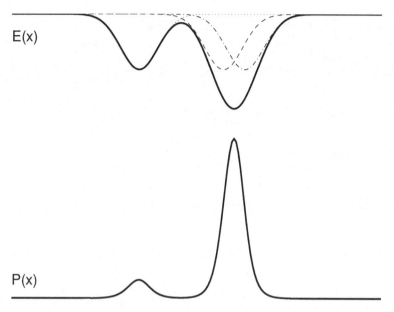

Figure 15.1. An energy landscape over a one-dimensional space. Each neuron adds a dimple (dotted line) to the energy landscape (solid line). b) The corresponding probability density. Where dimples overlap the corresponding probability density becomes sharper. Since the dimples decay to zero, the location of a sharp probability peak is not affected by distant dimples and multimodal distributions can be represented.

conditionally independent likelihood terms. This is trivially achieved by adding two energy landscapes[1].

Representing the Coefficients on the Basis Functions

To perform perception at video rates, the probability distributions over instantiation parameters need to be represented at about 30 frames per second. This seems difficult using relatively slow spiking neurons because it requires the real-valued multiplicative coefficients on the basis functions to be communicated accurately and quickly using all-or-none spikes. The trick is to realise that when a spike arrives at another neuron it produces a postsynaptic potential that is a smooth function of time. So from the perspective of the postsynaptic neuron, the spike has been convolved with a smooth temporal function. By adding a number of these smooth functions together,

---

1. We thank Zoubin Ghahramani for pointing out that another important operation, convolving a probability distribution with Gaussian noise, is a difficult non-linear operation on the energy landscape.

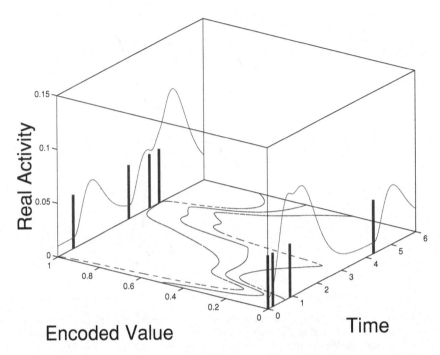

Figure 15.2. Two spiking neurons centered at 0 and 1 can represent the time-varying mean and standard deviation on a single spatial dimension. The spikes are first convolved with a temporal kernel and the resulting activity values are treated as exponents on Gaussian distributions centered at 0 and 1. The ratio of the activity values determines the mean and the sum of the activity values determines the inverse variance.

with appropriate temporal offsets, it is possible to represent any smoothly varying sequence of coefficient values on a basis function, and this makes it possible to represent the temporal evolution of probability distributions as shown in Figure 15.3. The ability to vary the location of a spike in the single dimension of time thus allows real-valued control of the representation of probability distributions over multiple spatial dimensions.

Our proposed use of spike timing to convey real values quickly and accurately does not require precise coincidence detection, sub-threshold oscillations, modifiable time delays, or any of the other paraphernalia that has been invoked to explain how the brain could make effective use of the single, real-valued degree of freedom in the timing of a spike (Hopfield, 1995).

The coding scheme we have proposed would be far more convincing if we could show how it was learned and could demonstrate that it was effective in a simulation. There are two ways to design a learning algorithm for such spiking neurons. We could work in the relatively low-dimensional space of the instantiation parameters and design the learning to produce the right representations and interactions

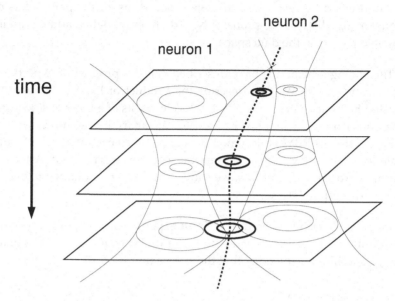

Figure 15.3. Spikes can be used to represent smoothly varying coefficients on basis functions in two (or more) spatial dimensions. Time flows from top to bottom. Each spike makes a contribution to the energy landscape that resembles an hourglass (thin lines). The waist of the hourglass corresponds to the time at which the spike has its strongest effect on some post-synaptic population. By moving the hourglasses in time, it is possible to get whatever temporal cross-sections are desired (thick lines) provided the temporal sampling rate is comparable to the time course of the effect of a spike.

between representations in this space. Or we could treat this space as an implicit emergent property of the network and design the learning algorithm to optimize some objective function in the much higher-dimensional space of neural activities in the hope that this will create representations that can be understood using the implicit space of instantiation parameters. We chose the latter approach.

A Learning Algorithm for Restricted Boltzmann Machines

Hinton (2000) describes a learning algorithm for probabilistic generative models that are composed of a number of experts. Each expert specifies a probability distribution over the visible variables and the experts are combined by multiplying these distributions together and renormalizing:

$$p(\mathbf{d}|\theta_1...\theta_n) = \frac{\Pi_m p_m(\mathbf{d}|\theta_m)}{\sum_{\mathbf{c}} \Pi_m p_m(\mathbf{c}|\theta_m)} \tag{15.1}$$

where $\mathbf{d}$ is a data vector in a discrete space, θ_m is all the parameters of individual model m, $p_m(\mathbf{d}|\theta_m)$ is the probability of $\mathbf{d}$ under model m, and $\mathbf{c}$ is an index over all possible vectors in the data space.

The coding scheme we have described is just a product of experts in which each spike is an expert. We first describe the Product of Experts learning rule for a restricted Boltzmann machine (RBM) which consists of a layer of stochastic binary visible units connected to a layer of stochastic binary hidden units with no intralayer connections. An RBM is designed for *i.i.d.* data so each unit adopts a single binary state for each data vector and temporal sequence is irrelevant. After explaining the learning procedure for RBM's, we show how it can be extended to deal with spiking units and temporal data.

In an RBM, each hidden unit, j, is an expert. When it is off, it specifies a uniform distribution over the states of the visible units. When it is on, its weight to each visible unit, i, specifies the log odds that the visible unit is on:

$$\log \frac{p(s_i = 1|s_j = 1)}{1 - p(s_i = 1|s_j = 1)} = w_{ij} \tag{15.2}$$

hence:

$$p(s_i = 1|s_j = 1) = \frac{1}{1 + \exp(-w_{ij})} \tag{15.3}$$

Multiplying the distributions specified by the different hidden units is achieved by adding the log odds of all the active hidden units:

$$p(s_i = 1) = \frac{1}{1 + \exp(-\sum_j w_{ij}s_j)} \tag{15.4}$$

Inference in an RBM is much easier than in a causal belief net because there is no explaining away. There is therefore no need to perform any iteration to determine the activites of the hidden units (compare the iteration required even for MAP estimation in the chapter by Olshausen in this book). The hidden states, s_j, are conditionally independent given the visible states, s_i, and the distribution of s_j is given by the standard logistic function:

$$p(s_j = 1) = \frac{1}{1 + \exp(-\sum_i w_{ij}s_i)} \tag{15.5}$$

Conversely, the hidden states of an RBM are *marginally* dependent so it is easy for an RBM to learn population codes in which units may be highly correlated. It is hard to do this in causal belief nets with one hidden layer because the generative model of a causal belief net assumes marginal independence.

An RBM can be trained by following the gradient of the log likelihood of the data. Taking logs and differentiating Eq. 15.1 gives:

$$\frac{\partial \log p(\mathbf{d}|\theta_1...\theta_n)}{\partial \theta_m} = \frac{\partial \log p_m(\mathbf{d}|\theta_m)}{\partial \theta_m} - \sum_{\mathbf{c}} p(\mathbf{c}|\theta_1...\theta_n)\frac{\partial \log p_m(\mathbf{c}|\theta_m)}{\partial \theta_m} \qquad (15.6)$$

The second term on the RHS of Eq. 15.6 is just the expected derivative of the log probability of an expert on fantasy data, $\mathbf{c}$, that is generated from the RBM. It is possible to get a noisy but unbiased estimate of this term by using Gibbs sampling to generate fantasies and then computing the derivatives of $\log p_m(\mathbf{c}|\theta_m)$ on these sampled fantasies. In Gibbs sampling, each variable draws a sample from its posterior distribution given the current states of the other variables. Given the data, the hidden units can all be updated in parallel using Eq. 15.5 because they are conditionally independent. This is a very important consequence of the product formulation. Given the hidden states, the visible units can then be updated in parallel using Eq. 15.4. So Gibbs sampling can alternate between parallel updates of the hidden and visible variables. To get unbiased fantasies from the RBM, it is necessary for the Markov chain to converge to the equilibrium distribution, so although an RBM is a *bona fide* generative model, it has the curious property that it is very hard work to generate samples from it.

There is a simple weight update procedure which follows the derivative of the log likelihood of the data (Hinton and Sejnowski, 1986):

$$\Delta w_{ij} = \epsilon \left(< s_i s_j >^0 - < s_i s_j >^\infty \right) \qquad (15.7)$$

where $< s_i s_j >^0$ is the expected value of $s_i s_j$ when data is clamped on the visible units and the hidden states are sampled from their conditional distribution given the data, and $< s_i s_j >^\infty$ is the expected value of $s_i s_j$ after prolonged Gibbs sampling that alternates between sampling from the conditional distribution of the hidden states given the visible states and vice versa.

This learning rule may not work well because it can take a long time to approach thermal equilibrium and the sampling noise in the estimate of $< s_i s_j >^\infty$ can swamp the gradient. Maximizing the log likelihood of the data is equivalent to minimizing the Kullback-Leibler divergence, $Q^0||Q^\infty$, between the data distribution, Q^0, and the equilibrium distribution of fantasies over the visible units, Q^∞, produced by the

RBM. Hinton (2000) shows that it is far more effective to minimize the *difference* between $Q^0||Q^\infty$ and $Q^1||Q^\infty$ where Q^1 is the distribution of the one-step reconstructions of the data that are produced by first picking binary hidden states from their conditional distribution given the data and then picking binary visible states from their conditional distribution given the hidden states. The exact gradient of this "contrastive divergence" is complicated because the distribution Q^1 depends on the weights but Hinton (2000) shows that this dependence can safely be ignored to yield a simple and effective learning rule for following the approximate gradient of the contrastive divergence:

$$\Delta w_{ij} = \epsilon \left(< s_i s_j >^0 - < s_i s_j >^1 \right) \tag{15.8}$$

Restricted Boltzmann Machines Through Time

Using a restricted Boltzmann machine, we can represent time by *spatializing* it, *i.e.* taking each visible unit, i, and hidden unit, j, and replicating them through time with the constraint that the weight $w_{ij\tau}$ between replica t of i and replica $t + \tau$ of j does not depend on t. To implement the desired temporal smoothing, we also force the weights to be a smooth function of τ that has the shape of the temporal kernel shown in Figure 15.4. The only remaining degree of freedom in the weights between replicas of i and replicas of j is the vertical scale of the temporal kernel and it is this scale that is learned. The replicas of the visible and hidden units still form a bipartite graph and the probability distribution over the hidden replicas can be inferred exactly without considering data that lies further into the future than the width of the temporal kernel.

One problem with the restricted Boltzmann machine when we spatialize time is that hidden units at one time step have no memory of their states at previous time steps; they only see the data. If we were to add undirected connections between hidden units at different time steps, then the architecture would return to a fully connected Boltzmann machine in which the hidden units are no longer conditionally independent given the data. A useful trick borrowed from Elman nets (Elman, 1990) is to allow the hidden units to see their previous states, but to treat these observations like data that cannot be modified by future hidden states. Thus, the hidden states may still be inferred independently without resorting to Gibbs sampling. The connections between hidden layer weights also follow the time course of the temporal kernel. These connections act as a predictive prior over the hidden units. It is important to note that these forward connections are not required for the network to model a sequence, but only for the purposes of extrapolating into the future.

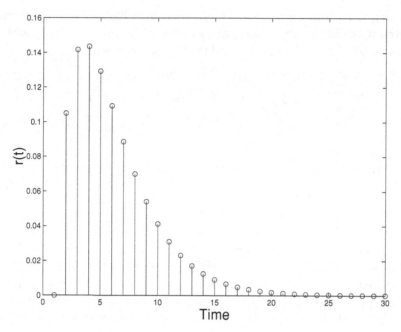

Figure 15.4: The form of the temporal kernel.

Now, the probability that $s_j(t) = 1$ given the states of the visible units is:

$$P(s_j(t) = 1) = \sigma \left(\sum_i w_{ij} h_i(t) + \sum_k w_{kj} h_k(t) \right) \tag{15.9}$$

where $h_i(t)$ is the convolution of the history of visible unit i with the temporal kernel, i.e.

$$h_i(t) = \sum_{\tau=0}^{\infty} s_i(t - \tau) r(\tau) \tag{15.10}$$

$h_k(t)$, the convolution of the hidden unit history, is computed similarly. [2] Learning the weights follows immediately from this formula for doing inference. In the positive phase, the visible units are clamped at each time step and the posterior of the hidden units conditioned on the data is computed (we assume zero boundary conditions for time before $t = 0$). Then, in the negative phase, we sample from the posterior of the

---

2. Computing the conditional probability distribution over the visible units given the hidden states is done in a similar fashion, with the caveat that the weights in each direction must be symmetric. Thus, the convolution is done using the reverse kernel.

hidden units, and compute the distribution over the visible units at each time step given these hidden unit states. In each phase, the correlations between the hidden and visible units are computed and the learning rule is:

$$\Delta w_{ij} = \sum_{t=0}^{\infty} \sum_{\tau=0}^{\infty} r(\tau) \left(\langle s_j(t) s_i(t-\tau) \rangle^0 - \langle s_j(t) s_i(t-\tau) \rangle^1 \right) \qquad (15.11)$$

Results

We trained this network on a sequence of 8x8 synthetic images of a Gaussian blob moving in a circular path. In the following diagrams, we display the time sequence of images as a matrix. Each row of the matrix represents a single image with its pixels stretched out into a vector in scanline order, and each column is the time course of a single pixel. The intensity of the pixel is represented by the area of the white patch. We used 20 hidden units. Figure 15.5a shows a segment (200 time steps) of the time series which was used in training. In this sequence, the period of the blob is 80 time steps.

Figure 15.5b shows how the trained model reconstructs the data after we sample from the hidden layer units. Once we have trained the model, it is possible to do forecasting by clamping visible layer units for a segment of a sequence and then doing iterative Gibbs sampling to generate future points in the sequence. Figure 15.5c shows that given 50 time steps from the series, the model can predict reasonably far into the future, before the pattern dies out.

One problem with these simulations is that we are treating the real valued intensities in the images as probabilities. While this works for the blob images, where the values can be viewed as the probabilities of pixels in a binary image being on, this is not true for more natural images.

Discussion

In our initial simulations, we used a causal sigmoid belief network (SBN) rather than a restricted Boltzmann machine. Inference in an SBN is *much* more difficult than in an RBM. It requires Gibbs sampling or severe approximations, and even if a temporal kernel is used to ensure that a replica of a hidden unit at one time has no connections to replicas of visible units at very different times, the posterior

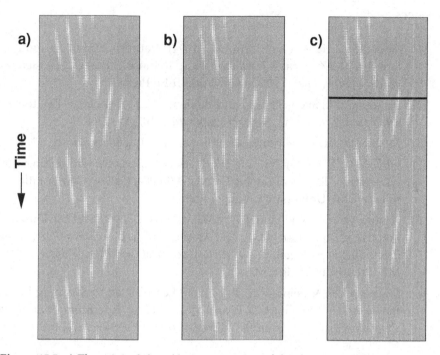

Figure 15.5. a) The original data, b) reconstruction of the data, and c) prediction of the data given 50 time steps of the sequence. The black line indicates where the prediction begins.

distribution of the hidden units still depends on data far in the future. The Gibbs sampling made our SBN simulations very slow and the sampling noise made the learning far less effective than in the RBM.

Although the RBM simulations seem closer to biological plausibility, they too suffer from a major problem. To apply the learning procedure, it is necessary to reconstruct the data from the hidden states and we do not know how to do this without interfering with the incoming datastream. In our simulations, we simply ignored this problem by allowing a visible unit to have both an observed value and a reconstructed value at the same time.

Acknowledgements

We thank Zoubin Ghahramani, Peter Dayan, Rich Zemel, Terry Sejnowski and Radford Neal for helpful discussions. This research was funded by grants from the Gatsby Foundation and NSERC.

References

[1] Anderson, C.H. & van Essen, D.C (1994). Neurobiological computational systems. In J.M Zureda, R.J. Marks, & C.J. Robinson (Eds.), *Computational Intelligence Imitating Life* 213-222. New York: IEEE Press.

[2] Bishop, C. M., Svens'en, M., and Williams, C. K. I. (1998). GTM: the generative topographic mapping. *Neural Computation*, **10**, 215–234.

[3] Elman, J. L. (1990). Finding structure in time. *Cognitive Science*, **14**, 179-211.

[4] Hinton, G. E. (2000) Training Products of Experts by Minimizing Contrastive Divergence. Technical Report GCNU 2000-004, Gatsby Computational Neuroscience Unit, University College London.

[5] Hinton, G. E., McClelland, J. L., & Rumelhart, D. E. (1986) Distributed representations. In Rumelhart, D. E. and McClelland, J. L., editors, *Parallel Distributed Processing: Explorations in the Microstructure of Cognition. Volume 1: Foundations*, MIT Press, Cambridge, MA.

[6] Hinton, G. E. & Sejnowski, T. J. (1986) Learning and relearning in Boltzmann machines. In Rumelhart, D. E. and McClelland, J. L., editors, *Parallel Distributed Processing: Explorations in the Microstructure of Cognition. Volume 1: Foundations*, MIT Press

[7] Hopfield, J. (1995). Pattern recognition computation using action potential timing for stimulus representation. *Nature*, **376**, 33-36.

[8] Kohonen, T. (1995). *Self-Organizing Maps*. Springer-Verlag, Berlin.

[9] Zemel, R.S., Dayan, P. & Pouget, A. (1998). Probabilistic Interpretation of Population Codes. *Neural Computation* **10**, 403-430.

[10] Zhang, K.-C., Ginzburg, I., McNaughton, B. L., & Sejnowski, T. J. (1998). Interpreting neuronal population activity by reconstruction: Unified framework with application to hippocampal place cells. *J. Neurophysiol.*.

16 Predictive Coding, Cortical Feedback, and Spike-Timing Dependent Plasticity

Rajesh P. N. Rao and Terrence J. Sejnowski

Introduction

One of the most prominent but least understood neuroanatomical features of the cerebral cortex is feedback. Neurons within a cortical area generally receive massive excitatory feedback from other neurons in the same cortical area. Some of these neurons, especially those in the superficial layers, send feedforward axons to higher cortical areas while others neurons, particularly those in the deeper layers, send feedback axons to lower cortical areas. What is the functional significance of these local and long-range feedback connections?

In this chapter, we explore the following two hypotheses: (a) feedback connections from a higher to a lower cortical area carry predictions of expected neural activity in the lower area, while the feedforward connections carry the differences between the predictions and the actual neural activity; and (b) recurrent feedback connections between neurons within a cortical area are used to learn, store, and predict temporal sequences of input neural activity. Together, these two types of feedback connections help instantiate a hierarchical spatiotemporal generative model of cortical inputs.

The idea that feedback connections may instantiate a hierarchical generative model of sensory inputs has been proposed previously in the context of the Helmholtz machine [14, 15]. However, feedback connections in the Helmholtz machine were used only during training and played no role in perception, which involved a single feedforward pass through the hierarchical network. On the other hand, the possibility of feedback connections carrying expectations of lower level activity and feedforward connections carrying error signals was first studied by MacKay in the context of his epistemological automata [24]. More recently, similar ideas have been suggested by

Pece [34] and Mumford [31] as a model for corticothalamic and cortical networks. The idea of using lateral or recurrent feedback connections for storing temporal dynamics has received much attention in the neural networks community [21, 19, 36] and in models of the hippocampus [28, 1]. However, in the case of cortical models, recurrent connections have been used mainly to amplify weak thalamic inputs in models of orientation [7, 42] and direction selectivity [17, 44, 29]. Recent results on synaptic plasticity of recurrent cortical connections indicate a dependence on the temporal order of pre- and postsynaptic spikes: synapses that are activated slightly before the postsynaptic cell fires are strengthened whereas those that are activated slightly after are weakened [26]. In this chapter, we explore the hypothesis that such a synaptic learning rule allows local recurrent feedback connections to be used for encoding and predicting temporal sequences. Together with corticocortical feedback, these local feedback connections could allow the implementation of spatiotemporal generative models in recurrent cortical circuits.

Spatiotemporal Generative Models

Figure 16.1A depicts the problem faced by an organism perceiving the external world. The organism does not have access to the hidden states of the world that are causing its sensory experiences. Instead, it must solve the "inverse" problem of *estimating* these hidden state parameters using only the sensory measurements obtained from its various sensing devices in order to correctly interpret and understand the external world [35]. Note that with respect to the cortex, the definition of an "external world" need not be restricted to sensory modalities such as vision or audition. The cortex may learn and use internal models of "extra-cortical" systems such as the various musculo-skeletal systems responsible for executing body movements [47].

Perhaps the simplest mathematical form one can ascribe to an internal model is to assume a *linear generative model* for the process underlying the generation of sensory inputs. In particular, at any time instant t, the state of the given input generating process is assumed to be characterized by a k-element *hidden state vector* $\mathbf{r}(t)$. Although not directly accessible, this state vector is assumed to generate a measurable and observable output $\mathbf{I}(t)$ (for example, an image of n pixels) according to:

$$\mathbf{I}(t) = U\mathbf{r}(t) + \mathbf{n}(t) \tag{16.1}$$

where U is a (usually unknown) generative (or measurement) matrix that relates the $k \times 1$ state vector $\mathbf{r}(t)$ to the $n \times 1$ observable output vector $\mathbf{I}(t)$, and $\mathbf{n}(t)$ is a Gaussian stochastic noise process with mean zero and a covariance matrix given by

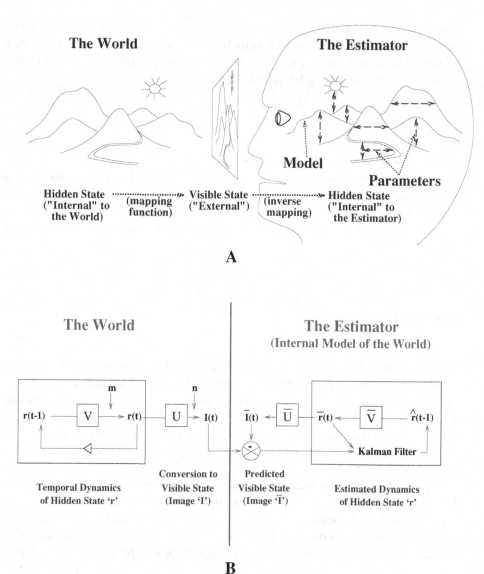

Figure 16.1. Internal Models and the Problem of Optimal Estimation of Hidden State
(A) The problem faced by an organism relying on an internal model of its environment
(from [33]). The underlying goal is to optimally estimate, at each time instant, the
hidden state of the environment given only the sensory measurements **I**. (B) depicts
a single-level Kalman filter solution to the estimation problem. The internal model is
encoded jointly by the state transition matrix $\overline{V}$ and the generative matrix $\overline{U}$, and the
filter uses this internal model to compute optimal estimates $\hat{\mathbf{r}}$ of the current state **r** of
the environment.

$\Sigma = E[\mathbf{n}\mathbf{n}^T]$ (E denotes the expectation operator and T denotes transpose). Note
that this is a sufficient description of **n** since a Gaussian distribution is completely
specified by its mean and covariance.

In addition to specifying how the hidden state of the observed process generates a spatial image, we also need to specify how the state itself changes with time t. We assume that the transition from the state $\mathbf{r}(t-1)$ at time instant $t-1$ to the state $\mathbf{r}(t)$ at the next time instant can be modeled as:

$$\mathbf{r}(t) = V\mathbf{r}(t-1) + \mathbf{m}(t-1) \tag{16.2}$$

where V is a (usually unknown) *state transition (or prediction) matrix* and $\mathbf{m}$ is a Gaussian noise process with mean $\overline{\mathbf{m}}(t)$ and covariance $\Pi = E[(\mathbf{m} - \overline{\mathbf{m}})(\mathbf{m} - \overline{\mathbf{m}})^T]$. In other words, the matrix V is used to characterize the dynamic behavior of the observed system over the course of time. Any difference between the actual state $\mathbf{r}(t)$ and the prediction from the previous time step $V\mathbf{r}(t-1)$ is modeled as the stochastic noise vector $\mathbf{m}(t-1)$.

Optimization Functions

The parameters $\mathbf{r}$, U, and V in the spatiotemporal generative model above can be estimated and learned directly from input data if we can define an appropriate optimization function with respect to $\mathbf{r}$, U, and V. For the present purposes, assume that we know the true values of U and V, and we therefore wish to find, at each time instant, an optimal estimate $\widehat{\mathbf{r}}(t)$ of the current state $\mathbf{r}(t)$ of the observed process using only the measurable inputs $\mathbf{I}(t)$.

Suppose that we have already computed a prediction $\overline{\mathbf{r}}$ of the current state $\mathbf{r}$ based on prior data. In particular, let $\overline{\mathbf{r}}(t)$ be the mean of the current state vector *before* measurement of the input data $\mathbf{I}$ at the current time instant t. The corresponding covariance matrix is given by $E[(\mathbf{r} - \overline{\mathbf{r}})(\mathbf{r} - \overline{\mathbf{r}})^T] = M$. A common optimization function whose minimization yields an estimate for $\mathbf{r}$ is the *least-squares criterion*:

$$J_1 = \sum_{i=1}^{n} \left(\mathbf{I}^i - U^i\mathbf{r}\right)^2 + \sum_{i=1}^{k}(\mathbf{r}^i - \overline{\mathbf{r}}^i)^2 = (\mathbf{I} - U\mathbf{r})^T(\mathbf{I} - U\mathbf{r}) + (\mathbf{r} - \overline{\mathbf{r}})^T(\mathbf{r} - \overline{\mathbf{r}}) \tag{16.3}$$

where the superscript i denotes the ith element or row of the superscripted vector or matrix. For example, in the case where $\mathbf{I}$ represents an image, the value for $\mathbf{r}$ that minimizes this quadratic function is the value that (1) yields the smallest sum of pixel-wise differences (squared residual errors) between the image $\mathbf{I}$ and its reconstruction $U\mathbf{r}$ obtained using the matrix U, and (2) is also as close as possible to the prediction $\overline{\mathbf{r}}$ computed from prior data.

The quadratic optimization function above is a special case of the more general *weighted least-squares criterion* [10, 35]:

$$J = (\mathbf{I} - U\mathbf{r})^T \Sigma^{-1} (\mathbf{I} - U\mathbf{r}) + (\mathbf{r} - \bar{\mathbf{r}})^T M^{-1} (\mathbf{r} - \bar{\mathbf{r}}) \tag{16.4}$$

The weighted least-squares criterion becomes meaningful when interpreted in terms of the stochastic model described in the previous section. Recall that the measurement equation 16.1 was characterized in terms of a Gaussian with mean zero and covariance Σ. Also, as given in the previous paragraph, $\mathbf{r}$ follows a Gaussian distribution with mean $\bar{\mathbf{r}}$ and covariance M. Thus, it can be shown that J is simply the sum of the negative log of the (Gaussian) probability of generating the data $\mathbf{I}$ given the state $\mathbf{r}$, and the negative log of the (Gaussian) prior probability of the state $\mathbf{r}$:

$$J = (-\log P(\mathbf{I}|\mathbf{r})) + (-\log P(\mathbf{r})) \tag{16.5}$$

The first term in the above equation follows from the fact that $P(\mathbf{I}|\mathbf{r}) = P(\mathbf{I}, \mathbf{r})/P(\mathbf{r}) = P(\mathbf{n}, \mathbf{r})/P(\mathbf{r}) = P(\mathbf{n})$, assuming $P(\mathbf{n}, \mathbf{r}) = P(\mathbf{n})P(\mathbf{r})$. Now, note that the *posterior* probability of the state given the the input data is given by (using Bayes theorem):

$$P(\mathbf{r}|\mathbf{I}) = P(\mathbf{I}|\mathbf{r})P(\mathbf{r})/P(\mathbf{I}) \tag{16.6}$$

By taking the negative log of both sides (and ignoring the term due to $P(\mathbf{I})$ since it is a fixed quantity), we can conclude that minimizing J is exactly the same as maximizing the posterior probability of the state $\mathbf{r}$ given the input data $\mathbf{I}$.

Predictive Coding

The optimization function J formulated in the previous section can be minimized to find the optimal value $\hat{\mathbf{r}}$ of the state $\mathbf{r}$ by setting $\frac{\partial J}{\partial \mathbf{r}} = 0$:

$$-U^T \Sigma^{-1} (\mathbf{I} - U\hat{\mathbf{r}}) + M^{-1}(\hat{\mathbf{r}} - \bar{\mathbf{r}}) = 0 \tag{16.7}$$

which yields:

$$(U^T \Sigma^{-1} U + M^{-1})\hat{\mathbf{r}} = M^{-1}\bar{\mathbf{r}} + U^T \Sigma^{-1}\mathbf{I} \tag{16.8}$$

Using the substitution $N(t) = (U^T \Sigma^{-1} U + M^{-1})^{-1}$ and rearranging the terms in the above equation, we obtain the following predictive coding equation (also known as the *Kalman filter* in optimal control theory [10]):

$$\hat{\mathbf{r}}(t) = \bar{\mathbf{r}}(t) + N(t)U^T \Sigma(t)^{-1}(\mathbf{I}(t) - U\bar{\mathbf{r}}(t)) \tag{16.9}$$

This equation is of the form:

New Estimate = Old Estimate + Gain × Sensory Residual Error   (16.10)

The gain matrix $K(t) = N(t)U^T \Sigma(t)^{-1}$ in Equation 16.9 determines the weight given to the sensory residual in correcting the old estimate $\bar{\mathbf{r}}$. Note that this gain can be interpreted as a form of "signal-to-noise" ratio: it is determined by the covariances Σ and M, and therefore effectively trades off the prior estimate $\bar{\mathbf{r}}$ against the sensory input $\mathbf{I}$ according to the *uncertainties* in these two sources. The Kalman filter estimate $\hat{\mathbf{r}}$ is in fact the *mean* of the Gaussian distribution of the state $\mathbf{r}$ *after* measurement of $\mathbf{I}$ [10]. The matrix N, which performs a form of divisive normalization, can likewise be shown to be the corresponding *covariance* matrix.

Recall that $\bar{\mathbf{r}}$ and M were the mean and covariance *before* measurement of $\mathbf{I}$. We can now specify how these quantities can be updated over time:

$$\bar{\mathbf{r}}(t) = V\hat{\mathbf{r}}(t-1) + \bar{\mathbf{m}}(t-1) \tag{16.11}$$
$$M(t) = VN(t-1)V^T + \Pi(t-1) \tag{16.12}$$

The above equations propagate the estimates of the mean and covariance ($\hat{\mathbf{r}}$ and N respectively) forward in time to generate the predictions $\bar{\mathbf{r}}$ and M for the next time instant. Figure 16.2A summarizes the essential components of the predictive coding model (see also Figure 16.1B).

Predictive Coding and Cortical Feedback

The cerebral cortex is usually characterized as a 6-layered structure, where layer 4 is typically the "input" layer and layer 5 is typically the "output" layer. Neurons in layers 2/3 generally project to layer 4 of "higher" cortical areas while the deeper layers, including layer 6, project back to the "lower" area (see Figure 16.2B). Further details and area-specific variations of these rules can be found in the review article by Van Essen [46].

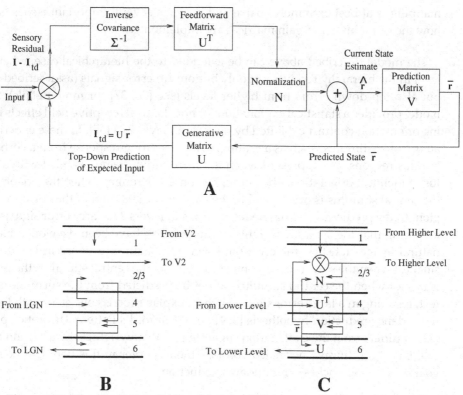

Figure 16.2. The Predictive Coding Model. (A) Schematic diagram of the predictive coding model. (B) The pattern of interlaminar connectivity in primary visual cortex (after [9]). (C) A possible mapping of the components of the predictive coding model onto cortical circuitry.

In the predictive coding model, one needs to predict one step into the future using Equation 16.11, obtain the next sensory input $\mathbf{I}(t)$, and then correct the prediction $\bar{\mathbf{r}}(t)$ using the sensory residual error $(\mathbf{I}(t) - U\bar{\mathbf{r}}(t))$ and the gain $K(t) = N(t)U^T\Sigma^{-1}$. This yields the corrected estimate $\hat{\mathbf{r}}(t)$, which is then used to make the next prediction $\bar{\mathbf{r}}(t+1)$.

This suggests the following mapping between the predictive coding model and cortical anatomy. Feedback connections from a higher cortical area to a lower area may carry the prediction $U\bar{\mathbf{r}}(t)$ to the lower area, while the feedforward connections may carry the prediction error $(\mathbf{I}(t) - U\bar{\mathbf{r}}(t))$. Here, $\mathbf{I}(t)$ is the input signal at the lowest level (for example, the lateral geniculate nucleus (LGN)). The deeper layer neurons, for example those in layer 6, are assumed to implement the feedback weights U while the connections to input layer 4 implement the synaptic weights U^T. Neurons in the "output" layer 5 maintain the current estimate $\hat{\mathbf{r}}(t)$ and the recurrent intracortical connections between neurons in layer 5 are assumed to implement the synaptic weights V. This suggested mapping is depicted in Figure 16.2C. Note that this mapping is at best extremely coarse and neglects several important issues, such as how the covariance and gain matrices are implemented.

The model described above can be extended to the hierarchical case, where each level in the hierarchy receives not only bottom-up error signals (as described above) but also top-down errors from higher levels (see [36, 37] for more details). Such a model provides a statistical explanation for nonclassical receptive field effects involving orientation contrast exhibited by neurons in layer 2/3 [37]. In these experiments, an oriented stimulus, such as a grating, evokes a strong response from a cortical cell but this response is suppressed when the surrounding region is filled with a stimulus of identical orientation. The neural response is strongest when the orientation of the central stimulus is orthogonal to the stimulus orientation of the surrounding region. In the predictive coding model, neurons in layers 2/3 carry error signals. Thus, assuming that the synaptic weights of the network have been developed based on natural image statistics, the error (and hence the neural response in layers 2/3) is smallest when the surrounding context can predict the central stimulus; the response is largest when the central stimulus cannot be predicted from the surrounding context, resulting in a large error signal. Such an explanation is consistent with Barlow's redundancy reduction hypothesis [3, 4] and Mumford's Pattern Theoretic approach [32]. It differs from the explanation suggested by Wainwright, Schwartz, and Simoncelli based on divisive normalization (see their chapter in this book), although the goal in both approaches is redundancy reduction.

Spike-Timing Dependent Plasticity and Predictive Sequence Learning

The preceding section sketched a possible mapping between cortical anatomy and an algorithm for predictive coding. An important question then is whether there exists neurophysiological evidence supporting such a mapping. In this section, we focus specifically on the hypothesis, put forth in the previous section, that recurrent intracortical connections between neurons in layer 5 implement the synaptic weights V that are used in the predictive coding model to encode temporal sequences of the state vector $\mathbf{r}(t)$.

Recent experimental results suggest that recurrent excitatory connections between cortical neurons are modified according to a spike-timing dependent Hebbian learning rule: synapses that are activated slightly before the cell fires are strengthened whereas those that are activated slightly after are weakened [26] (see also [22, 48, 8, 1, 20, 41, 43]). Such a time-sensitive learning rule is especially well-suited for learning temporal sequences [1, 28, 38].

To investigate how such a timing-dependent learning rule could allow predictive learning of sequences, we used a two-compartment model of a cortical neuron consisting of a dendrite and a soma-axon compartment. The compartmental model was based on a previous study that demonstrated the ability of such a model to reproduce a range of cortical response properties [25]. To study synaptic plasticity in this model, excitatory postsynaptic potentials (EPSPs) were elicited at different time delays with respect to postsynaptic spiking by presynaptic activation of a single excitatory synapse located on the dendrite. Synaptic currents were calculated using a kinetic model of synaptic transmission [18] with model parameters fitted to whole-cell recorded AMPA (α-amino-3-hydroxy-5-methyl-4-isoxazole proprionic acid) currents (see Methods for more details). Other inputs representing background activity were modeled as sub-threshold excitatory and inhibitory Poisson processes with a mean firing rate of 3 Hz. Synaptic plasticity was simulated by incrementing or decrementing the value for maximal synaptic conductance by an amount proportional to the temporal-difference in the postsynaptic membrane potential at time instants $t + \Delta t$ and t for presynaptic activation at time t [38]. The delay parameter Δt was set to 5 ms for these simulations; similar results were obtained for other values in the 5–15 ms range.

Figure 16.3A shows the results of pairings in which the postsynaptic spike was triggered 5 ms after and 5 ms before the onset of the EPSP respectively. While the peak EPSP amplitude was increased 58.5% in the former case, it was decreased 49.4% in the latter case, qualitatively similar to experimental observations [26]. The critical window for synaptic modifications in the model was examined by varying the time interval between presynaptic stimulation and postsynaptic spiking (with $\Delta t = 5$ ms). As shown in Figure 16.3B, changes in synaptic efficacy exhibited a highly asymmetric dependence on spike timing similar to physiological data [8]. Potentiation was observed for EPSPs that occurred between 1 and 12 ms before the postsynaptic spike, with maximal potentiation at 6 ms. Maximal depression was observed for EPSPs occurring 6 ms after the peak of the postsynaptic spike and this depression gradually decreased, approaching zero for delays greater than 10 ms. As in rat neocortical neurons [26], *Xenopus* tectal neurons [48], and cultured hippocampal neurons [8], a narrow transition zone (roughly 3 ms in the model) separated the potentiation and depression windows.

To see how a network of model neurons can learn to predict sequences using the learning mechanism described above, consider the simplest case of two excitatory neurons N1 and N2 connected to each other, receiving inputs from two separate input neurons I1 and I2 (Figure 16.4A). Suppose input neuron I1 fires before input neuron I2, causing neuron N1 to fire (Figure 16.4B). The spike from N1 results in a sub-threshold EPSP in N2 due to the synapse S2. If input arrives from I2 any time between 1 and 12 ms after this EPSP and the temporal summation of these two EPSPs causes N2 to fire, the synapse S2 will be strengthened. The synapse S1, on the other hand, will be weakened because the EPSP due to N2 arrives a few milliseconds after N1 has fired. Thus, on a subsequent trial, when input I1 causes neuron N1 to fire,

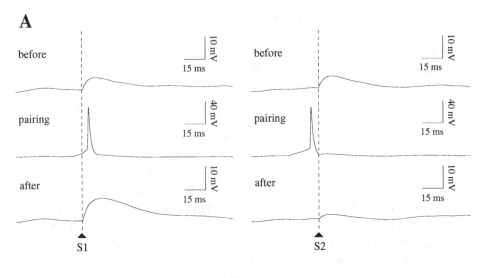

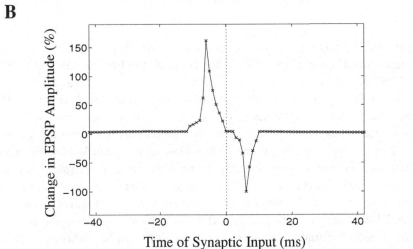

Figure 16.3. Synaptic Plasticity in a Model Neocortical Neuron. (from [39]) (**A**) (Left Panel) The response at the top (labeled "before") is the EPSP invoked in the model neuron due to a presynaptic spike (S1) at an excitatory synapse. Pairing this presynaptic spike with postsynaptic spiking after a 5 ms delay ("pairing") induces long-term potentiation as revealed by an enhancement in the peak of the EPSP evoked by presynaptic simulation alone ("after"). (Right Panel) If presynaptic stimulation (S2) occurs 5 ms after postsynaptic firing, the synapse is weakened resulting in a corresponding decrease in peak EPSP amplitude. (**B**) Critical window for synaptic plasticity obtained by varying the delay between presynaptic stimulation and postsynaptic spiking (negative delays refer to cases where presynaptic stimulation occurred before the postsynaptic spike).

it in turn causes N2 to fire several milliseconds *before* input I2 occurs due to the potentiation of the recurrent synapse S2 in previous trial(s) (Figure 16.4C). Input neuron I2 can thus be inhibited by the predictive feedback from N2 just before the occurrence of imminent input activity (marked by an asterisk in Figure 16.4C). This

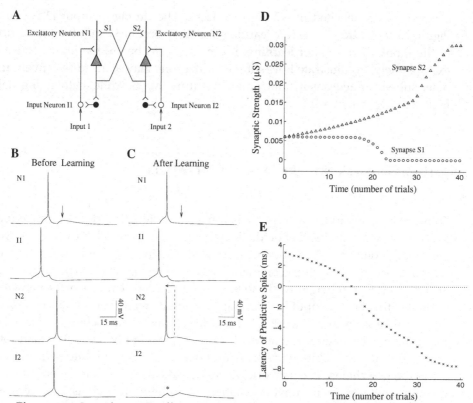

Figure 16.4. Learning to Predict using Spike-Timing Dependent Hebbian Plasticity.
(from [39]) (**A**) A simple network of two model neurons N1 and N2 recurrently connected via excitatory synapses S1 and S2. Sensory inputs are relayed to the two model neurons by input neurons I1 and I2. Feedback from N1 and N2 inhibit the input neurons via inhibitory interneurons (darkened circles). (**B**) Activity in the network elicited by the input sequence I1 followed by I2. Notice that N2 fires after its input neuron I2 has fired. (**C**) Activity in the network elicited by the same input sequence after 40 trials of learning. Notice that due to the strengthening of synapse S2, neuron N2 now fires several milliseconds before the time of expected input from I2 (dashed line), allowing it to inhibit I2 (asterisk). On the other hand, synapse S1 has been weakened, thereby preventing re-excitation of N1 (downward arrows show the corresponding decrease in EPSP). (**D**) Potentiation and depression of synapses S1 and S2 respectively during the course of learning. Synaptic strength was defined as maximal synaptic conductance in the kinetic model of synaptic transmission (see Methods). (**E**) Latency of the predictive spike in neuron N2 during the course of learning measured with respect to the time of input spike in I2 (dotted line). Note that the latency is initially positive (N2 fires after I2) but later becomes negative, reaching a value of up to 7.7 ms before input I2 as a consequence of learning.

inhibition prevents input I2 from further exciting N2. Similarly, a positive feedback loop between neurons N1 and N2 is avoided because the synapse S1 was weakened in previous trial(s) (see arrows in Figures 16.4B and 16.4C). Figure 16.4D depicts the process of potentiation and depression of the two synapses as a function of the number of exposures to the I1-I2 input sequence. The decrease in latency of the predictive spike elicited in N2 with respect to the timing of input I2 is shown in Figure 16.4E. Notice that before learning, the spike occurs 3.2 ms after the occurrence of the input whereas after learning, it occurs 7.7 ms before the input. This simple example helps to illustrate how subsets of neurons may learn to selectively trigger other subsets of neurons in anticipation of future inputs while maintaining stability in the recurrent network.

Comparisons to Awake Monkey Visual Cortex Data

To facilitate comparison with published neurophysiological data, we have focused specifically on the problem of predicting moving visual stimuli. We used a network of recurrently connected excitatory neurons (as shown in Figure 16.5A) receiving retino-topic sensory input consisting of moving pulses of excitation (8 ms pulse of excitation at each neuron) in the rightward and leftward directions. The task of the network was to predict the sensory input by learning appropriate recurrent connections such that a given neuron in the network can fire a few milliseconds before the arrival of its input pulse of excitation. The network was comprised of two parallel chains of neurons with mutual inhibition (dark arrows) between corresponding pairs of neurons along the two chains. The network was initialized such that within a chain, a given excitatory neuron received both excitation and inhibition from its predecessors and successors. This is shown in Figure 16.5B for a neuron labeled '0'. Inhibition at a given neuron was mediated by an inhibitory interneuron (dark circle) which received excitatory connections from neighboring excitatory neurons (Figure 16.5B, lower panel). The interneuron received the same input pulse of excitation as the nearest excitatory neuron. Maximum conductances for all synapses were initialized to small positive values (dotted lines in Figure 16.5C) with a slight asymmetry in the recurrent excitatory connections for breaking symmetry between the two chains. The initial asymmetry elicited a single spike slightly earlier for neurons in one chain than neurons in the other chain for a given motion direction, allowing activity in the other chain to be inhibited.

To evaluate the consequences of synaptic plasticity, the network of neurons was exposed alternately to leftward and rightward moving stimuli for a total of 100 trials. The excitatory connections (labeled 'EXC' in Figure 16.5B) were modified according to the spike-timing dependent Hebbian learning rule in Figure 16.3B while the excitatory connections onto the inhibitory interneuron (labeled 'INH') were modified according to an asymmetric anti-Hebbian learning rule that reversed the polarity of the rule in Figure 16.3B [6].

The synaptic conductances learned by two neurons (marked N1 and N2 in Figure 16.5A) located at corresponding positions in the two chains after 100 trials of

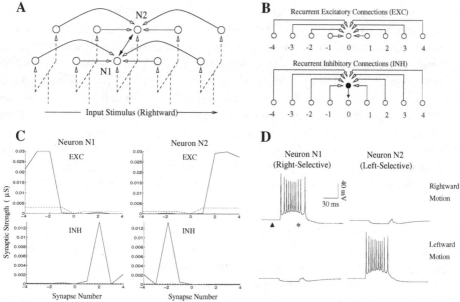

Figure 16.5. Emergence of Direction Selectivity in the Model. (A) A model network consisting of two chains of recurrently connected neurons receiving retinotopic inputs. A given neuron receives recurrent excitation and recurrent inhibition (white-headed arrows) as well as inhibition (dark-headed arrows) from its counterpart in the other chain. **(B)** Recurrent connections to a given neuron (labeled '0') arise from 4 preceding and 4 succeeding neurons in its chain. Inhibition at a given neuron is mediated via a GABAergic interneuron (darkened circle). **(C)** Synaptic strength of recurrent excitatory (EXC) and inhibitory (INH) connections to neurons N1 and N2 before (dotted lines) and after learning (solid lines). Synapses were adapted during 100 trials of exposure to alternating leftward and rightward moving stimuli. **(D)** Responses of neurons N1 and N2 to rightward and leftward moving stimuli. As a result of learning, neuron N1 has become selective for rightward motion (as have other neurons in the same chain) while neuron N2 has become selective for leftward motion. In the preferred direction, each neuron starts firing several milliseconds before the actual input arrives at its soma (marked by an asterisk) due to recurrent excitation from preceding neurons. The dark triangle represents the start of input stimulation in the network.

exposure to the moving stimuli are shown in Figure 16.5C (solid line). As expected from the learned asymmetric pattern of connectivity, neuron N1 was found to be selective for rightward motion while neuron N2 was selective for leftward motion (Figure 16.5D). Moreover, when stimulus motion is in the preferred direction, each neuron starts firing a few milliseconds before the time of arrival of the input stimulus at its soma (marked by an asterisk) due to recurrent excitation from preceding neurons. Conversely, motion in the non-preferred direction triggers recurrent inhibition from preceding neurons as well as inhibition from the active neuron in the corresponding position in the other chain.

Similar to complex cells in primary visual cortex, model neurons are direction selective throughout their receptive field because at each retinotopic location, the corresponding neuron in the chain receives the same pattern of asymmetric excitation and inhibition from its neighbors as any other neuron in the chain. Thus, for a given neuron, motion in any local region of the chain will elicit direction selective responses due to recurrent connections from that part of the chain. This is consistent with previous modeling studies [11] suggesting that recurrent connections may be responsible for the spatial-phase invariance of complex cell responses. Assuming a 200 μm separation between excitatory model neurons in each chain and utilizing known values for the cortical magnification factor in monkey striate cortex [45], one can estimate the preferred stimulus velocity of model neurons to be 3.1°/s in the fovea and 27.9°/s in the periphery (at an eccentricity of 8°). Both of these values fall within the range of monkey striate cortical velocity preferences (1°/s to 32 °/s) [46, 23].

The model predicts that the neuroanatomical connections for a direction selective neuron should exhibit a pattern of asymmetrical excitation and inhibition similar to Figure 16.5C. A recent study of direction selective cells in awake monkey V1 found excitation on the preferred side of the receptive field and inhibition on the null side consistent with the pattern of connections learned by the model [23]. For comparison with this experimental data, spontaneous background activity in the model was generated by incorporating Poisson-distributed random excitatory and inhibitory alpha synapses on the dendrite of each model neuron. Post stimulus time histograms (PSTHs) and space-time response plots were obtained by flashing optimally oriented bar stimuli at random positions in the cell's activating region. As shown in Figure 16.6, there is good qualitative agreement between the response plot for a direction-selective complex cell and that for the model. Both space-time plots show a progressive shortening of response onset time and an increase in response transiency going in the preferred direction: in the model, this is due to recurrent excitation from progressively closer cells on the preferred side. Firing is reduced to below background rates 40-60 ms after stimulus onset in the upper part of the plots: in the model, this is due to recurrent inhibition from cells on the null side. The response transiency and shortening of response time course appears as a slant in the space-time maps, which can be related to the neuron's velocity sensitivity (see [23] for more details).

Conclusions

This chapter reviewed the hypothesis that (i) feedback connections between cortical areas instantiate probabilistic generative models of cortical inputs, and (ii) recurrent feedback connections within a cortical area encode the temporal dynamics associated with these generative models. We formalized this hypothesis in terms of a predictive coding framework and suggested a possible implementation of the predictive coding

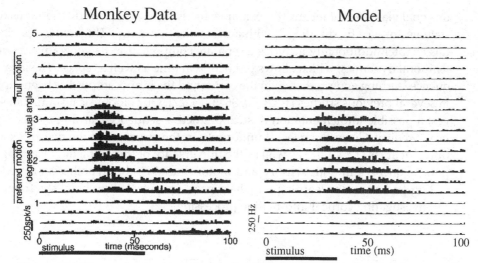

Figure 16.6. Comparison of Monkey and Model Space-Time Response Plots. (Left) Sequence of PSTHs obtained by flashing optimally oriented bars at 20 positions across the 5°-wide receptive field (RF) of a complex cell in alert monkey V1 (from [23]). The cell's preferred direction is from the part of the RF represented at the bottom towards the top. Flash duration = 56 ms; inter-stimulus delay = 100 ms; 75 stimulus presentations. (Right) PSTHs obtained from a model neuron after stimulating the chain of neurons at 20 positions to the left and right side of the given neuron. Lower PSTHs represent stimulations on the preferred side while upper PSTHs represent stimulations on the null side.

model within the laminar structure of the cortex. At the biophysical level, we showed that recent results on spike-timing dependent plasticity in recurrent cortical synapses are consistent with our suggested roles for cortical feedback. Data from model simulations were shown to be similar to electrophysiological data from awake monkey visual cortex.

An important direction for future research is exploring hierarchical models of spatiotemporal predictive coding based on spike-timing dependent sequence learning at multiple levels. A related direction of research is elucidating the role of spike timing in predictive coding. The chapter by Ballard, Zhang, and Rao in this book investigates the hypothesis that cortical communication may occur via synchronous volleys of spikes. The spike-timing dependent learning rule appears to be especially well-suited for learning synchrony [20, 1], but the question of whether the same learning rule allows the formation of multi-synaptic chains of synchronously firing neurons remains to be ascertained.

The predictive coding model is closely related to models based on sparse coding (see the chapters by Olshausen and Lewicki) and to competitive/divisive normalization models (see the chapters by Piepenbrock and Wainwright, Schwartz, and Simoncelli). These models share the goal of redundancy reduction but attempt to achieve this goal via different means (for example, by using sparse prior distributions on the state vector $\mathbf{r}$ or by dividing it with a normalization term). The model described in this chapter additionally includes a separate component in its generative model for temporal dynamics, which allows prediction in time as well as space. The idea of sequence learning and prediction in the cortex and the hippocampus has been explored in several previous studies [1, 28, 30, 36, 5, 13, 27]. Our biophysical simulations suggest a possible implementation of such predictive sequence learning models in cortical circuitry. Given the general uniformity in the structure of the neocortex across different areas [12, 40, 16] as well as the universality of the problem of learning temporal sequences in both sensory and motor domains, the hypothesis of predictive coding and sequence learning may help provide a unified probabilistic framework for investigating cortical information processing.

Acknowledgments

This work was supported by the Alfred P. Sloan Foundation and Howard Hughes Medical Institute. We thank Margaret Livingstone, Dmitri Chklovskii, David Eagleman, and Christian Wehrhahn for discussions and comments.

References

[1]   L. F. Abbott and K. I. Blum, "Functional significance of long-term potentiation for sequence learning and prediction," *Cereb. Cortex* **6**, 406-416 (1996).

[2]   L. F. Abbott and S. Song, "Temporally asymmetric Hebbian learning, spike timing and neural response variability," in *Advances in Neural Info. Proc. Systems 11*, M. S. Kearns, S. A. Solla and D. A. Cohn, Eds. (MIT Press, Cambridge, MA, 1999), pp. 69–75.

[3]   H. B. Barlow, "Possible principles underlying the transformation of sensory messages," in W. A. Rosenblith, editor, *Sensory Communication*, pages 217–234. Cambridge, MA: MIT Press, 1961.

[4]   H. B. Barlow, "What is the computational goal of the neocortex?" in C. Koch and J. L. Davis, editors, *Large-Scale Neuronal Theories of the Brain*, pages 1–22. Cambridge, MA: MIT Press, 1994.

[5]   H. Barlow, "Cerebral predictions," *Perception* **27**, 885-888 (1998).

[6]   C. C. Bell, V. Z. Han, Y. Sugawara, and K. Grant, "Synaptic plasticity in a cerebellum-like structure depends on temporal order," *Nature* **387**, 278-281 (1997).

[7] R. Ben-Yishai, R. L. Bar-Or, and H. Sompolinsky, "Theory of orientation tuning in visual cortex," *Proc. Natl. Acad. Sci. U.S.A.* **92**, 3844-3848 (1995).

[8] G. Q. Bi and M. M. Poo, "Synaptic modifications in cultured hippocampal neurons: Dependence on spike timing, synaptic strength, and postsynaptic cell type," *J. Neurosci.* **18**, 10464-10472 (1998).

[9] J. Bolz, C. D. Gilbert, and T. N. Wiesel, "Pharmacological analysis of cortical circuitry," *Trends in Neurosciences*, 12(8):292–296, 1989.

[10] A. E. Bryson and Y.-C. Ho. *Applied Optimal Control.* New York: John Wiley and Sons, 1975.

[11] F. S. Chance, S. B. Nelson, and L. F. Abbott, "Complex cells as cortically amplified simple cells," *Nature Neuroscience* **2**, 277-282 (1999).

[12] O. D. Creutzfeldt, "Generality of the functional structure of the neocortex," *Naturwissenschaften* **64**, 507-517 (1977).

[13] J. G. Daugman and C. J. Downing, "Demodulation, predictive coding, and spatial vision," *J. Opt. Soc. Am. A* **12**, 641-660 (1995).

[14] P. Dayan, G.E. Hinton, R.M. Neal, and R.S. Zemel, "The Helmholtz machine," *Neural Computation*, 7:889–904 (1995).

[15] P. Dayan and G. E. Hinton, "Varieties of Helmholtz machine," *Neural Networks* 9(8), 1385-1403 (1996).

[16] R. J. Douglas, K. A. C. Martin, and D. Whitteridge, "A canonical microcircuit for neocortex," *Neural Computation* **1**, 480-488 (1989).

[17] R. J. Douglas, C. Koch, M. Mahowald, K. A. Martin, and H. H. Suarez, "Recurrent excitation in neocortical circuits," *Science* **269**, 981-985 (1995).

[18] A. Destexhe, Z. F. Mainen, and T. J. Sejnowski, "Kinetic models of synaptic transmission," in *Methods in Neuronal Modeling*, C. Koch and I. Segev, Eds. (MIT Press, Cambridge, MA, 1998).

[19] J. L. Elman, "Finding structure in time," *Cognitive Science* **14**, 179-211 (1990).

[20] W. Gerstner, R. Kempter, J. L. van Hemmen, and H. Wagner, "A neuronal learning rule for sub-millisecond temporal coding," *Nature* **383**, 76-81 (1996).

[21] M. I. Jordan, "Attractor dynamics and parallelism in a connectionist sequential machine," in *Proceedings of the Annual Conf. of the Cog. Sci. Soc.*, pp. 531-546 (1986).

[22] W. B. Levy and O. Steward, "Temporal contiguity requirements for long-term associative potentiation/depression in the hippocampus," *Neuroscience* **8**, 791-797 (1983).

[23] M.S. Livingstone, "Mechanisms of direction selectivity in macaque V1," *Neuron*, 20:509–526 (1998).

[24] D. M. MacKay, "The epistemological problem for automata," in *Automata Studies*, pages 235–251. Princeton, NJ: Princeton University Press, 1956.

[25] Z. F. Mainen and T. J. Sejnowski, "Influence of dendritic structure on firing pattern in model neocortical neurons," *Nature* **382**, 363-366 (1996).

[26] H. Markram, J. Lubke, M. Frotscher, and B. Sakmann, "Regulation of synaptic efficacy by coincidence of postsynaptic APs and EPSPs," *Science* **275**, 213-215 (1997).

[27] M. R. Mehta and M. Wilson, "From hippocampus to V1: Effect of LTP on spatiotemporal dynamics of receptive fields," in *Computational Neuroscience, Trends in Research 1999*, J. Bower, Ed. (Elsevier Press, Amsterdam, 2000).

[28] A. A. Minai and W. B. Levy, "Sequence learning in a single trial," in *Proceedings of the 1993 INNS World Congress on Neural Networks* II, (Erlbaum, NJ, 1993), pp. 505-508.

[29] P. Mineiro and D. Zipser, "Analysis of direction selectivity arising from recurrent cortical interactions," *Neural Comput.* **10**, 353-371 (1998).

[30] P. R. Montague and T. J. Sejnowski, "The predictive brain: Temporal coincidence and temporal order in synaptic learning mechanisms," *Learning and Memory* **1**, 1-33 (1994).

[31] D. Mumford, "On the computational architecture of the neocortex. II. The role of cortico-cortical loops," *Biological Cybernetics*, 66:241–251 (1992).

[32] D. Mumford, "Neuronal architectures for pattern-theoretic problems," in C. Koch and J. L. Davis, editors, *Large-Scale Neuronal Theories of the Brain*, pages 125–152. Cambridge, MA: MIT Press, 1994.

[33] R. C. O'Reilly. *The LEABRA model of neural interactions and learning in the neocortex*. PhD thesis, Department of Psychology, Carnegie Mellon University, 1996.

[34] A. E. C. Pece, "Redundancy reduction of a Gabor representation: a possible computational role for feedback from primary visual cortex to lateral geniculate nucleus," in I. Aleksander and J. Taylor, editors, *Artificial Neural Networks 2*, pages 865–868. Amsterdam: Elsevier Science, 1992.

[35] R. P. N. Rao, "An optimal estimation approach to visual perception and learning," *Vision Research* **39**, 1963-1989 (1999).

[36] R. P. N. Rao and D. H. Ballard, "Dynamic model of visual recognition predicts neural response properties in the visual cortex," *Neural Computation* **9**, 721-763 (1997).

[37] R. P. N. Rao and D. H. Ballard, "Predictive coding in the visual cortex: A functional interpretation of some extra-classical receptive field effects," *Nature Neuroscience* **2**, 79-87 (1999).

[38] R. P. N. Rao and T. J. Sejnowski, "Predictive sequence learning in recurrent neocortical circuits", in *Advances in Neural Information Processing Systems 12*, S. A. Solla and T. K. Leen and K.-R. Müller, Eds. (MIT Press, Cambridge, MA, 2000), pp. 164-170.

[39] R. P. N. Rao and T. J. Sejnowski, "Spike-timing-dependent Hebbian plasticity

as Temporal Difference learning," *Neural Computation* **13**, 2221-2237, (2001).

[40] T. J. Sejnowski, "Open questions about computation in cerebral cortex," in *Parallel Distributed Processing: Explorations in the Microstructure of Cognition, vol. 2*, J. L. McClelland *et al.*, editors (MIT Press, Cambridge, MA, 1986), pp. 372-389.

[41] T. J. Sejnowski, "The book of Hebb," *Neuron* **24**(4), 773-776 (1999).

[42] D. C. Somers, S. B. Nelson, and M. Sur, "An emergent model of orientation selectivity in cat visual cortical simple cells," *J. Neurosci.* **15**, 5448-5465 (1995).

[43] S. Song, K. D. Miller, and L. F. Abbott, "Competitive Hebbian learning through spike-timing dependent synaptic plasticity," *Nature Neuroscience* **3**, 919–926 (2000).

[44] H. Suarez, C. Koch, and R. Douglas, "Modeling direction selectivity of simple cells in striate visual cortex with the framework of the canonical microcircuit," *J. Neurosci.* **15**, 6700-6719 (1995).

[45] R. B. Tootell, E. Switkes, M. S. Silverman, and S. L. Hamilton, "Functional anatomy of macaque striate cortex. II. Retinotopic organization," *J. Neurosci.* **8**, 1531-1568 (1988).

[46] D.C. Van Essen, "Functional organization of primate visual cortex," in A. Peters and E.G. Jones, editors, *Cerebral Cortex*, volume 3, pages 259–329. New York, NY: Plenum, 1985.

[47] D. M. Wolpert, Z. Ghahramani, and M. I. Jordan, "An internal model for sensorimotor integration," *Science*, 269:1880–1882 (1995).

[48] L. I. Zhang, H. W. Tao, C. E. Holt, W. A. Harris, and M. M. Poo, "A critical window for cooperation and competition among developing retinotectal synapses," *Nature* **395**, 37-44 (1998).

Contributors

Dana H. Ballard
Department of Computer Science
University of Rochester
Rochester, New York, USA

Andrew D. Brown
Gatsby Computational
Neuroscience Unit
University College London
London, England, UK

James M. Coughlan
Smith-Kettlewell Eye Research Institute
San Francisco, California, USA

David J. Fleet
Xerox Palo Alto Research Center
Palo Alto, California, USA

William T. Freeman
Artificial Intelligence Laboratory
MIT
Cambridge, Massachusetts, USA

Federico Girosi
Center for Biological
and Computational Learning
Artificial Intelligence Laboratory
MIT
Cambridge, Massachusetts, USA

John Haddon
University of California
Berkeley, California, USA

Geoffrey E. Hinton
Department of
Computer Science
University of Toronto
Toronto, Canada

Robert A. Jacobs
Department of Brain
and Cognitive Sciences
and the Center for Visual Science
University of Rochester
Rochester, New York, USA

Daniel Kersten
Department of Psychology
University of Minnesota
Minneapolis, Minnesota, USA

Michael Landy
Department of Psychology
New York University
New York, New York, USA

Michael S. Lewicki
Computer Science Department and
Center for the Neural Basis of Cognition
Carnegie Mellon University
Pittsburgh, USA

Laurence T. Maloney
Center for Neural Science
New York University
New York, New York, USA

Pascal Mamassian
Department of Psychology
University of Glasgow
Glasgow, Scotland, UK

Jean-Pierre Nadal
Laboratoire de Physique Statistique
Ecole Normale Supérieure
Paris, France

Bruno A. Olshausen
Dept. of Psychology and
Center for Neuroscience
University of California
Davis, California, USA

Constantine P. Papageorgiou
Center for Biological
and Computational Learning
Artificial Intelligence Laboratory
MIT
Cambridge, Massachusetts, USA

Egon C. Pasztor
MIT Media Lab
Cambridge, Massachusetts, USA

Christian Piepenbrock
Epigenomics
Berlin, Germany

Jonathan Pillow
Center for Neural Science
New York University
New York, New York, USA

Tomaso Poggio
Center for Biological
and Computational Learning
Artificial Intelligence Laboratory
MIT
Cambridge, Massachusetts, USA

Rajesh P. N. Rao
Department of Computer Science
and Engineering
University of Washington
Seattle, Washington, USA

Paul Schrater
Department of Psychology
University of Minnesota
Minneapolis, Minnesota, USA

Odelia Schwartz
Center for Neural Science
New York University
New York, New York, USA

Terrence J. Sejnowski
Department of Biology
University of California
at San Diego &
The Salk Institute for
Biological Studies
La Jolla, California, USA

Eero P. Simoncelli
Center for Neural Science, and
Courant Inst. of Math. Sciences
New York University
New York, New York, USA

Martin J. Wainwright
Stochastic Systems Group
Laboratory for Information
& Decision Systems
MIT
Cambridge, Massachusetts, USA

Yair Weiss
Computer Science Division
University of California
Berkeley, California, USA

A.L. Yuille
Smith-Kettlewell Eye Research Institute
San Francisco, California, USA

Richard S. Zemel
Department of Computer Science
University of Toronto
Toronto, Canada

Zuohua Zhang
Department of Computer Science
University of Rochester
Rochester, New York, USA

Index

Printed in the United States
By Bookmasters